Manual of Neonatal Respiratory Care

Edited by

Sunil K. Sinha, M.D., Ph.D.
Consultant in Paediatrics and Neonatology
Director of Neonatology
South Cleveland Hospital
Middlesbrough, United Kingdom

and

Steven M. Donn, M.D.
Professor of Pediatrics
Interim Director, Division of Neonatal-Perinatal Medicine
Medical Director, Holden Neonatal Intensive Care Unit
University of Michigan Health System
Ann Arbor, Michigan, USA

Futura Publishing
Company, Inc.
Armonk, NY

Library of Congress Cataloging-in-Publication Data
Manual of neonatal respiratory care/edited by Sunil K. Sinha and Steven M. Donn.
   p. cm.
   includes bibliographical references and index.
   ISBN 0-87993-444-1
   1. Respiratory therapy for newborn infants. I. Sinha, Sunil K., M.D., Ph.D.
II. Donn, Steven M.
   [DNLM: 1. Respiration Disorders—therapy—Infant, Newborn. 2. Intensive
Care, Neonatal—methods. 3. Respiratory Therapy—Infant, Newborn.
4. Ventilators, Mechanical. WS 280 M294 1999]
RJ312.M36 1999
618.92'206—dc21   99-039510
                                              CIP

Copyright 2000
Futura Publishing Company, Inc.

Published by
Futura Publishing Company, Inc.
135 Bedford Road
Armonk, New York 10504

LC #: 99-039510
ISBN #: 0-87993-444-1

Every effort has been made to ensure that the information in this book is as up to date
and as accurate as possible at the time of publication. However, due to the constant
developments in medicine, neither the author, nor the editor, nor the publisher can
accept any legal or any other responsibility for any errors or omissions that may occur.

All rights reserved.
No part of this book may be translated or reproduced in any form without written
permission of the publisher.

Printed in the United States of America.

Printed on acid-free paper.

*To yesterday's patients, who made
possible today's treatments and
brighter tomorrows.*

Contributors

Namasivayam Ambalavanan, M.D. *Assistant Professor of Pediatrics, Division of Neonatology, University of Alabama at Birmingham Medical Center, Birmingham, Alabama, USA*

Jeanette M. Asselin, M.S., R.R.T. *Department of Respiratory Therapy, Children's Hospital of Oakland, Oakland, California, USA*

Kenneth P. Bandy, R.R.T. *Technical Director, Department of Critical Care Support Services, University of Michigan Health System, Ann Arbor, Michigan, USA*

Daniel G. Batton, M.D. *Director of Neonatology, William Beaumont Hospital, Royal Oak, Michigan, USA*

J. Harry Baumer, F.R.C.P., F.R.C.P.C.H. *Consultant Paediatrician, Derriford Hospital, Plymouth, Devon, UK*

Michael A. Becker, R.R.T. *Clinical Specialist, Department of Critical Care Support Services, C.S. Mott Children's Hospital, University of Michigan Health System, Ann Arbor, Michigan, USA*

Graham Bernstein, M.D. *Associate Clinical Professor of Pediatrics, School of Medicine, University of California, San Diego; Sharp Mary Birch Women's Hospital, Children's Hospital and Health Center, San Diego, California, USA*

Vinod K. Bhutani, M.D. *Professor of Pediatrics, Department of Newborn Medicine, Pennsylvania Hospital, Philadelphia, Pennsylvania, USA*

J. Bert Bunnell, Sc.D. *Chairman and Chief Technical Officer, Bunnell Incorporated, Salt Lake City, Utah, USA*

Waldemar A. Carlo, M.D. *Professor of Pediatrics, Director of Neonatology, University of Alabama at Birmingham Medical Center, Birmingham, Alabama, USA*

Robert L. Chatburn, R.R.T. *Associate Professor of Pediatrics, Case Western Reserve University, Director of Respiratory Care, University Hospitals of Cleveland, Cleveland, Ohio, USA*

Malcolm L. Chiswick, M.D., F.R.C.P., F.R.C.P.C.H., D.C.H. *Professor of Paediatrics and Child Health, University of Manchester, Consultant Paediatrician, Neonatal Medical Unit, St. Mary's Hospital for Women and Children, Manchester, UK*

Reese H. Clark, M.D. *Professor of Pediatrics, Division of Neonatology, Duke University Medical Center, Durham, North Carolina, USA*

Jonathan M. Davis, M.D. *Professor of Pediatrics, Director of Neonatology, Winthrop-University Hospital, Mineola, New York, USA*

Mary K. Dekeon, R.R.T. *Clinical Specialist, Department of Critical Care Support Services, C.S. Mott Children's Hospital, University of Michigan Health System, Ann Arbor, Michigan, USA*

Steven M. Donn, M.D. *Professor of Pediatrics, Interim Director, Division of Neonatal-Perinatal Medicine, Medical Director, Holden Neonatal Intensive Care Unit, C.S. Mott Children's Hospital, University of Michigan Health System, Ann Arbor, Michigan, USA*

David J. Durand, M.D. *Staff Neonatologist, Children's Hospital of Oakland, Oakland, California, USA*

Roger G. Faix, M.D. *Professor of Pediatrics, Division of Neonatal-Perinatal Medicine, C.S. Mott Children's Hospital, University of Michigan Health System, Ann Arbor, Michigan, USA*

S. David Ferguson, M.A., F.R.C.P., F.R.C.P.C.H. *Consultant Paediatrician, Royal Gwent Hospital, Gwent, Wales, UK*

David J. Field, F.R.C.P., F.R.C.P.C.H., D.C.H., D.M. *Professor of Neonatal Medicine, Department of Child Health, Leicester Royal Infirmary, Leicester, UK*

Alistair R. Fielder, F.R.C.P., F.R.C.S., F.R.C.Ophth. *Professor of Ophthalmology, Imperial College School of Medicine, Academic Unit of Ophthalmology, The Western Eye Hospital, London, UK*

Neil N. Finer, M.D. *Professor of Pediatrics, Director of Neonatology, Unversity of California, San Diego Medical Center, San Diego, California, USA*

David S. Foley, M.D. *Research Fellow, Department of Surgery, University of Michigan Health System, Ann Arbor, Michigan, USA*

Molly R. Gates, M.S., R.N.C. *Neonatal Outreach Coordinator, Department of Nursing, C.S. Mott Children's Hospital, University of Michigan Health System, Ann Arbor, Michigan, USA*

Dale R. Gerstmann, M.D. *Staff Neonatologist, Utah Valley Regional Medical Center, Provo, Utah, USA*

Jay P. Goldsmith, M.D. *Chairman of Pediatrics, Division of Neonatology, Ochsner Clinic and Alton Ochsner Medical Foundation, New Orleans, Louisiana, USA*

Anne Greenough, M.D., F.R.C.P., F.R.C.P.C.H., D.C.H. *Professor of Clinical Respiratory Physiology, Department of Paediatrics, Guy's, King's, and St. Thomas' School of Medicine, King's College Hospital, London, UK*

Cheryll K. Hagus, E.M.B.A., R.R.T. *Assistant Professor of Respiratory Care, School of Health Professions, Southwest Texas State University, San Marcos, Texas, USA*

Ronald B. Hirschl, M.D. *Associate Professor of Surgery, Division of Pediatric Surgery, C.S. Mott Children's Hospital, University of Michigan Health System, Ann Arbor, Michigan, USA*

Martin Keszler, M.D. *Professor of Pediatrics, Division of Neonatology, Georgetown University Medical Center, Washington, D.C., USA*

Susan Kidd, M.R.C.P. *Research Fellow in Neonatal Paediatrics, Simpson Memorial Maternity Pavilion, Edinburgh, Scotland, UK*

Lawrence R. Kuhns, M.D. *Professor of Radiology, Division of Pediatric Radiology, C.S. Mott Children's Hospital, University of Michigan Health System, Ann Arbor, Michigan, USA*

Mary E. Linton, R.N., M.S., N.N.P. *Neonatal Nurse Practitioner, Holden Neonatal Intensive Care Unit, C.S. Mott Children's Hospital, University of Michigan Health System, Ann Arbor, Michigan, USA*

M. Jeffrey Maisels, M.D. *Chairman of Pediatrics, William Beaumont Hospital, Royal Oak, Michigan; Clinical Professor of Pediatrics, University of Michigan Medical School, Ann Arbor, Michigan; and Wayne State University, Detroit, Michigan, USA*

Marie C. McGettigan, M.D. *Staff Neonatologist, Department of Pediatrics, Division of Neonatology, Ochsner Clinic and Alton Ochsner Medical Foundation, New Orleans, Louisiana, USA*

Neil McIntosh, F.R.C.P., F.R.C.P.E., F.R.C.P.C.H., D.Sc. (Med.) *Professor of Paediatrics, Department of Child Life and Health, University of Edinburgh, Edinburgh, Scotland, UK*

Gopi Menon, M.R.C.P., F.R.C.P.C.H. *Consultant in Neonatal Paediatrics, Simpson Memorial Maternity Pavilion, Edinburgh, Scotland, UK*

Anthony D. Milner, M.D., F.R.C.P., F.R.C.P.C.H., D.C.H. *Professor of Neonatology, Department of Paediatrics, Guy's, King's, and St. Thomas' School of Medicine, St. Thomas' Hospital, London, UK*

Colin J. Morley, M.A., D.C.H., M.D., F.R.C.P., F.R.C.P.C.H. *Professor of Paediatrics, Director of Neonatal Medicine, Royal Women's Hospital, Carlton, Melbourne, Victoria, Australia*

Martha Nelson, M.D. *Clinical Instructor of Pediatrics, Division of Neonatal-Perinatal Medicine, C.S. Mott Children's Hospital, University of Michigan Health System, Ann Arbor, Michigan, USA*

Jill M. Neubert, R.N., M.S., N.N.P. *Neonatal Nurse Practitioner, Holden Neonatal Intensive Care Unit, C.S. Mott Children's Hospital, University of Michigan Health System, Ann Arbor, Michigan, USA*

Joanne J. Nicks, R.R.T. *Infant Product Manager, Bird Products Corporation, Thermo Respiratory Group, Palm Springs, California, USA*

Donald M. Null, Jr., M.D. *Professor of Pediatrics, Medical College of Pennsylvania/Hahnemann University School of Medicine, Director, Division of Neonatology, Allegheny General Hospital, Pittsburgh, Pennsylvania, USA*

Jeffrey M. Perlman, M.B. *Professor of Pediatrics, Division of Neonatal-Perinatal Medicine, The University of Texas Southwestern Medical Center, Dallas, Texas, USA*

Christian F. Poets, M.D. *Department of Pediatric Pulmonology, Hannover Medical School, Hannover, Germany*

Contributors

Charles A. Pohl, M.D. *Clinical Assistant Professor, Department of Pediatrics, Division of Neonatology, Jefferson Medical College of Thomas Jefferson University, Philadelphia, Pennsylvania, USA*

Tonse N. K. Raju, M.D. *Professor of Pediatrics, Division of Neonatology, University of Illinois at Chicago Medical Center, Chicago, Illinois, USA*

Jan Reiss, M.R.C.P. *Research Fellow in Neonatal Paediatrics, Simpson Memorial Maternity Pavilion, Edinburgh, Scotland, UK*

Janet M. Rennie, M.A., M.D., F.R.C.P, F.R.C.P.C.H, D.C.H. *Consultant and Senior Lecturer in Neonatal Medicine, King's College Hospital, London, UK*

Sam W. J. Richmond, F.R.C.P, F.R.C.P.C.H. *Consultant in Paediatrics, Neonatal Unit, Sunderland Royal Infirmary, Sunderland, UK*

N. R. C. Roberton, M.A, M.B, F.R.C.P. *Retired Paediatrician, Broadford, Isle of Skye, Scotland, UK*

Robert E. Schumacher, M.D. *Associate Professor of Pediatrics, Division of Neonatal-Perinatal Medicine, C.S. Mott Children's Hospital, University of Michigan Health System, Ann Arbor, Michigan, USA*

Sunil K. Sinha, M.D., Ph.D., F.R.C.P, F.R.C.P.C.H. *Consultant in Paediatrics and Neonatology, Director of Neonatology, South Cleveland Hospital, Middlesbrough, UK*

Emidio M. Sivieri, M.S. *Section on Newborn Pediatrics, Pennsylvania Hospital, Philadelphia, Pennsylvania, USA*

David P. Southall, M.D., F.R.C.P., F.R.C.P.C.H. *Professor of Paediatrics, Academic Department of Paediatrics, University of Keele, North Staffordshire Hospital Centre, Stoke on Trent, UK*

Alan R. Spitzer, M.D. *Professor of Pediatrics, Division of Neonatology, Jefferson Medical College of Thomas Jefferson University, Philadelphia, Pennsylvania, USA*

Kim K. Tekkanat, M.D. *Fellow in Neonatal-Perinatal Medicine, Department of Pediatrics, C.S. Mott Children's Hospital, University of Michigan Health System, Ann Arbor, Michigan, USA*

Win Tin, M.R.C.P., F.R.C.P.C.H. *Consultant in Paediatrics and Neonatology, South Cleveland Hospital, Middlesbrough, UK*

Dharmapuri Vidyasagar, M.D. *Professor of Pediatrics, Director of Neonatology, University of Illinois at Chicago Medical Center, Chicago, Illinois, USA*

Christine A. Walker, M.R.C.P, F.R.C.P.C.H. *Consultant in Community Health, Northampton General Hospital, Northampton, UK*

Unni Wariyar, M.D., F.R.C.P., F.R.C.P.C.H. *Consultant in Paediatrics and Neonatology, Royal Victoria Infirmary Hospital, Newcastle-upon-Tyne, UK*

Thomas E. Wiswell, M.D. *Professor of Pediatrics, Division of Neonatology, Jefferson Medical College of Thomas Jefferson University, Philadelphia, Pennsylvania, USA*

Jonathan P. Wyllie, F.R.C.P., F.R.C.P.C.H. *Consultant in Paediatrics and Neonatology, South Cleveland Hospital, Middlesbrough, UK*

Foreword

The respiratory care of newborn infants has a short and rich history of striking success and innovation. As with most medical advances, one class of patients (the intermediate to large-sized preterm infant) has benefited without question. In contrast, the highest risk patients (the very low birthweight preterm and term infants with severe respiratory failure) have improved survival but considerable morbidity. Much of this morbidity can be attributed either directly or indirectly to mechanical ventilation. Drs. Sinha and Donn have edited *Manual of Neonatal Respiratory Care* to achieve a remarkable uniformity of style and content on a wide range of subjects that touch on all aspects of the respiratory management of the newborn. The emphasis on basic principles of physiology, techniques, and information about equipment provides a remarkable compendium of information that will be valuable to all who provide care for infants. The outline format will be particularly useful for the day-to-day review of strategies for respiratory care of infants.

The inexperienced practitioner will be surprised by the number of strategies and variety of equipment used for infant ventilation. The diversity and continued development of more technically complex infant ventilators might suggest that ventilating infants is difficult and unsuccessful. The contrary is true for the majority of preterm or term infants without severe disease. Any of the techniques or equipment described in this manual will yield good outcomes if used appropriately. The new innovations are targeted to infants with severe respiratory failure from multiple causes and to very preterm infants at risk of chronic lung disease. The diversity of equipment and techniques demonstrate a lack of consensus in the field about how best to provide respiratory care for these high risk infants. This manual includes particularly strong chapters on gas exchange, pulmonary mechanics, and assessments of cardiopulmonary function, among others.

The *art* of ventilating the infant is based on careful application of the principles of assessment outlined in these chapters. The user of this excellent manual will best serve patients by recognizing that optimal ventilatory management of infants blends accurate clinical assessment, effective technique, and a touch of the *art* of respiratory management.

ALAN H. JOBE, M.D., Ph.D.
Professor of Pediatrics
Children's Hospital Medical Center
Division of Pulmonary Biology
Cincinnati, Ohio, USA

Preface

Developments in the field of neonatology over the past 30 years have produced phenomenal advances in the care of newborns with respiratory failure. Neonatal respiratory care comprises a fascinating blend of basic science and clinical research, in one of the fastest growing areas of medicine. The first reports of the successful use of mechanical ventilation to treat respiratory disorders in newborns were published in the mid-1960s. These reports were followed by the widespread implementation of mechanical ventilation during the 1970s. The developments of high-frequency ventilation and extracorporeal life support dominated the 1980s. During the 1990s, the use of surfactant replacement therapy and synchronized ventilation became standard. These advances have rendered the neonatal intensive care unit a source of both medical wonders and technological nightmares.

The explosion of technology has also dramatically changed the management of neonatal respiratory failure. Gone are the "cookbook" days when all infants placed on ventilators were handled the same way. Clinicians now have a wide range of diagnostic and therapeutic tools to customize management in a disease-specific manner. Yet, the choices can be overwhelming at times, especially for the young and inexperienced clinician.

This volume has been developed as a readily available source of information for those providing intensive respiratory care to the newborn. It was our intent to provide a simple, yet comprehensive, manual that covers virtually all aspects of neonatal respiratory care, including: lung development, function, and pathophysiology; principles of mechanical ventilation; available diagnostic and therapeutic equipment; strategies for treating the various respiratory disorders; alternative treatments for intractable respiratory failure; outcomes; and ethical considerations in the care of infants with severe problems. We have also included a section with clinical case studies in order to illustrate the application of various principles to bedside care. We have chosen an outline format that is clinically focused to facilitate "bedside" applicability.

We hope that the material contained in this volume will be helpful to all those who come into contact with neonatal intensive care units, including medical students, house officers, respiratory therapists, nurses, nurse practitioners, fellows, pediatricians, and neonatologists. The contributors to this book are a distinguished group of health care professionals who are leaders in their respective fields. We are greatly indebted to them for giving their time and effort to this project.

Several individuals deserve recognition for the contributions made in the production of this manual. Our respective secretaries, Vicky Cowley and Susan Peterson, did a fantastic job in coordinating the assemblage and organization of 83 chapters, written by 63 contributors from three continents. Steven Korn, Chairman of the Board of Futura Publishing Company, Inc., provided strong encouragement for this project. Our colleagues at both South Cleveland Hospital and the University of Michigan Health System have been most supportive, not only through their substantive contributions to the content, but also in making it possible for us to continue to bring new devices and ideas to the practice of neonatology.

Finally, we would like to give special thanks to our families. We appreciate the personal sacrifices they made while we were busy putting this book together, and we hope they will share our sense of pride and achievement in the finished product.

SUNIL K. SINHA, M.D., Ph.D.
Middlesbrough, UK

STEVEN M. DONN, M.D.
Ann Arbor, Michigan, USA

Abbreviations Used in This Book

A   alveolar
a   arterial
a/A   arterial/alveolar ratio
A-aDO$_2$ alveolar-arterial oxygen tension gradient
ACT   activated clotting time
A/C   assist/control
ADP   adenosine diphosphate
ALTE   apparent life-threatening event
AM   morning
AMP   adenosine monophosphate
Ao   aortic
AOE   antioxidant enzymes
AOI   apnea of infancy
AOP   apnea of prematurity
ARDS   adult respiratory distress syndrome
ATP   adenosine triphosphate
ATPS   ambient temperature and pressure, saturated with water vapor

BAER   brainstem audiometric evoked responses
BPD   bronchopulmonary dysplasia
BPM (bpm)   beats or breaths per minute
BR   breath rate
BTPS   body temperature and pressure, saturated with water vapor

C   compliance
°C   degrees Celsius (Centigrade)
C$_{20}$ compliance over last 20% of inflation
CaO$_2$ arterial oxygen content
C$_D$ or C$_{DYN}$ dynamic compliance
C$_L$ compliance
C$_{ST}$ static compliance
cAMP   cyclic adenosine monophosphate
CBF   cerebral blood flow
CBG   capillary blood gas
cc   cubic centimeter
CDH   congenital diaphragmatic hernia

CDP	continuous distending pressure
cGMP	cyclic guanosine monophosphate
CHD	congenital heart disease
CLD	chronic lung disease
cm	centimeter
cm H_2O	centimeters of water
CMV	conventional mechanical ventilation
CNS	central nervous system
CO	cardiac output
CO_2	carbon dioxide
COHb	carboxyhemoglobin
CPAP	continuous positive airway pressure
CPR	cardiopulmonary resuscitation
CPT	chest physiotherapy
CRP	C-reactive protein
CSF	cerebrospinal fluid
CT	computed tomography
CV	conventional ventilation
CVP	central venous pressure
CXR	chest x-ray (radiograph)
D	end-diastole
DIC	disseminated intravascular coagulation
dL	deciliter
DPPC	dipalmitoylphosphatidylcholine
D_5W	dextrose 5% in water
E	elastance
ECG	electrocardiogram
ECLS	extracorporeal life support
ECMO	extracorporeal membrane oxygenation
EDRF	endothelial-derived relaxing factor
EEG	electroencephalogram
EF	ejection fraction
EMG	electromyogram
EMLA	eutectic mixture of Lidocaine and Prilocaine
ERV	expiratory reserve volume
ET	endotracheal
$ETCO_2$	end-tidal carbon dioxide
ETCPAP	endotracheal continuous positive airway pressure
ETT	endotracheal tube

F or f	frequency
F or Fr	French
FDA	Food and Drug Administration (USA)
F_IO_2	fraction of inspired oxygen
FiO_2	fraction of inspired oxygen
FRC	functional residual capacity
FTA	fluorescent treponemal antibody
F-V	flow-volume loop
G	gravida
g	gauge
g	gram
GA	gestational age
GER	gastroesophageal reflux
GERD	gastroesophageal reflux disease
gm	gram
GTP	guanosine triphosphate
h or hr	hour
Hb	hemoglobin
HbA	adult hemoglobin
HbF	fetal hemoglobin
HbO_2	oxygenated hemoglobin
HFJV	high-frequency jet ventilation
HFO	high-frequency oscillation
HFOV	high-frequency oscillatory ventilation
HFV	high-frequency ventilation
HMD	hyaline membrane disease
Hg	mercury
Hgb	hemoglobin
H_2O	water
HR	heart rate
Hz	Hertz
I	inertance
IC	inspiratory capacity
I:E	inspiratory:expiratory ratio
Ig	immunoglobulin
IMV	intermittent mandatory ventilation
iNO	inhaled nitric oxide
IPPV	intermittent positive pressure ventilation

IRV	inspiratory reserve volume
IUGR	intrauterine growth retardation
IV	intravenous
IVH	intraventricular hemorrhage
IVS	interventricular septum
IVSD	interventricular septum at diastole
IVSS	interventricular septum at systole
K	constant
°K	degrees Kelvin
kDa	kilodalton
kg	kilogram
kPa	kilopascal
L	liter
LA	left atrium
LBW	low birthweight
LCD	liquid crystalline display
LED	light-emitting diode
LOS	length of stay
LPA	left pulmonary artery
LPM (lpm)	liters per minute
LV	left ventricle
LVEDD	left ventricular end-diastolic dimension
LVID	left ventricular internal diameter
LVIDD	left ventricular internal diameter at diastole
LVIDS	left ventricular internal diameter at systole
m	meter
MAP	mean arterial pressure
MAS	meconium aspiration syndrome
mcg	microgram
MD	minute distance
mEq	milliequivalent
MetHb	methemoglobin
mg	milligram
MIC	mean inhibitory concentration
min	minute
mL (ml)	milliliter
mm	millimeter
MMV	mandatory minute ventilation

mo	month
mOsm	milliosmoles
MPA	main pulmonary artery
MRI	magnetic resonance imaging
MSAF	meconium-stained amniotic fluid
msec	millisecond
MV	minute ventilation
NEC	necrotizing enterocolitis
NICU	neonatal intensive care unit
NO	nitric oxide
NO_2	nitrogen dioxide
NOS	nitric oxide synthase
O_2	oxygen
OI	oxygenation index
P	para
P	pressure
ΔP	change in pressure
P_{50}	point of 50% saturation of hemoglobin with oxygen
Paw	airway pressure
$\bar{P}aw$	mean airway pressure
P_E	elastic pressure
P_{H2O}	partial pressure of water vapor
P_I	inertial pressure
P_I	inspiratory pressure
P_{IP}	intrapleural pressure
P_{N2}	partial pressure of nitrogen
P_R	resistive pressure
P_{ST}	static pressure
P_{TP}	transpulmonary pressure
PvO_2	partial pressure of oxygen, venous
$PACO_2$	partial pressure of carbon dioxide, alveolar
$PaCO_2$	partial pressure of carbon dioxide, arterial
PAO_2	partial pressure of oxygen, alveolar
PaO_2	partial pressure of oxygen, arterial
PB	periodic breathing
PC	pressure control
PCA	postconceptional age
PCO_2	partial pressure (tension) of carbon dioxide

PDA	patent ductus arteriosus
PEEP	positive end-expiratory pressure
PFCs	perfluorocarbons
PFC	persistent fetal circulation
PG	prostaglandin
PGE_2	prostaglandin E_2
PIE	pulmonary interstitial emphysema
PIP	peak inspiratory pressure
PL	pressure limit
PLV	partial liquid ventilation
PMA	postmenstrual age
PMA	pre-market approval (USA)
PO	*per os*, by mouth
PPHN	persistent pulmonary hypertension of the newborn
ppm	parts per million
PRBCs	packed red blood cells
PRVC	pressure-regulated volume control
PS	pressure support
psig	pounds per square inch gauge
PSV	pressure support ventilation
PT	prothrombin time
PUFA	polyunsaturated fatty acids
P-V	pressure-volume loop
PV-IVH	periventricular-intraventricular hemorrhage
PVL	periventricular leukomalacia
$\dot{Q}$	perfusion
q	every
R	resistance
r	radius
R_{AW}	airway resistance
R_E	expiratory resistance
R_I	inspiratory resistance
RDS	respiratory distress syndrome
REM	rapid eye movement
ROP	retinopathy of prematurity
RPA	right pulmonary artery
RR	respiratory rate
RV	reserve volume

RV	residual volume
RV	right ventricle
RVOT	right ventricular outflow tract
RVR	rate-volume ratio
S	end-systole
$S_{1\ (2,3,4)}$	first (second, third, fourth) heart sound
SaO_2	arterial oxygen saturation
SAVI	synchronized assisted ventilation of infants
SpO_2	pulse oximetry saturation
SvO_2	venous oxygen saturation
sec	second
sGC	soluble guanylate cyclase
SIDS	sudden infant death syndrome
SIMV	synchronized intermittent mandatory ventilation
SOD	superoxide dismutase
SP	surfactant protein
sq	square
STPD	standard temperature and pressure, dry
SV	stroke volume
SVC	superior vena cava
T	temperature
$TcPCO_2$	transcutaneous carbon dioxide tension
$TcPO_2$	transcutaneous oxygen tension
T_E or T_e	expiratory time
T_I or T_i	inspiratory time
TBW	total body water
TCPLV	time-cycled, pressure-limited ventilation
TCT	total cycle time
TGV	thoracic gas volume
TGV	total gas volume
THAM	tris-hydroxyaminomethane
TLC	total lung capacity
TLV	total liquid ventilation
TPN	total parenteral nutrition
TRH	thyroid-releasing hormone
TTN, TTNB	transient tachypnea of the newborn
U	units
UAC	umbilical artery catheter

V	volume
$\dot{V}$	flow
$\ddot{V}$	rate of change of flow
V_A	alveolar space
V_A	anatomic volume
$\dot{V}_A$	alveolar ventilation
V_A	alveolar volume
$\dot{V}_{CO2}$	carbon dioxide elimination
V_D	dead space volume
V_E	minute volume (expired)
V_T	tidal volume
V_{TE}	expired tidal volume
V_{TI}	inspired tidal volume
VAPS	volume assured pressure support
VC	vital capacity
VC	volume control
VCF	velocity of circumferential fiber shortening
VCV	volume-controlled ventilation
VDRL	venereal disease research laboratory
VIVE	variable inspiratory and variable expiratory flow
VLBW	very low birthweight
$\dot{V}/\dot{Q}$	ventilation/perfusion matching
VS	volume support
VSD	ventricular septal defect
VTI	velocity-time interval
WBC	white blood cell
wks	weeks
yrs	years

Contents

Contents

xxv

Contents

Contents

SECTION I

Lung Development and Normal Pulmonary Physiology

Chapter 1

Development of the Respiratory System

Vinod K. Bhutani

I. Introduction

  A. Prenatal development of the respiratory system is not complete until sufficient gas exchange surface has formed to support the newborn at birth.

  B. Pulmonary vasculature must also achieve sufficient capacity to transport carbon dioxide and oxygen through the lungs.

  C. Gas exchange surface must be structurally stable, functional, and elastic to require minimal effort for ventilation and to be responsive to the metabolic needs of the infant.

  D. Structural maturation of the airways, chest wall, and respiratory muscles and neural maturation of respiratory control are integral to the optimal function of the gas exchange "unit."

  E. Respiratory system development continues after birth and well into childhood (Table 1).

Table 1
Magnitude of Lung Development: From Fetal Age to Adulthood

	30 Wks	*Term*	*Adult*	*Fold Increase After Term PCA*
Surface area: sq m	0.3	4.0	100	23
Lung volume: mL	25	200	5000	23
Lung weight: g	25	50	800	16
Alveoli: number	Few	50 m	300 m	6
Alveolar diameter: μm	32	150	300	10
Airway branching: number	24	24	24	0

PCA = postconceptual age.

F. Fundamental processes that impact on respiratory function
   1. Ventilation and distribution of gas volumes
   2. Gas exchange and transport
   3. Pulmonary circulation
   4. Mechanical forces that initiate breathing and those that impede airflow
   5. Organization and control of breathing

Table 2
Stages of Prenatal and Postnatal Structural Lung Development

Phase	Post-Conceptional Age	Length: Terminal Bronchiole to Pleura	Lung Development
Embryonic	0–7 weeks	<0.1 mm	Budding from the foregut
Pseudoglandular	8–16 weeks	0.1 mm	Airway division commences and terminal bronchioles formed
Canalicular	17–27 weeks	0.2 mm	3 generations of respiratory bronchioles Primitive saccules formation with type I and II epithelial cells Capillarization
Saccular	28–35 weeks	0.6 mm	Transitional alveolar ducts formed; three generations of saccules
Alveolar	>36 weeks	11 mm	Terminal saccules formed; true alveoli appear
Postnatal	2 months	175 mm	5 generations of alveolar ducts; alveoli form with septation
Early childhood	6–7 years	400 mm	Airways remodeled; alveolar sac budding occurs

3

II. Lung Development

A. Background. The lung's developmental design is based upon the functional goal of allowing air and blood to interface over a vast surface area and an extremely thin yet intricately organized tissue barrier. The developmental maturation is such that growth (a quantitative phenomenon) progresses separately from maturation (a qualitative phenomenon). A tension skeleton composed of connective tissue fibers determines the mechanical properties of the lungs: axial, peripheral, and alveolar septal.

1. Axial connective tissue fibers have a centrifugal distribution from the hilum to the branching airways.
2. Peripheral fibers have a centripetal distribution from the pleura to within the lungs.
3. Alveolar septal fibers connect the axial and peripheral fibers.

B. Functional anatomy (Table 2)

1. Fetal lung development takes place in seven phases.
2. Demarcations are not exact but arbitrary with transition and progression occurring between each.
3. Little is known about the effects of antenatal steroids on the transition and maturation of fetal lung development.

C. Factors that impact fetal lung growth

1. Physical, hormonal, and local factors play a significant role (Table 3).
2. The physical factors play a crucial role in the structural development and influence size and capacity of the lungs.
3. Hormonal influences may be either stimulatory or inhibitory.

D. Fetal lung fluid and variations in lung development. Production, effluence, and physiology are dependent on physiologic control of fetal lung fluid.

1. Production – secretion commences in mid-gestation, during canalicular phase and composition distinctly differs from fetal plasma and amniotic fluid (Table 4).
2. Distending pressure – daily production rate of 250-300 mL/24 h results in distending pressure of 3-5 cm H_2O within the respiratory system. This hydrostatic pressure seems to be crucial for fetal lung

Table 3
Factors that Influence Fetal Lung Maturation

Physical	Hormonal	Local
Fetal respiration	Glucocorticoids	cAMP
Fetal lung fluid	Prolactin	Methylxanthines
Thoracic volume (FRC)	Insulin	
	Sex hormones	

FRC = functional residual capacity; cAMP = cyclic adenosine monophosphate.

Table 4
Chemical Features of Fetal Fluids

	Osmolality mOsm/L	*Protein g/dL*	*pH*	*Sodium mEq/L*	*Potassium mEq/L*	*Chloride mEq/L*	*Bicarbonate mEq/L*
Fetal lung fluid	300	0.03	6.27	140	6.3	144	2.8
Fetal plasma	290	4.1	7.34	140	4.8	107	24
Amniotic fluid	270	0.1–0.7	7.07	110	7.1	94	18

development and the progressive bifurcations of the airways and development of terminal saccules.

3. Fetal breathing – during fetal breathing movements, tracheal egress of lung fluid (up to 15 mL/h) during expiration (compared to minimal loss during fetal apnea) ensures that lung volume remains

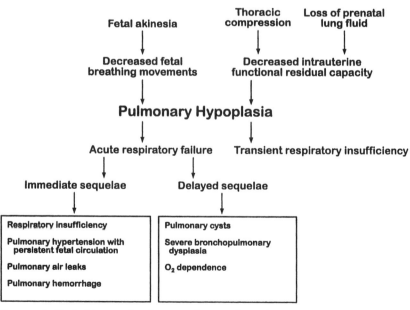

Figure 1. Probable mechanisms and sequelae of pulmonary development during prolonged amniotic leak. (Modified from Bhutani VK, Abbasi S, Weiner S: Neonatal pulmonary manifestations due to prolonged amniotic leak. Am J Perinatol 1986; 3:225, ©Thieme Medical Publishers, with permission.)

at about 30 mL/kg (equivalent to the functional residual capacity, FRC). Excessive egress has been associated with pulmonary hypoplasia (Figure 1), whereas tracheal ligation has been associated with pulmonary hyperplasia.

III. Upper Airway Development

A. Airways are heterogeneous, conduct airflow, and do not participate in gas exchange. Starting as the upper airways (nose, mouth, pharynx, and larynx), they lead to the trachea. From here, the cartilaginous airways taper to the small bronchi and then to the membranous airways and the last branching, the terminal bronchioles (Table 5). The lower airways and the gas exchange area commence with the respiratory bronchioles. The upper airways are not rigid, but are distensible, extensible, and compressible. The branching is not symmetrical and dichotomous but irregular. The lumen is not circular and subject to rapid changes in cross-sectional area and diameter because of a variety of extramural, mural, and intramural factors.

B. Anatomy – includes the nose, oral cavity, palate, pharynx, larynx, hyoid bone, and extrathoracic trachea.

C. Function – to conduct, humidify, warm (or cool) to body temperature, filter air into the lungs. Also help to separate functions of respiration and feeding as well as share in the process of vocalization.

Table 5
Classification, Branching, and Lumen Size of Adult Human Airways

Branch Order	Name	Number	Diameter (mm)	Cross-sectional Area (cm^2)
0	Trachea	1	18	2.54
1	Main bronchi	2	12.2	2.33
2	Lobar bronchi	4	8.3	2.13
3	Segmental bronchi	8	5.6	2.00
4	Subsegmental bronchi	16	4.5	2.48
5–10	Small bronchi	32–1,025	3.5–1.3	3.11–13.4
11–14	Bronchioles	2,048–8,192	1.09–0.74	19.6–69.4
15	Terminal bronchiole	32,768	0.66	113
16–18	Respiratory bronchioles	65,536–262,144	0.54–0.47	180–534
19–23	Alveolar ducts	524,288–8,388,608	0.43	944–11,800
24	Alveoli	300,000,000	0.2	2.8 m^2

D. Patency control – stable pressure balance between collapsing forces (inherent viscoelastic properties of the structures and that of the constricting tone) and the dilator forces of supporting musculature help to maintain upper airway patency. Negative pressure in the airways, neck flexion, and changes in the head and neck posture narrow the airways. Both intrinsic and extrinsic muscles of the upper airway can generate dilator forces, such as flaring of the alae nasi.

IV. Lower Airway Development

A. Anatomy
1. Conducting airways of the intrathoracic trachea
2. Respiratory gas exchange portions of terminal and respiratory bronchioles and alveolar ducts

B. Function of airway smooth muscle
1. Tone is evident early in fetal life and plays significant role in controlling airway lumen.
2. In presence of respiratory barotrauma, there appears to be a propensity for airway reactivity, perhaps a component of the smooth muscle hyperplasia seen in bronchopulmonary dysplasia (BPD).
3. Patency control – excitatory and inhibitory innervations lead to bronchoconstriction or dilatation, respectively.
4. Narrow airways – narrowing of the airways leads to increased resistance to airflow, an increased resistive load during breathing, and thereby an increased work of breathing and wasted caloric expenditure. Clinical factors associated with airway narrowing are listed in Table 6.

V. Thoracic and Respiratory Muscle Development

A. Anatomy
1. Three groups of skeletal muscles are involved in respiratory function.
   a. Diaphragm
   b. Intercostal and accessory muscles
   c. Abdominal muscles
2. These comprise the respiratory pump that helps conduct the air in and out of the lungs.
3. During quiet breathing, the primary muscle for ventilation is the diaphragm.
4. The diaphragm is defined by its attachments to the skeleton.
   a. That part attached to the lumbar vertebral regions is the crural diaphragm.
   b. That part attached to the lower six ribs is the costal diaphragm.
   c. Both converge and form a single tendon of insertion.

Table 6
Clinical Conditions Associated with Narrowing of the Airways

Airway inflammation	• Mucosal edema • Excessive secretions • Inspissation of secretions • Tracheitis
Bronchoconstriction	• Reactive airways • Exposure to cold, dry air • Exposure to bronchoconstricting drugs
Bronchomalacia	• Prolonged mechanical ventilation • Congenital • Secondary to vascular abnormality
Trauma	• Foreign body • Mucosal damage from ventilation, suction catheters • Subglottic stenosis
Congenital	• Choanal stenosis • High arched palate
Chemical	• Aspiration of gastric contents • Hyper-/hypo-osmolar fluid in the airways

5. Innervation of the diaphragm is by alpha motor neurons of the 3rd through 5th cervical segments, the phrenic nerve.

6. Attached to the circumference of the lower thoracic cage, its contraction pulls the muscle downward, displaces the abdomen outwards, and lifts up the thoracic cage.

7. In the presence of a compliant thoracic cage, relative to the lungs, the thoracic cage is pulled inward (sternal retraction).

8. The concomitant pressure changes during inspiration are reduction of intrapleural pressure and an increase in the intraabdominal pressure.

B. Respiratory contractile function

1. Strength, endurance, and the inherent ability to resist fatigue may assess the performance of the respiratory muscles.

2. Strength is determined by the intrinsic properties of the muscle (such as its morphologic characteristics and types of fibers).

3. Clinically, strength may be measured by the pressures generated at the mouth or across the diaphragm at specific lung volumes during a static inspiratory or expiratory maneuver.

4. Endurance capacity of a respiratory muscle depends on the properties of the system as well as the energy availability of the muscles.

5. Clinically, endurance is defined as the capacity to maintain either maximal or submaximal levels of ventilation under isocapnic conditions. It may be standardized either as maximal ventilation for

Table 7
Postnatal Maturation of the Lung

	Number of Alveoli	Surface Area (sq.m)	Respiratory Rate (per minute)
Birth	24,000,000	2.8	45 (35–55)
5–6 mo	112,000,000	8.4	27 (22–31)
~1 yr	129,000,000	12.2	19 (17–23)
~3 yr	257,000,000	22.2	19 (16–25)
~5 yr	280,000,000	32.0	18 (14–23)
Adult	300,000,000	75	15 (12–18)

duration of time, or ventilation maintained against a known resistive load, or sustained ventilation at a specific lung volume (elastic load). It is also determined with respect to a specific ventilatory target and the time to exhaustion (fatigue).

6. Respiratory muscles fatigue when energy consumption exceeds energy supply.
7. Fatigue is likely to occur when work of breathing is increased, strength is reduced, or inefficiency results so that energy consumption is affected.
8. Hypoxemia, anemia, decreased blood flow to muscles, and depletion of energy reserves alter energy availability.
9. Clinical manifestations of respiratory muscle fatigue are progressive hypercapnia or apnea.

C. Postnatal maturation
1. Lung size, surface area, and volume grow in an exponential manner for about 2 months after term gestation.
2. Control of breathing (feedback control through chemoreceptors and stretch receptors), and the neural maturation of the respiratory centers also appear to coincide with maturation at about 2 months postnatal age.
3. Beyond this age, lung volumes continue to increase during infancy, slowing during childhood but still continuing to grow structurally into early adolescence (Table 7).
4. It is this biologic phenomenon that provides a scope of recovery for infants with BPD.
5. In health, the increasing lung volume and cross-sectional area of the airways is associated with a reduction in the normal respiratory rate.

Chapter 2

Spontaneous Breathing

Emidio M. Sivieri, Vinod K. Bhutani

I. **Introduction**

   A. Air, like liquid, moves from a region of higher pressure to one with lower pressure.

   B. During breathing and just prior to inspiration, no gas flows because the gas pressure within the alveoli is equal to atmospheric pressure.

   C. For inspiration to occur, alveolar pressure must be less than atmospheric pressure.

   D. For expiration to occur, alveolar pressure must be higher than atmospheric pressure.

   E. Thus, for inspiration to occur, the gradient in pressures can be achieved either by lowering the alveolar pressure ("negative," "natural," spontaneous breathing) or, raising the atmospheric pressure ("positive," "pressure," mechanical breathing).

   F. The clinical and physiologic implications of forces that influence inspiration and expiration are discussed in this section.

II. **Signals of Respiration**

   A. Each respiratory cycle can be described by the measurement of three signals: driving pressure (P), volume (V), and time (Figure 2).

   B. The rate of change in volume over time defines flow ($\dot{V}$).

   C. The fundamental act of spontaneous breathing results from the generation of P, the inspiratory driving force needed to overcome the elastic, flow-resistive, and inertial properties of the entire respiratory system in order to initiate $\dot{V}$.

   1. This relationship has been best described by Röhrer using an equation of motion in which the driving pressure (P) is equal to the sum of elastic (P_E), resistive (P_R), and inertial pressure (P_I) components, thus:

$$P = P_E + P_R + P_I$$

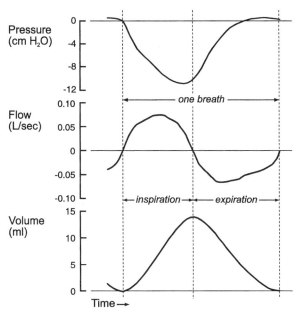

Figure 2. Graphic representation of a respiratory cycle demonstrating pressure, flow, and volume waveforms. Volume is obtained by integration (area under the curve) of the flow signal. (Modified from Bhutani VK, Sivieri EM, Abbasi S: Evaluation of pulmonary function in the neonate. In Polin RA, Fox WW [Eds.]: *Fetal and Neonatal Physiology, 2nd Edition.* Philadelphia, W.B. Saunders, 1998, p. 1144, with permission.)

2. In this relationship, the elastic pressure is assumed to be proportional to volume change by an elastic constant (E) representing the elastance (or elastic resistance) of the system.

3. The resistive component of pressure is assumed proportional to airflow by a resistive constant (R) representing inelastic airway and tissue resistances.

4. In addition, the inertial component of pressure is assumed to be proportional to gas and tissue acceleration ($\ddot{V}$) by an inertial constant (I). Therefore:

$$P = EV + R\dot{V} + I\ddot{V}$$

5. This is a linear, first order model in which the respiratory system is treated as a simple mechanical system (Figure 3), where applied pressure P causes gas to flow through a tube (the respiratory airways) which is connected to a closed elastic chamber (alveoli) of volume (V). In this ideal model E, R, and I are assumed to be

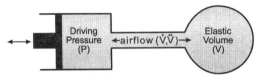

Figure 3. Linear, first order model of the respiratory system, where applied pressure causes gas to flow through a tube connected to an elastic chamber.

constants in a linear relationship between driving pressure and volume.

6. Under conditions of normal breathing frequencies (relatively low airflow and tissue acceleration) the inertance term is traditionally considered negligible, therefore:

$$P = EV + R\dot{V}$$

7. In respiratory terminology, elastance is usually replaced by compliance (C), which is a term used to represent the expandability or distensibility of the system. Since compliance is simply the reciprocal of elastance, the equation of motion can be rewritten as:

$$P = V/C + R\dot{V}$$

8. This simplified form of the Röhrer equation is the basis for most evaluations of pulmonary mechanics where measurements of P, V, and $\dot{V}$ are used to compute the various components of respiratory system compliance, resistance, and work of breathing.

D. One can further study the nonlinear nature of the respiratory system using more advanced nonlinear models and by analyzing two-dimensional graphic plots of P-V, V-$\dot{V}$, and P-$\dot{V}$ relationships.

E. Because the inherent nature of the respiratory signals is to be variable (especially in premature infants), it is imperative that the signals are measured in as steady state as feasible and over a protracted period of time (usually 2–3 minutes).

III. Driving Pressure

A. During spontaneous breathing, the driving pressure required to overcome elastic, airflow-resistive, and inertial properties of the respiratory system is the result of intrapleural pressure (P_{IP}) changes generated by the respiratory muscles (Figure 4).

B. During a respiratory cycle both the intrapleural and alveolar pressures change.

1. Just before the commencement of an inspiratory cycle, the intrapleural pressure is subatmospheric (−3 to −6 cm H_2O) because of the elastic recoil effect of the lung.

2. At this time, the alveolar pressure is atmospheric (zero), because

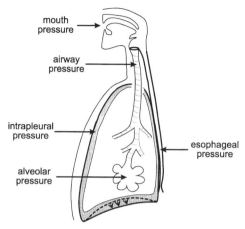

Figure 4. Schematic representation of components of respiratory pressures used in pulmonary function studies. Esophageal pressure approximates intrapleural pressure. (Modified from Bhutani VK, Sivieri EM, Abbasi S: Evaluation of pulmonary function in the neonate. In Polin RA, Fox WW [Eds.]: *Fetal and Neonatal Physiology, 2nd Edition.* Philadelphia, W.B. Saunders, 1998, p. 1153, with permission.)

there is no airflow and thus no pressure drop along the conducting airways.

3. During a spontaneous inspiration, forces generated by the respiratory muscles cause the intrapleural pressure to further decrease, producing a concomitant fall in alveolar pressure so as to initiate a driving pressure gradient which forces airflow into the lung.

4. During a passive expiration, the respiratory muscles are relaxed and the intrapleural pressure becomes less negative.

5. Elastic recoil forces in the now expanded lung and thorax cause alveolar pressure to become positive and thus the net driving pressure forces air to flow out of the lungs.

6. With forced expiration, the intrapleural pressure rises above atmospheric pressure.

7. The magnitude of the change in the alveolar pressure depends on the airflow rate and the airway resistance, but usually varies between 1–2 cm H_2O below and above atmospheric pressure during inspiration and expiration, respectively.

8. This range of alveolar pressure change can be markedly increased with air trapping or airway obstruction.

B. The following are some physiologic observations of changes in intrapleural pressure during spontaneous breathing:

1. Under some conditions respiratory airflow is zero or very close to zero:
   a. During tidal breathing, airflow is zero at end-inspiration and end-expiration where it reverses direction (Figure 5).
   b. During slow static inflation, airflow can be approximated as zero.
   c. In both cases, the resistive component of driving pressure as described above is zero or $R\dot{V} = 0$ and P_{IP} is equal to elastic pressure only:

$$P_{IP} = P_E = V/C$$

2. The elastic component of intrapleural pressure can be estimated on the pressure tracing by connecting with straight lines the points of zero flow at end-expiration and end-inspiration (Figure 5). The vertical segment between this estimated elastic pressure line and the measured intrapleural pressure (solid line) represents the resistive pressure component (Figure 6).
3. Resistive pressure is usually maximal at points of peak airflow, which usually occurs during mid-inspiration and mid-expiration.

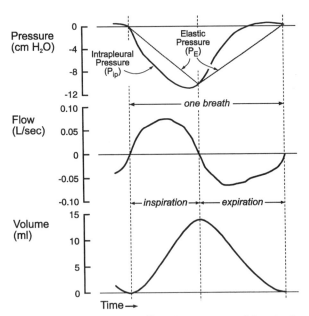

Figure 5. During tidal breathing, airflow is zero at end-inspiration and end-expiration, where it reverses direction. The pressure difference between these two points represents the net elastic pressure at end-inspiration. The elastic component of intrapleural pressure at other points can be approximated by a straight line connecting points of zero flow.

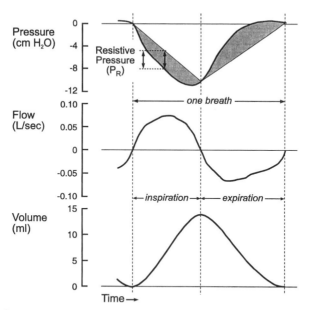

Figure 6. The elastic component of intrapleural pressure can be estimated on the pressure tracing by connecting points of zero flow at end-expiration and end-inspiration with a straight line. The vertical distance between this estimate and the measured intrapleural pressure is the resistive pressure component.

4. Transpulmonary pressure (P_{TP}) is the differential between intrapleural pressure and alveolar pressure. This is the portion of the total respiratory driving pressure which is attributed to inflation and deflation of the lung specifically.

C. With mechanical ventilation, of course, the driving pressure is provided by the ventilator. In contrast to spontaneous breathing, where a negative change in intrapleural pressure is the driving pressure for inspiration, the mechanical ventilator applies a positive pressure to an endotracheal tube. Nonetheless, in both cases there is a positive pressure gradient from the mouth to the alveoli. In both cases, the transpulmonary pressure gradient is in the same direction.

IV. Factors that Impact Mechanics of Airflow
Factors that influence the respiratory muscles and respiratory mechanics have an effect on how air flows in and out of the lungs. These are characterized by physical, physiologic, and pathophysiologic considerations.

A. Physical factors
1. The pattern of airflow is affected by the physical properties of the gas molecules, the laminar or turbulent nature of airflow, and the

15

dimensions of the airways, as well as the other effects described by the Poiseuille equation (see Chapter 4).

2. The elastic properties of the airway, the transmural pressure on the airway wall, and structural features of the airway wall also determine the mechanics of airflow.

3. In preterm newborns, the airways are narrower in diameter and result in a higher resistance to airflow. Also, the increased airway compliance increases the propensity for airway collapse or distension. If a higher transmural pressure is generated during tidal breathing (as in infants with bronchopulmonary dysplasia [BPD], or, during positive pressure ventilation), the intrathoracic airways are likely to be compressed during expiration (Figure 7).

4. During forced expiration, the more compliant airways are also likely to be compressed in the presence of a high intrathoracic pressure.

5. Increased distensibility of airways, as when exposed to excessive end-distending pressure, can result in increased and wasted dead space ventilation.

6. Turbulence of gas flow, generally not an issue in a healthy individual, can lead to a need for a higher driving pressure in the sick preterm infant with structural airway deformations as encountered in those with BPD.

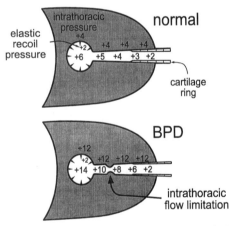

Figure 7. Schematic comparison of normal and abnormal airflow. Infant with bronchopulmonary dysplasia (BPD) has higher transmural pressure generated during tidal breathing and thoracic airways are likely to be compressed during expiration, resulting in a flow limitation. (Modified from Bhutani VK, Sivieri EM: Physiological principles for bedside assessment of pulmonary graphics. In Donn SM [Ed.]: *Neonatal and Pediatric Pulmonary Graphics: Principles and Clinical Applications.* Armonk, NY, Futura Publishing Co., 1998, p. 63, with permission.)

B. Physiologic
1. The tone of the tracheobronchial smooth muscle provides a mechanism to stabilize the airways and prevent collapse.
2. An increased tone as a result of smooth muscle hyperplasia or a hyper-responsive smooth muscle should lead to a bronchospastic basis of airflow limitation.
3. The bronchomalacic airway may be destabilized in the presence of tracheal smooth muscle relaxants.
4. The effect of some of the other physiologic factors, such as the alveolar duct sphincter tone, are not yet fully understood.

C. Pathophysiologic
1. Plugging of the airway lumen, mucosal edema, cohesion, and compression of the airway wall lead to alterations in tracheobronchial airflow.
2. Weakening of the airway walls secondary to the structural airway barotrauma and the consequent changes of tracheobronchomalacia also result in abnormal airflow patterns.
3. BPD-related airflow effects have also been previously described.

V. Lung Volumes

Ventilation is a cyclic process of inspiration and expiration. Total or minute ventilation (MV) is the volume of air expired each minute. The volume of air moved in or out during each cycle of ventilation is the tidal volume (V_T) and is a sum of the air in the conducting zone (V_D, or dead space) and the respiratory zone (V_A, or alveolar space). Thus,

$$MV = (V_A + V_D) \times frequency$$

The process of spontaneous breathing generally occurs at about mid total lung capacity such that about two-thirds of the total capacity is available as reserve.

A. Ventilatory volumes
1. V_T: volume of air inspired with each breath
2. MV: product of frequency (F, the number of tidal volumes taken per minute) and V_T
3. V_D: volume in which there is no gas exchange
   a. Dead space refers to the volume within the respiratory system that does not participate in gas exchange and is often the most frequent and unrecognized cause for hypercapnia.
   b. It is composed of several components.
      (1) Anatomic dead space is the volume of gas contained in the conducting airway.
      (2) Alveolar dead space refers to the volume of gas in areas of "wasted ventilation," that is, in alveoli that are ventilated poorly or are underperfused.

(3) The total volume of gas that is not involved in gas exchange is called the physiologic dead space. It is the sum of the anatomic and alveolar dead space.

c. In a normal person, the physiologic dead space should be equal to the anatomic dead space. For this reason, some investigators refer to physiologic dead space as pathological dead space.

d. Several factors can modify the dead space volume.

(1) Anatomic dead space increases as a function of airway size and the airway compliance. Because of the interdependence of the alveoli and airways, anatomic dead space increases as a function of lung volume. Similarly, dead space increases as a function of body height, bronchodilator drugs, and diseases such as BPD, tracheomegaly, and oversized artificial airways.

(2) Anatomic dead space is decreased by reduction of the size of the airways, as occurs with bronchoconstriction, tracheomalacia, or a tracheostomy.

4. Alveolar volume ($\dot{V}_A$): volume in which gas exchange occurs.

$$V_A = V_T - V_D$$

5. Alveolar ventilation (V_A): product of frequency and V_A.

B. Lung reserve volumes
Reserve volumes represent the maximal volume of gas that can be moved above or below a normal tidal volume (Figure 8). These values

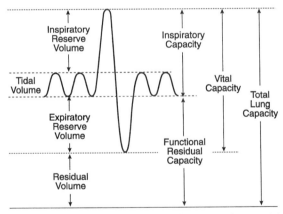

Figure 8. Graphic representation of lung volumes and capacities. (Modified from Bhutani VK, Sivieri EM: Physiological principles for bedside assessment of pulmonary graphics. In Donn SM [Ed.]: *Neonatal and Pediatric Pulmonary Graphics: Principles and Clinical Applications.* Armonk, NY, Futura Publishing Co., 1998, p. 67, with permission.)

reflect the balance between lung and chest wall elasticity, respiratory strength, and thoracic mobility.

1. Inspiratory reserve volume (IRV) is the maximum volume of gas that can be inspired from the peak of tidal volume.
2. Expiratory reserve volume (ERV) is the maximum volume of gas that can be expired after a normal tidal expiration. Therefore, the reserve volumes are associated with the ability to increase or decrease tidal volume. Normal lungs do not collapse at the end of the maximum expiration.
3. The volume of gas that remains is called the residual volume (RV).

C. Lung capacities

The capacity of the lungs can be represented in four different ways: total lung capacity, vital capacity, inspiratory capacity, and functional residual capacity (Figure 8).

1. Total lung capacity (TLC) is the amount of gas in the respiratory system after a maximal inspiration. It is the sum of all four lung volumes. The normal values as well as the values of static lung volumes for term newborns are shown below in Table 8.
2. Vital capacity (VC) is the maximal volume of gas that can be expelled from the lungs after a maximal inspiration. As such, the vital capacity is the sum of IRV + TV + ERV. Inspiratory capacity (IC) is the maximal volume of gas that can be inspired from the resting end-expiration level; therefore it is the sum of TV + IRV.
3. Functional residual capacity (FRC) is the volume of gas in the lung when the respiratory system is at rest; that is, the volume in the lung at the end of a normal expiration that is in continuity with the airways. The size of the FRC is determined by the balance of two opposing forces:
   a. Inward elastic recoil of the lung tending to collapse the lung
   b. Outward elastic recoil of the chest wall tending to expand the lung. FRC is the volume of gas above which a normal tidal

Table 8
Lung Volumes in Term Newborns*

Ventilatory Volumes *Normal Values for Term Newborns*		*Static Lung Volumes* *Normal Values for Term Newborns*	
V_T	5–8 mL/kg	RV	10–15 mL/kg
F	40–60 breaths/min	FRC	25–30 mL/kg
V_D	2–2.5 mL/kg	TGV	30–40 mL/kg
MV	200–480 mL/min/kg	TLC	50–90 mL/kg
$\dot{V}_A$	60–320 mL/min/kg	VC	35–80 mL/kg

* See text for definition of abbreviations.

volume oscillates. A normal FRC avails optimum lung mechanics and alveolar surface area for efficient ventilation and gas exchange.

4. ERV: volume of air (residual volume) remaining in the respiratory system at the end of the maximum possible expiration

$$RV = FRC - ERV$$

D. It is important to note that thoracic gas volume (TGV) is the total amount of gas in the lung (or thorax) at end-expiration. This value differs from FRC and the difference would indicate the magnitude of air trapping.

Chapter 3

Pulmonary Gas Exchange

Vinod K. Bhutani

I. **Introduction**

   A. Independent pulmonary gas exchange to replace the maternal placental gas exchange mechanism needs to be established within the first few minutes of birth.

   B. In order to effect this transition, several physiologic changes occur
   1. Adjustments in circulation
   2. Pulmonary mechanics
   3. Gas exchange
   4. Acid-base status
   5. Respiratory control

   C. Upon transition, gas exchange takes place through an air-liquid interphase of alveolar epithelium with alveolar gas in one compartment and blood in the other (vascular) compartment. An understanding of gas laws, alveolar ventilation, and pulmonary vasculature are important in facilitating optimal pulmonary gas exchange.

II. **Brief Outline of Cardiopulmonary Adaptations**

   A. Prior to birth, the fetus is totally dependent on the placenta (Figure 9) and has made cardiopulmonary adjustments for optimal delivery of oxygen, whereas the maternal physiology has been adapted to maintain fetal normocapnia.

   B. The salient features and sequence of events that occur during fetal to neonatal transition are listed in Table 9.

III. **Application of Gas Laws for Pulmonary Gas Exchange**

   A. There are fundamental laws of physics that pertain to the behavior of gases and thereby impact on gas exchange.

   B. An understanding of these laws is also specifically pertinent to the clinician in his/her ability not only to measure and interpret blood gas values but also to evaluate the impact on gas exchange during clinical

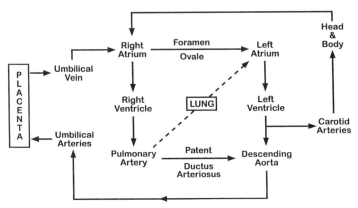

Figure 9. Schematic representation of fetal circulation. (From Bhutani VK: Extrauterine adaptations in the newborn. Sem Perinatol 1997; 1:1-12, with permission.)

conditions of hypothermia, high altitude, and use of gas mixtures of varying viscosities and densities.

C. A brief description of the pertinent and clinically relevant gas laws is listed in Table 10.

D. One of the most fundamental and widely used relationships to describe pulmonary gas exchange is summarized as:

$$P_ACO_2 = 863(\dot{V}_{CO2}/\dot{V}_A)$$

where, in a steady state and with negligible inspired carbon dioxide, the alveolar pressure of carbon dioxide (P_ACO_2) is proportional to the ratio of the rates of carbon dioxide elimination ($\dot{V}_{CO2}$) and alveolar ventilation ($\dot{V}_A$). This equation helps to summarize several of the gas laws. The applications of the laws are thus:

1. P_ACO_2: when measured in dry gas as a percentage, Dalton's law needs to be applied to convert the value to partial pressure. The partial pressure of carbon dioxide, rather than its percentage composition, is the significant variable because Henry's law of solubility states that the gas is physically dissolved in liquid and in equilibrium with the gas phase at the same partial pressure.

2. 863: this peculiar number is derived from the need to standardize measurements from body temperature (310°K) to standard pressure and temperature (760 mm Hg · 273°K). Based on the product 310 × (760/273), we obtain the value 863 (in mmHg) providing the constant for the relationship in the above equation.

3. $\dot{V}_{CO2}/\dot{V}_A$: These values are measured at ambient temperature and pressure, saturated with water vapor (ATPS). Carbon dioxide output needs to be converted to STPD (standard temperature, pressure, dry) using Boyle's and Charles's laws, while alveolar venti-

Table 9
Salient Features of Extrauterine Cardiopulmonary Adaptations

Parameter	Mother (2nd Trimester)	Fetus (Before Labor)	Newborn (Before 1st Breath)	Newborn (At about 6 Hours)
PaO_2	80–95 torr	<25 torr in pulmonary artery	16–18 torr	80–95 torr
$PaCO_2$	~34 torr	40–42 torr	45–65 torr	34 torr
pH	~7.45	7.35–7.40	7.10–7.30	7.35–7.40
Pulmonary blood flow	Equivalent to cardiac output	13–25% cardiac output	~25% cardiac output	90–100% cardiac output
Shunts	Placental shunts	Placental shunts Foramen ovale Ductus arteriosus	Foramen ovale Ductus arteriosus Intrapulmonary shunts	Foramen ovale closed Ductus arteriosus usually closed Intrapulmonary shunts
Pulmonary mechanics	Air-filled lungs Hyperventilation	Liquid-filled FRC at 30 mL/kg	Air and fluid (16–19 mL/kg) in the lungs	Air-filled FRC at 30 mL/kg
Control of respiration	Progesterone-mediated hyperventilation	Fetal breathing dependent more on stretch receptors than on chemoreceptors.	First breath initiated by nonspecific respiratory stimuli such as proprioceptive feedback.	Rhythmic respiratory cycles based on chemoreceptor and stretch receptor feedback.

FRC = functional residual capacity.

Table 10
Laws that Describe Gas Behavior

Law	Description
Boyle's law	At constant temperature (T), a given volume (V) of gas varies inversely to the pressure (P) to which it is subjected.
Charles's law	Gas expands as it is warmed and shrinks as it is cooled.
Dalton's law	The total pressure exerted by a mixture of gases is equal to the sum of the partial pressure of each gas.
Amagat's law	The total volume of a mixture of gases is equal to the sum of the partial volume of each gas at the same temperature and pressure.
Henry's law	At constant temperature, any gas physically dissolves in a liquid in proportion to its partial pressure, although the solubility coefficient decreases with increasing temperature and differs from one gas to another.
Graham's law	The rate of diffusion of a gas is inversely proportional to the square root of its density.
Fick's law	The transfer of solute by diffusion is directly proportional to the cross-sectional area available for diffusion and to the difference in concentration per unit distance perpendicular to that cross section.
Ideal gas equation	Summation of above laws: $PV = nRT$, where R is a numerical constant
Van der Waals's equation	Refinement of the ideal gas equation based upon the attractive forces between molecules and upon the volume occupied by the molecules.
Barometric pressure and altitude	The decrease in barometric pressure is not linear with increasing altitude; weather, temperature, density of atmosphere, acceleration of gravity, etc. influence it.

lation has to be corrected to BTPS (body temperature, pressure, and saturated with water vapor).

IV. **Development of Pulmonary Vasculature**
   A. The main pulmonary artery develops from the embryonic left sixth arch.
      1. The sixth arches appear at about 32 days after conception (5 mm embryo stage) and give branches to the developing lung bud.
      2. Branches from the aorta that supply the lung bud and the right arch disappear subsequently.
      3. By 50 days (18 mm embryo stage), the adult pattern of vascularization has commenced.
   B. Before the main pulmonary veins are developed, the vessels drain into the systemic circulation of the foregut and trachea.
      1. These connections are lost as the main pulmonary vein develops.
      2. A primitive pulmonary vein appears as a bud from the left side of the atrial chamber at about 35 days.
      3. Starting as a blind capillary, it bifurcates several times to connect with the developing lung bud.
      4. Subsequently, the first two branches are resorbed to form the left atrium at about the 7th week.
   C. The branches of the pulmonary arterial system maintain a position next to the bronchial structures as both develop during the glandular and canalicular stages of lung development.
   D. By 16 weeks, there is a complete set of vessels that lead to the respiratory bronchioles, terminal bronchioles, and the terminal sacs.

V. **Onset of Pulmonary Gas Exchange**
   A. The physiologic processes that facilitate the onset of postnatal pulmonary gas exchange (described in the series of events depicted in Figure 10).
      1. The effect of ventilation on reducing pulmonary vascular resistance (A)
      2. The effect of acidosis correction to enhance pulmonary blood flow (B)
      3. The effect of driving pressure and successful establishment of respiration during first breaths to achieve an optimal functional residual capacity (C)
      4. The effect of driving pressure to maintain optimal tidal volume and achieve the least work of breathing (D)
   B. These events highlight the other series of biochemical and physiologic events that concurrently occur to successfully establish and maintain the matching of ventilation to perfusion.
   C. Maladaptations delay transition to adequate pulmonary gas exchange.
   D. Though it has been well established that a newborn is more likely to

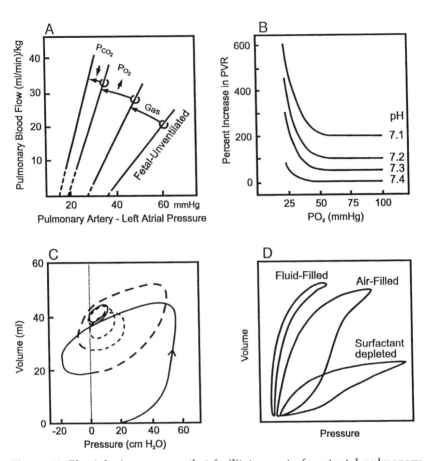

Figure 10. Physiologic processes that facilitate onset of postnatal pulmonary gas exchange. **A.** Effect of ventilation on reducing pulmonary vascular resistance (PVR). **B.** Effects of acidosis correction on reducing PVR. **C.** First breaths and establishment of optimal functional residual capacity. **D.** Effect of driving pressure to maintain optimal tidal volume and work of breathing. (Modified from Bhutani VK: Differential diagnosis of neonatal respiratory disorders. In Spitzer AR [Ed.]: *Intensive Care of the Fetus and Neonate.* St. Louis, Mosby-Year Book, 1996, p. 500, with permission.)

have events that lead to hypoxemia or maintain adequate oxygenation with an inability to compensate hemodynamically, it has also been realized that a newborn is more tolerant of hypoxemia than an adult. Reasons for occurrences of hypoxemic events:

1. Reduced FRC relative to the oxygen consumption
2. Presence of intrapulmonary shunts that lead to $\dot{V}/\dot{Q}$ mismatching

3. A high alveolar-arterial oxygen gradient

E. Hypercapnia that results from an inability to maintain adequate alveolar ventilation in the face of mechanical loads also results in lower alveolar oxygen tension.

F. From a hemodynamic perspective, impaired oxygen delivery may occur because of:

1. Low P_{50} values due to high oxygen affinity of the fetal hemoglobin
2. Increased blood viscosity
3. Lower myocardial response to a volume or pressure load
4. Inadequate regional redistribution of the cardiac output

G. The relationship between arterial oxygen and carbon dioxide values and how these relate to hypoxemia and respiratory failure are shown in Figure 11.

H. The effect of oxygen inhalation on the composition of alveolar and blood gas tensions is shown in Table 11.

VI. Optimal Pulmonary Gas Exchange

A. Failure to establish optimal pulmonary gas exchange leads to either oxygenation or ventilation failure.

B. Factors that impact on adequacy of neonatal gas exchange (especially a preterm newborn) are listed in Table 12.

C. Respiratory failure can initially lead to increased respiratory effort in an attempt at compensation, followed by an inability to ventilate, or apnea.

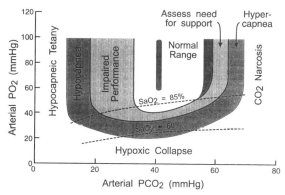

Figure 11. The relationship between alveolar oxygen and carbon dioxide values and how these relate to hypoxemia and respiratory failure. (Modified from Bhutani VK: Differential diagnosis of neonatal respiratory disorders. In Spitzer AR [Ed.]: *Intensive Care of the Fetus and Neonate*. St. Louis, Mosby-Year Book, 1996, p. 501, with permission.)

Table 11
Effect of Oxygen Inhalation (100%) on Composition
of Alveolar and Blood Gas Tensions

	Inspired Dry Gas		*Alveolar Gas*		*End Pulmonary Capillary Blood*		*Arterial Blood*		*End-Systemic Capillary Blood*	
	Air	O_2	*Air*	O_2	*Air*	O_2	*Air*	O_2	*Air*	O_2
P_{O2}, torr	159.1	760	104	673	104	673	100	640	40	53.5
P_{CO2}, torr	0.3	0	40	40	40	40	40	40	46	46
P_{H2O}, torr	0.0	0	47	47	47	47	47	47	47	47
P_{N2}, torr	600.6	0	569	0	569	0	573	0	573	0
P_{total}, torr	760	760	760	760	760	760	760	727	706	146.5*
O_2Sat (%)					98	100	98	100	75	85.5

* What happens to the total gas tension when a baby breathes 100% oxygen: the total venous gas tension is now at 146.5 torr.

D. The concurrent changes in arterial oxygen and carbon dioxide gas tensions during both health and disease are shown in Figure 11.

VII. Physiologic Principles to Improve Pulmonary Gas Exchange

A. The physiologic principles that may be utilized to improve oxygenation, enhance carbon dioxide elimination, and establish ventilation at

Table 12
Factors that Impact on Adequacy of Neonatal Gas Exchange

Factors for Gas Exchange	*Impact of Prematurity*
Neural control of respiration	Immaturity
Mechanical loads: elastic and resistive	High chest wall to lung compliance ratio
Stability of end-expiratory lung volume	Compliant airways with pre-end-expiratory closure of airways
Ventilation/perfusion matching	Reactive pulmonary vasculature
Hemoglobin dissociation curve properties	Fetal hemoglobin characteristics
Match cardiac output to oxygen consumption	High neonatal oxygen consumption
Ability to maintain alveolar ventilation	Propensity for respiratory muscle fatigue

optimal FRC (and thereby with the least barotrauma) are listed in Figure 10 A, B, C, D.

B. The clinically relevant interventional strategies are crucial to achieve optimal gas exchange.

C. It is also valuable to be reminded that, in a healthy newborn, gas tensions are maintained in a narrow range by exquisitely sensitive feedback mechanisms of chemoreceptors and stretch receptors.

D. Moreover, during fetal development the maternal physiology is significantly altered to maintain fetal normocapnia and neutral acid-base status.

E. Thus, as clinicians assume control of the newborn's ventilation with supportive technologies, the road map for optimal pulmonary gas exchange needs to be "quality controlled" from physiologic perspectives and with the least amount of barotrauma.

Chapter 4

Pulmonary Mechanics

Emidio M. Sivieri, Vinod K. Bhutani

I. Introduction

   A. The structural and physiologic characteristics of the neonatal respiratory system are unique and may act as impediments for normal respiration.

   B. These mechanical characteristics are the elastic and resistive properties of the respiratory system and the forces that cause airflow.

   C. The energy for ventilating the lungs is supplied by the active contraction of the respiratory muscles, and this is required to overcome the elastic recoil of the lungs and the frictional resistance to airflow in the conducting airways.

II. Elastic Properties

   A. The elastic properties of the lung parenchyma are dependent on the elasticity of pulmonary tissues, gas exchange spaces, smooth muscle, connective tissue, and the vascular tissue. Equally important as tissue elasticity is the recoil effect from surface tension forces at the alveolar liquid-air interface. The elastic properties of the airway depend on the smooth muscle, tissue properties, and fibrocartilaginous structure, whereas the elastic properties of the thorax depend on the rib cage, intercostal muscle, the diaphragm, and tissues of the chest wall. These forces are interdependent, maintain a complex balance, and are influenced by the respiratory cycle and position of the body.

   B. Elasticity is the property of matter such that if a system is disturbed by stretching or expanding it, the system will tend to return to its original position when all external forces are removed. Like a spring, the tissues of the lungs and thorax stretch during inspiration, and when the force of contraction (respiratory muscular effort) is removed, the tissues return to their resting position. The resting position or lung volume is established by a balance of elastic forces. At rest, the elastic recoil forces of the lung tissues equal exactly those of the chest wall and diaphragm. This occurs at the end of every normal expiration when the respiratory muscles are relaxed, and the volume remaining in the lungs is the functional residual capacity (FRC).

C. The visceral pleura of the lung is separated from the parietal pleura of the chest wall by a thin film of fluid creating a potential space between the two structures. In a normal newborn at the end of expiration, the mean pressure in this space (i.e., the intrapleural pressure) is 3–6 cm H_2O below atmospheric pressure. This pressure results from the equal and opposite retractile forces of the lungs and chest wall and varies during the respiratory cycle, becoming more negative during active inspiration and more positive during expiration. During normal breathing the pressure within the lungs is dependent on the airway and tissue frictional resistive properties in response to airflow. Because there is no net movement of air at end-expiration and at end-inspiration, pressure throughout the lung at these times is in equilibrium with atmospheric air.

D. Lung compliance

1. If pressure is sequentially decreased (made more subatmospheric) around the outside of an excised lung, the lung volume increases.

2. When the pressure is removed from around the lung, it returns to its resting volume.

3. This elastic behavior of the lungs is characterized by the pressure-volume curve (Figure 12A). Note that the pressure-volume curve during inspiration is different from that during expiration.

4. This difference is typical of non-ideal elastic systems and is called the hysteresis of the system.

5. The ratio of change in lung volume to change in distending pressure defines the compliance of the lungs:

$$\text{Lung compliance} = \frac{\Delta \text{ lung volume}}{\Delta P_{TP}}$$

where transpulmonary pressure (P_{TP}) is the net driving pressure to expand the lungs only and is defined as the difference between alveolar pressure and intrapleural pressure. Intrapleural pressure cannot easily be measured directly, but it can be approximated by measuring the intraesophageal pressure.

6. By definition, lung compliance is a static characteristic obtained while the respiratory system is in a passive state and there is no airflow.

a. This can be achieved in infants by numerous, well-proven, static techniques.

b. Using special dynamic techniques, lung compliance can also be measured during uninterrupted spontaneous breathing or mechanical ventilation.

c. Compliance obtained in this manner is termed dynamic compliance.

7. Although the pressure-volume relationship of the lung is not linear over the entire lung volume range, the compliance (of slope $\Delta V/\Delta P$) may be close to linear over the normal range of tidal volumes beginning at FRC (Figure 12F). Thus, for a given change in pressure, tidal volume will increase in proportion to lung compliance, or $\Delta V = C\Delta P$.

31

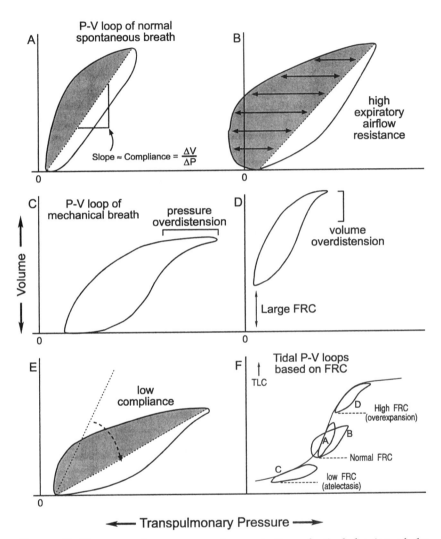

Figure 12. Pressure-volume curves demonstrating elastic behavior of the lungs. **A.** Normal spontaneous breath. **B.** High expiratory airflow resistance. **C.** Mechanical breath with pressure overdistension. **D.** Mechanical breath with volume overdistension and large functional residual capacity. **E.** Low compliance with clockwise shift of axis. **F.** Tidal pressure-volume loops based on the functional residual capacity. (Modified from Bhutani VK, Sivieri EM: Physiological principles for bedside assessment of pulmonary graphics. In Donn SM [Ed.]: *Neonatal and Pediatric Pulmonary Graphics: Principles and Clinical Applications.* Armonk, NY, Futura Publishing Co., 1998, p. 70, with permission.)

    a. As lung compliance is decreased, the lungs are stiffer and more difficult to expand.

    b. When lung compliance is increased, the lung becomes easier to distend, and is thus more compliant.

8. Lung compliance and pressure-volume relationships are determined by the interdependence of elastic tissue elements and alveolar surface tension. Tissue elasticity is dependent on elastin and collagen content of the lung.

9. A typical value for lung compliance in a young healthy newborn is 1.5–2.0 mL/cm H_2O/kg.

    a. This value is dependent on the size of the lung (mass of elastic tissue).

    b. As may be expected, the compliance of the lung increases with development as the tissue mass of the lung increases.

    c. When comparing values between different subjects, lung compliance should be normalized for lung volume by dividing by the FRC. This ratio is called the specific lung compliance.

10. The surface-active substance (surfactant) lining the alveoli of the lung has a significant physiologic function.

    a. Surfactant lowers surface tension inside the alveoli, thereby contributing to lung stability by reducing the pressure necessary to expand the alveoli.

    b. Alveolar type II cells contain osmophilic lamellar bodies that are associated with the transformation of surfactant.

    c. Impaired surface activity, as occurs in those premature infants with respiratory distress syndrome (RDS), typically results in lungs that are stiff (low compliance) and prone to collapse (atelectasis).

11. In bronchopulmonary dysplasia (BPD), the areas of fibrosis and scarring lead to a reduction in the lung compliance. In these conditions, the baby has to generate a higher driving pressure to achieve a similar tidal volume or else hypoventilation would occur.

E. Total respiratory system compliance

  1. If the driving pressure is measured across the entire respiratory system (the transthoracic pressure), then for a given volume change we obtain the compliance of the combined lung and chest wall together:

$$\text{Total compliance} = \frac{\Delta \text{ lung volume}}{\Delta \text{ transthoracic pressure}}$$

where, in a passive respiratory system, transthoracic pressure is the differential between alveolar and atmospheric pressure.

  2. In a newborn connected to a mechanical ventilator, the transthoracic pressure can be measured simply as the airway pressure applied at the mouth or endotracheal tube.

F. Chest wall compliance
1. Like the lung, the chest wall is elastic.
2. If air is introduced into the pleural cavity, the lungs will collapse inward and the chest wall will expand outward.

$$\text{Chest wall compliance} = \frac{\Delta \text{ volume}}{\Delta \text{ intrathoracic pressure}}$$

where the intrathoracic pressure is the pressure differential across the chest wall to atmosphere. Because it is difficult to measure chest wall pressure directly, chest wall compliance may be measured indirectly where:

Elastance of the respiratory system = Elastance of lungs +

elastance of chest wall

Thus,

$$\frac{1}{\text{total lung compliance}} = \frac{1}{\text{lung compliance}} + \frac{1}{\text{chest wall compliance}}$$

3. As previously discussed, there is a balance of elastic recoil forces at rest (end of expiration) such that the lungs maintain a stable FRC (Figure 13).

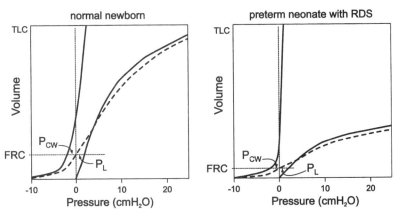

Figure 13. Balance of elastic recoil at rest to maintain stable functional residual capacity. **Left.** Normal newborn. Chest wall compliance is higher than that of the adult. **Right.** Preterm newborn with RDS. Chest wall is even more compliant and aggravated by disease state; FRC is lower. (Modified from Bhutani VK, Sivieri EM: Physiological principles for bedside assessment of pulmonary graphics. In Donn SM [Ed.]: *Neonatal and Pediatric Pulmonary Graphics: Principles and Clinical Applications.* Armonk, NY, Futura Publishing Co., 1998, p. 72, with permission.)

  a. In the newborn, the chest wall compliance is higher than that of the adult.

  b. The chest wall becomes more compliant at earlier stages of gestation.

  c. Even if the lungs have a normal elastic recoil and compliance, the FRC will be lowered because the chest wall would be unable to balance the elastic forces.

  d. The preterm newborn is therefore destined to have a lower FRC and this state is aggravated if the FRC is lowered further because of disease states.

III. Resistive Properties

A. Nonelastic properties of the respiratory system characterize its resistance to motion.

B. Since motion between two surfaces in contact usually involves friction or loss of energy, resistance to breathing occurs in any moving part of the respiratory system.

C. These resistances would include frictional resistance to airflow, tissue resistance, and inertial forces.

  1. Lung resistance results predominantly (80%) from airway frictional resistance to airflow.

  2. Tissue resistance (19%) and inertia (1%) also influence lung resistance.

D. Airflow through the airways requires a driving pressure generated by changes in alveolar pressure.

E. When alveolar pressure is less than atmospheric pressure (during spontaneous inspiration), air flows into the lung; when alveolar pressure is greater than atmospheric pressure, air flows out of the lung.

F. By definition, resistance to airflow is equal to the resistive component of driving pressure (P_R) divided by the resulting airflow ($\dot{V}$), thus:

$$\text{Resistance} = \frac{P_R}{\dot{V}}$$

G. When determining pulmonary resistance (tissue and airway), the resistive component of the measured transpulmonary pressure is used as the driving pressure (Figure 14).

H. To obtain airway resistance alone, the differential between alveolar pressure and atmospheric pressure is used as the driving pressure.

I. Under normal tidal breathing conditions, there is a linear relationship between airflow and driving pressure.

  1. The slope of the flow vs. pressure curve increases as the airways narrow, indicating that the patient with airway obstruction has a greater resistance to airflow.

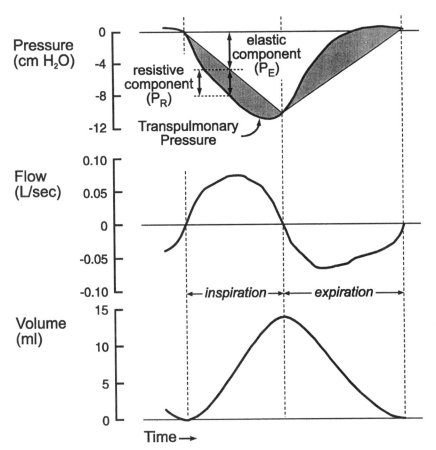

Figure 14. The relative elastic and resistive components of transpulmonary pressure recorded from a typical single spontaneous breath. Pulmonary resistance is determined from simultaneous measures of the resistive component of pressure and the flow signal.

2. The resistance to airflow is greatly dependent on the size of the airway lumen.

3. According to Poiseuille's law, the pressure (ΔP) required to achieve a given flow ($\dot{V}$) for a gas having viscosity η and flowing through a rigid and smooth cylindrical tube of length L and radius r is given as:

$$\Delta P = \frac{\dot{V}8\eta L}{\pi r^4}$$

Therefore, resistance to airflow is defined as:

$$\frac{\Delta P}{\dot{V}} = \frac{8 \eta L}{\pi r^4}$$

4. Thus, the resistance to airflow increases by a power of four with any decrease in airway diameter.

5. Because the newborn airway lumen is approximately half that of the adult, the neonatal airway resistance is about 16-fold that of the adult. Normal airway resistance in a term newborn is approximately 20–40 cm $H_2O/L/s$, which is about 16-fold the value observed in adults (1–2 cm $H_2O/L/s$).

J. Nearly 80% of the total resistance to airflow occurs in large airways up to about the fourth to fifth generation of bronchial branching.

1. The patient usually has large airway disease when resistance to airflow is increased.

2. Since the smaller airways contribute a small proportion of total airway resistance, they have been designated as the "silent zone" of the lung, in which airway obstruction can occur without being readily detected.

IV. Inertial Properties

Inertial forces are generally considered negligible for normal tidal breathing and when considering a linear model of respiration. However, with use of high airflow mechanical ventilation, high-frequency ventilation, and in severe airway disease, inertial forces need to be considered.

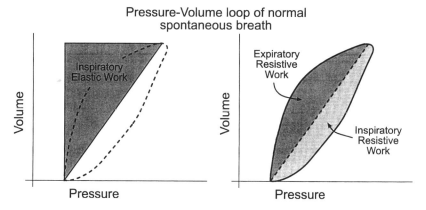

Pressure-Volume loop of normal spontaneous breath

Figure 15. Work of breathing is calculated as the area under the pressure versus volume curve (shaded areas).

Table 13
Mean Normal Values of Neonatal Pulmonary Function During the First Month

Author	Study year	GA (wks)	Age (days)	V_T (mL/kg)	FRC (mL/kg)	C_{DYN} (mL/cm H$_2$O)	R (cm H$_2$O/L/sec)
Berglund/Karlberg	1956	Term	7		27		
Cook et al.	1957	Term	1–6	5.3		5.2	29
Swyer et al.	1960	Term	1–11	6.7		4.9	26
Polgar	1961	Term	1–17		52.6	5.7	18.8
Strang/McGrath	1962	Term	1–6		49.5		
Nelson et al.	1963	Preterm	1–16		38.7		
		Term	2–4		27		
Feather/Russell	1974	Term	1–3			3.7	42
Ronchetti et al.	1975	34	4–28		29.5		
Taeusch et al.	1976	Term	4–6	7.2		3.7	
Adler/Wohl	1978	Term	2–5			3.5	
Mortola et al.	1984	Term	1–4	6.2		3.8	
Taussig et al.	1982	Term	1–9		31.4		
Migdal et al.	1987	34	1–28			2.4	
		Term	1–29			3.2	
Anday et al.	1987	28–30	2–3	5.9		2.0	50 exp
			5–7	6.6		2.3	70 exp
Gerhardt et al.	1987	31–36	3–30		16.7	2.2	87 exp
		Term	6–16		17.1	3.6	58 exp
Abbasi/Bhutani	1990	28–34	2–3	6.3		2.4	54
Sivieri et al.	1995	27–40	2–30		23.4		
		26–37	2–30		21.5 RDS		
		23–32	1–22		18.9 BPD		

GA = gestational age; V_T = tidal volume; FRC = functional residual capacity; C_{DYN} = dynamic lung compliance; R = pulmonary resistance; exp = expiratory; RDS = infants with respiratory distress syndrome; BPD = infants who developed bronchopulmonary dysplasia.

V. Work of Breathing

A. True work of breathing may be expressed as the energy required by the respiratory muscles in moving a given tidal volume of air into and out of the lungs. For obvious reasons, this type of work is difficult to determine accurately, whereas the actual mechanical work done by or on the lungs is much easier to measure. The mechanical work expended in compressing or expanding a given volume is obtained from the integral product of the applied pressure and the resulting volume change or:

$$Work = \int PdV$$

B. This value is simply the area under the applied pressure vs. volume curve for any gas. Therefore, by integrating the transpulmonary pressure curve over volume, the pulmonary work of breathing is easily calculated (Figure 15). This mechanical work can be partitioned into elastic and resistive components.

  1. Elastic work is that portion needed to overcome elastic resistance to inflate the lungs. Under normal conditions this work is stored as potential energy and is used in restoring the system to its resting volume.

  2. Resistive work is that portion needed to overcome airway and tissue frictional resistances. The hysteresis of the pressure-volume relationship represents the resistive work of breathing and can be further partitioned into inspiratory and expiratory components.

C. Normally, the elastic energy stored during inspiration is sufficient to provide the work needed to overcome expiratory frictional resistance.

  1. In babies with obstructive airway disease, the expiratory component of resistive work of breathing is increased (Figure 12B).

  2. The units of work of breathing correspond to the units of pressure

Table 14
Calculated Respiratory Parameters

	Units	Adult	Newborn	Newborn RDS	Newborn BPD
Pulmonary compliance	mL/cm H$_2$O/kg	2.5–3	2 2.5	<0.6	<1.0
Chest wall compliance	mL/cm H$_2$O	<1	>4	—	—
Pulmonary resistance	cm H$_2$O/L/sec	1–2	20–40	>40	>150
Resistive work	gm-cm/kg	<10	20–30	30–40	>40

RDS = respiratory distress syndrome; BPD = bronchopulmonary dysplasia.

times volume (cm $H_2O \bullet L$), or equivalently, force times distance ($Kg \bullet m$), and is usually expressed as the work per breath or respiratory cycle.

VI. Some Reference Values

   A. Table 13 lists values of neonatal pulmonary function parameters during the first month from several investigators collected over several decades of work in this area.
   B. Calculated values of both elastic and resistive properties determined in adult and term newborns are listed in Table 14. These are compared with values obtained in infants with RDS and BPD.

Suggested Reading (Chapters 1–4)

Bancalari E: Pulmonary function testing and other diagnostic laboratory procedures in neonatal pulmonary care. In Thibeault DW, Gary GA (Eds.): *Neonatal Pulmonary Care, 2nd Edition.* East Norwalk, CT, Appleton-Century Crofts, 1986, pp. 195-234.

Bhutani VK, Sivieri EM: Physiological principles for bedside assessment of pulmonary graphics. In Donn SM (Ed.): *Neonatal and Pediatric Pulmonary Graphics: Principles and Clinical Applications.* Armonk, NY, Futura Publishing Co., 1998, pp. 57-79.

Bhutani VK, Shaffer TH, Vidyasager D (Eds.): *Neonatal Pulmonary Function Testing: Physiological, Technical and Clinical Considerations.* Ithaca, NY, Perinatology Press, 1988.

Bhutani VI, Sivieri EM, Abbasi S: Evaluation of Pulmonary Function in the Neonate. In Polin RA, Fox WW (Eds.): *Fetal and Neonatal Physiology, 2nd Edition.* Philadelphia, W.B. Saunders Co., 1998, pp. 1143-1164.

Comroe JH, Forster RE, Dubois AB, et al: *Clinical Physiology and Pulmonary Function Tests, 2nd Edition.* Chicago, Year Book Medical Publishers, 1971.

Comroe JH. *Physiology of Respiration, 2nd Edition.* Chicago, Year Book Medical Publishers, 1974.

Polgar G, Promadhat V: *Pulmonary Function Testing in Children.* Philadelphia, WB Saunders Co., 1971.

Rodarte JR, Rehder K: Dynamics of respiration. In Geiger SR (Ed.): *Handbook of Physiology, Section 3: The Respiratory System*, Macklem PT, Mead J (Volume Eds.), Volume III, Mechanical of Breathing, Part I, Fishman AP (Section Ed.). Bethesda, American Physiological Society, 1986, pp. 131-144.

Stocks J, Sly PD, Tepper RS, Morgan WJ (Eds.): *Infant Respiratory Function Testing.* New York, Wiley-Liss, 1996.

West JB: *Respiratory Physiology: The Essentials.* Oxford, UK, Blackwell Scientific Publications, 1974.

SECTION II

Assessment of Cardiopulmonary Function

Chapter 5

Clinical Examination

N.R.C. Roberton

I. **Normal Physical Findings**

    A. Respiratory rate 40–60 breaths/min

        1. Irregular with pauses ≤5 seconds in rapid eye movement (REM) sleep

        2. Regular in non-REM sleep, rate 5–10 breaths/min slower than in REM sleep or when awake

        3. No dyspnea

        4. No intercostal retractions

        5. No subcostal retractions

        6. No grunting (an expiratory noise produced by sudden relaxation of the laryngeal adductors at the end of expiration)

    B. Pulse rate 120–160 beats/min

        1. Sinus arrhythmia is rare in the newborn.

        2. Pulses easy to feel; some reduction in leg pulses common in newborns ≤48 hours old

    C. First and second heart sounds are often single; S_2 splits by 48 hours in 75% of newborns.

    D. Murmurs are common in the first few days.

    E. Perfusion (capillary time ≤3 sec)

II. **Clinical Examination of Cardiorespiratory System**

    A. The four classic components should be followed.

        1. Observation

        2. Palpation

        3. Percussion

        4. Auscultation

        5. Of these, in the newborn, the most useful and important is observation, both visual and auditory.

        6. Cardinal signs of respiratory distress

            a. Intercostal, subcostal, and substernal retractions

      b. Nasal flaring

      c. Expiratory grunting

      d. Tachypnea >60 breaths/min

      e. Cyanosis

III. **Observation**

    A. Respiratory rate

      1. Rates >60 breaths/min are abnormal.

      2. Very fast rates may have a better prognosis as they occur in more mature babies with a good respiratory pump able to sustain the tachypnea.

      3. Slow irregular rates <30 breaths/min with or without gasping are ominous.

    B. Remember that tachypnea is a very nonspecific finding and can be caused by:

      1. Pulmonary disease

      2. Cardiac disease

      3. Sepsis

      4. Anemia

      5. Any cause of metabolic acidemia

      6. Fever

      7. Central nervous system (CNS) pathology

      8. Stress (e.g., after feeding or crying)

IV. **Dyspnea**

    A. Distortion of the chest by the powerful attempts of the muscles of respiration to expand noncompliant lungs is one of the most significant findings in parenchymal lung disease.

    B. With anemia, acidemia, cyanotic heart disease, and fever, there is often tachycardia without dyspnea.

    C. Preterm babies (<1.50 kg) in non-REM sleep when muscle tone is low show mild intercostal and subcostal retractions.

    D. Other features of dyspnea include:

      1. Flaring of the alae nasi

      2. "See-saw" respiration, abdominal expansion (from diaphragmatic contraction) at the same time as sternal retractions

      3. Intercostal and subcostal retractions

      4. Suprasternal retractions

V. **Interaction with Positive Pressure Ventilation**

    A. In the early stages of severe lung disease, especially respiratory distress syndrome (RDS), the baby may breathe out of phase with the ventilator. This compromises oxygenation and increases the risk of air leaks.

B. In ventilated babies, a sign of recovery is that they breathe faster than the ventilator and this becomes part of the weaning process as the ventilator rate is turned down with or without one of the support modes of ventilation.

C. In both situations, it is important to count the ventilator rate as well as the baby's spontaneous ventilation rate.

D. In the acute phase of the disease (<24 hours), an attempt should be made to assess whether the baby is breathing asynchronously with the ventilator.

E. If the baby's condition has deteriorated rapidly, is the chest moving at all with the ventilator? If not, it may suggest a blocked or dislodged endotracheal tube.

VI. **Apnea and Gasping**
When counting the respiratory rate, note whether there are any pauses lasting more than 5 seconds, or whether there are any gasping respirations (both very abnormal), as opposed to normal sighs (deep inspirations against the normal background respiratory pattern).

VII. **General Appearance**

A. Does the baby look ill or well? Multiple factors to assess are:
1. Level of activity
2. Eye opening
3. Posture
4. Edema
5. Perfusion
6. Cyanosis

B. Edema – leaky capillaries in ill babies lead to subcutaneous edema as well as pulmonary edema

C. Perfusion
1. Pallor (capillary refill time >3 seconds)
2. Nonspecific illness
3. Anemia
4. Hypotension
5. Shock (septic or other)
6. Visible veins in skin (especially in preterm)
   a. Hypercapnia
   b. Nonspecific severe illness with shock (e.g., extensive hemorrhage)

D. Cyanosis
1. Assessed from lips, mucous membranes (peripheral cyanosis – common and rarely significant)
2. Difficult in nonwhite races (even in mucosa)
3. Cyanosis results from >5.0 g/dL desaturated hemoglobin.
   a. Seen in normally oxygenated polycythemic babies
   b. Difficult to see in very anemic babies
4. In an oxygen-enriched environment, oxygen may be absorbed through the skin making the baby look pink although central cyanosis may be present.

E. Because clinical signs of hypoxemia are unreliable, if in doubt, SpO_2 should be initially checked by oximetry (quick and easy) and hypoxemia should be confirmed by arterial blood gas analysis.

VIII. Clubbing – may be seen in babies with chronic lung disease >1 month old.

IX. Other Systems

A. Abdomen
1. Distention
   a. Enlarged liver – heart failure
   b. Liver pushed down by overventilated chest
   c. Liver pushed down by tension pneumothorax
   d. Retention of urine secondary to drugs, CNS disease
2. Scaphoid – strongly suggests congenital diaphragmatic hernia (CDH)

B. Central nervous system
1. Seizures
2. Tense fontanelle
3. Abnormal tone
4. Abnormal level of consciousness (e.g., irritability, lethargy, coma)

X. Auditory Observations

A. Listen to the baby. If the baby is crying vigorously, he/she is unlikely to be seriously ill. Three important auditory clues:
1. Grunting – a pathognomonic feature of neonatal lung disease
2. Stridor, usually inspiratory
   a. Upper airway problems (e.g., laryngomalacia)
   b. Glottic and subglottic injury or edema postintubation
   c. Local trauma following over-vigorous laryngeal instrumentation

3. "Rattle" – the bubbling of gas through secretions in the orophar-ynx. Often an ominous sign in a baby with severe CNS injury as well as lung disease.

XI. Palpation

A. Not usually of great help. The following may be noted:
1. Mediastinal shift (trachea, apical beat) with air leak, diaphrag-matic hernia, collapse (consolidation)
2. Tense abdomen (tension pneumothorax or pneumoperitoneum)
3. Subcutaneous emphysema
4. Pulses
   a. Should be checked in all four limbs if there is any suspicion of cardiac disease and documented by blood pressure mea-surements
   b. Bounding pulses are a feature of an increased cardiac output often with a left-to-right shunt. In the preterm infant this may be the first sign of a patent ductus arteriosis (PDA).
5. Cardiac precordial activity
6. Thrills – very rare in the neonatal period; if present, always significant

XII. Percussion

A. Increased resonance may be seen with a pneumothorax and occa-sionally with severe pulmonary interstitial emphysema (PIE).

B. Decreased resonance accompanies pleural effusions.

C. Decreased resonance with marked collapse/consolidation:
1. Pneumonia
2. Endotracheal tube (ETT) in one bronchus

D. Decreased resonance with CDH

XIII. Auscultation

A. Always use the small neonatal stethoscope. It can be difficult to apply to the chest of a preterm newborn in a way that excludes extraneous noise, and trial and error will identify whether the bell or diaphragm is best in a given situation. Use whichever gives the best acoustic seal.

B. Another problem is that babies, particularly preterm ones, wiggle when the stethoscope is placed on the chest, making cardiac exam-ination difficult. The trick is to hold the pre-warmed stethoscope in the same place and after 10–15 seconds the baby habituates to the stimulus and lies still.

C. Breath sounds are widely conducted through the upper torso of the newborn and the smaller the baby, the greater the conduction. Even with the neonatal stethoscope head it is difficult to be certain about where air is going. Two common (and very serious) auscultation mistakes:

1. Failing to realize during mechanical ventilation that air is going in and out of the stomach rather than the lungs
2. Failing to realize that only one lung is being ventilated (particularly if there is some mediastinal shift)

XIV. **Air Entry**

   A. The breath sounds in newborns with normal lungs can be heard in both inspiration and expiration, being slightly louder and longer in inspiration. In other words, part of the expiratory phase, which is physiologically longer, is silent.
   B. A general reduction in air entry is heard with:
      1. Any severe lung disease (e.g., RDS)
      2. Occluded endotracheal tube
   C. Unilateral decrease in air entry – any unilateral lung disease, which will usually require a chest radiograph for further evaluation
      1. Pneumonia
      2. Air leak
      3. Effusion
      4. Misplaced ETT

XV. **Other Sounds**

   A. There should be no rales or crepitations (discontinuous sounds) and no rhonchi (continuous sounds). The other common sound heard on auscultating the chest of a preterm baby is water bubbling in the ventilator tubing in which it has condensed. Clearly, it is impossible to do a successful clinical examination under these circumstances. The tubing should be transiently disconnected from the ventilator circuit and emptied.
   B. Crepitations occur in:
      1. Pneumonia
      2. Aspiration
      3. Heart failure (PDA and other)
      4. Massive pulmonary hemorrhage
      5. Chronic lung disease
      6. Meconium aspiration (stickier and louder)
   C. Rhonchi occur in:
      1. Retained secretions during mechanical ventilation
      2. Meconium aspiration
      3. Chronic lung disease

D. None of these findings is specific. They indicate a lung disease that requires further evaluation, initially by radiography.

E. Bowel sounds in the chest are a specific finding of CDH.

XVI. Cardiac Auscultation

A. Heart sounds – the ready availability of echocardiography has blunted the need for sophisticated auscultatory diagnostic skills for the newborn. The following, however, should always be noted:

  1. S_1 and S_2 are usually single in the first 24–48 hours, with splitting of S_2 present in 75% of babies by 48 hours.

  2. A gallop rhythm (S_3 and S_4) is always abnormal, usually indicating heart failure.

B. Innocent murmurs are very common in the first 24–48 hours; characteristics include:

  1. Grade 1–2/6 midsystolic at the left sternal edge

  2. No ejection clicks

  3. Occur in babies with normal pulses (especially femoral – document by blood pressure measurements)

  4. Occur in babies with an otherwise normal clinical examination

C. Significant murmurs are more likely to be heard >48 hours of age; their features include:

  1. Pansystolic ± diastolic ± thrills

  2. Grade 3/6 or more and harsh

  3. Best heard at upper left sternal edge (e.g., PDA)

  4. Abnormal S_2 (not splitting) ± gallop rhythm

  5. Early or midsystolic click

  6. Decreased femoral pulses with murmur heard at back

  7. Other signs of illness (heart failure, shock, and cyanosis)

D. Any baby with these features needs urgent evaluation (chest x-ray, ECG, and echocardiogram). The absence of murmurs or auscultatory abnormality in the first 48–72 hours does not exclude serious or even fatal heart disease.

XVII. Transillumination (see Chapter 66)

A. A bright light source applied to the chest wall can be a very useful and effective way of detecting a collection of intrapleural air – typically a pneumothorax, but large cysts, severe PIE, or marked lobar emphysema may also transilluminate. To be effective, the light source has to be very bright (ideally, a fiberoptic source), the room around the baby needs to be very dark, and some experience is required to differentiate the normal 0.5–0.1 cm halo of light around the probe from increased transillumination from a small collection of air. In cases where the whole hemithorax lights up, the diagnosis is easy.

B. The technique is more useful in smaller babies in whom the light is transmitted into the pleural cavity much more easily than with term babies with a thick layer of subcutaneous fat.

XVIII. Blood Pressure

A. The readily available automatic blood pressure recording devices now make this a routine part of the assessment of all newborns.

B. Attention to the following details is important:

1. Baby is quiet and has not recently been crying
2. Cuff covers 75% of the distance between the axilla and the elbow
3. Bladder virtually encircles the arm
4. A similar cuff size if appropriate for the upper arm and the calf
5. In ill preterm babies, the oscillometric device may overestimate the true blood pressure, and if there is any doubt about systolic pressure accuracy, direct measurement from an indwelling arterial catheter may be indicated.

Suggested Reading

Cartlidge PHT, Rutter N: Percutaneous oxygen delivery to the preterm infant. Lancet 1988; I:315-317.

Elder DE, Roberton NRC: Clubbing due to neonatal lung disease. Acta Paediatr Scand 1989; 78:631-632.

Greenough A, Greenall F: Observation of spontaneous respiratory interaction with artificial ventilation. Arch Dis Child 1988; 63:168-171.

Chapter 6

Radiography

Lawrence R. Kuhns

I. **Plain Radiography**
   A. Indications
      1. Respiratory distress
      2. Abnormal blood gases
      3. Air leaks
         a. Pneumothorax
         b. Pulmonary interstitial emphysema (PIE)
         c. Pneumomediastinum
         d. Pneumopericardium
      4. Meconium below the vocal cords
      5. Sepsis/pneumonia
      6. Possible cardiac disease
      7. Bronchopulmonary dysplasia
      8. Suspected thoracic anomaly
         a. Congenital diaphragmatic hernia
         b. Cystic adenomatoid malformation
         c. Esophageal atresia/tracheoesophageal fistula
      9. The following procedures:
         a. Intubation
         b. Thoracentesis/thoracostomy
         c. Chest tube removal
         d. Vascular catheter placement
   B. Patient considerations
      1. Postmature newborn: coarse, irregular asymmetric pulmonary opacities are seen in infants with meconium aspiration or pneumonia (Figure 16).
      2. Term newborn: mild respiratory distress is often associated with transient tachypnea of the newborn (Figure 17). Mild haziness is seen, especially in the right lung. Fluid is in the right minor fissure. This haziness clears by 24 hours of age.

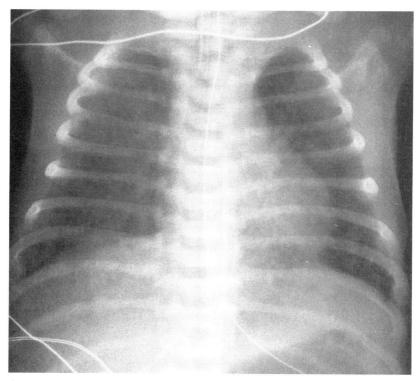

Figure 16. Patchy lung opacities are seen in the right lung and left lower lobe. They are quite symmetric. This patient had meconium aspiration.

3. Premature newborn: respiratory distress and abnormal blood gases are associated with surfactant deficiency, which presents with a fine salt and pepper or "ground glass" appearance throughout both lungs on the chest radiograph (Figure 18). A small radiographic focal spot of 0.3 mm or less and high detail screen film combination must be used to detect the fine reticulogranular appearance of surfactant deficiency (RDS).

4. Very premature newborn: respiratory distress is associated with immature lung, which presents as a fine hazy appearance on the chest radiograph. An enlarged heart suggests a patent ductus arteriosus.

5. Newborn of any gestational age with sudden onset of severe dyspnea
   a. PIE may occur with streaks of air seen dissecting toward the pulmonary hilum on either side.
   b. PIE may dissect into the mediastinum to produce a pneumome-

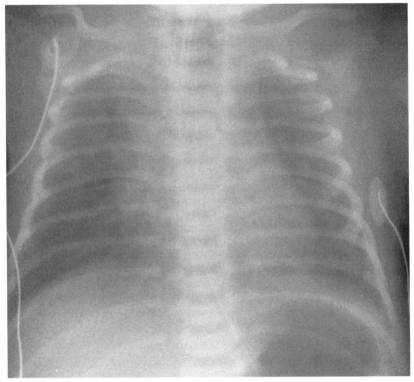

Figure 17. There is a fine haziness in the right lung and left lower lobe in this term infant with mild dyspnea, which resolved quickly. Follow-up radiographs 24 hours later should be completely negative if the patient has transient tachypnea of the newborn.

diastinum, or the PIE may rupture into the pleura to produce a pneumothorax. A pneumomediastinum can be detected on a cross-table lateral radiograph with the patient supine. A pneumothorax can be confirmed using a cross-table radiograph with the patient in a decubitus position (Figure 19, A, B).

6. Infant over 2 weeks of age with dyspnea and CO_2 retention: bronchopulmonary dysplasia should be suspected. Thick-walled cyst-like areas are seen in both lungs (Figure 20).

II. Indications for Chest Computed Tomography in the Newborn

A. Lung lesion seen on intrauterine sonography, even if the postnatal chest radiograph is negative (e.g., cystic adenomatoid malformation)

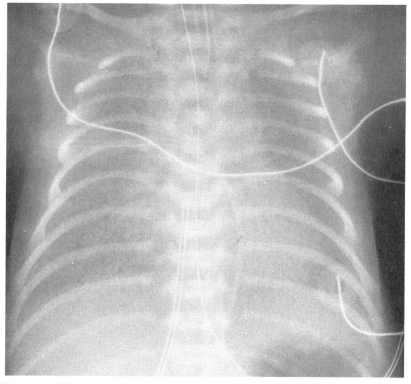

Figure 18. There is symmetrical, bilateral reticulogranularity of both lungs in this 34-week gestational age infant, indicating surfactant deficiency and respiratory distress syndrome.

    B. Better delineation of an abnormality seen on postnatal chest radiograph (e.g., lobar emphysema or sequestration)

    C. Suspected vascular ring or sling with airway obstruction

III. Indications for Chest Magnetic Resonance Imaging in the Newborn

    A. Pulmonary sequestration (to show the vascular supply from below the diaphragm, as well as the relationship of the sequestration to the diaphragm)

    B. Complex congenital heart disease where there is insufficient information from the echocardiogram (e.g., situs abnormalities)

    C. Anomalous venous return

    D. Evaluation of presence and size of the pulmonary arteries when they cannot be delineated by cardiac catheterization

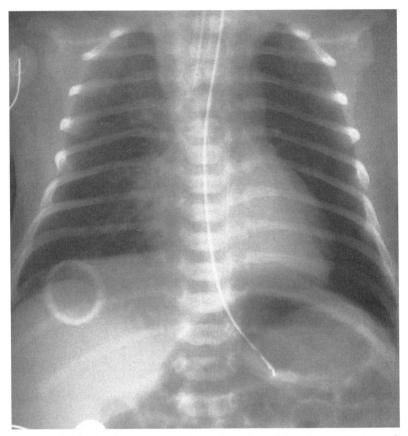

Figure 19. A. The left lung appears hyperlucent on this anteroposterior radiograph with the baby supine. There appears to be a left lower lobe collapse. (*continued*)

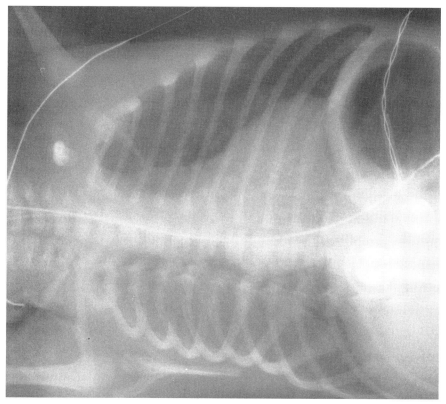

Figure 19. B. A cross-table radiograph is obtained with the baby in the right lateral decubitus position (right side down). A pneumothorax is now detectable on the left. Note the lung edge on the left, outlined by air.

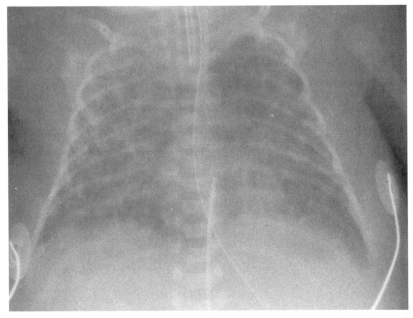

Figure 20. Diffuse bilateral coarse cyst-like changes are seen in this infant with bronchopulmonary dysplasia.

Suggested Reading

DiPietro MA: A radiologic atlas of neonatal emergencies. In Donn SM, Faix RG (Eds.): *Neonatal Emergencies.* Mount Kisco, NY, Futura Publishing Co., 1991, pp. 123-206.

Chapter 7

Interpretation of Blood Gases

David J. Durand

I. **Physiology of Blood Gases**

    A. Oxygenation. The movement of O_2 from the alveoli into the blood is dependent on the matching of ventilation and perfusion. Ventilation/perfusion matching is abnormal if:

        1. Pulmonary blood flows past unventilated alveoli (intrapulmonary shunt). In newborns, this is typically caused by atelectasis. The treatment for atelectasis is positive pressure, which opens previously unventilated alveoli and decreases intrapulmonary shunting.

        2. Blood flows right-to-left through the foramen ovale or patent ductus arteriosus (extrapulmonary shunt). This sort of extrapulmonary shunt is typically caused by elevated pulmonary vascular resistance (pulmonary hypertension) and can be treated by decreasing pulmonary vascular resistance (e.g., with inhaled nitric oxide).

    B. Ventilation. The movement of CO_2 from the blood into the alveoli is dependent on alveolar ventilation. Alveolar ventilation is the product of alveolar volume and respiratory rate. Thus, any change in ventilatory strategy which results in an increase in alveolar volume and/or respiratory frequency will improve ventilation and decrease $PaCO_2$.

    C. Acid-base status

        1. The pH of arterial blood is determined primarily by:

            a. $PaCO_2$

            b. Lactic acid, produced by anaerobic metabolism

            c. Buffering capacity, particularly the amount of bicarbonate in the blood

        2. Metabolic acidosis is reflected in an increased base deficit, also termed decreased base excess.

        3. Increase in $PaCO_2$ causes a decrease in pH, or respiratory acidosis. If $PaCO_2$ remains persistently elevated, the pH will gradually return to normal as a result of a compensatory metabolic alkalosis.

        4. Most extremely low birthweight infants have immature renal tubular function in the first week of life and spill bicarbonate in the urine, leading to a metabolic acidosis. Administration of extra base in the intravenous fluids will correct this.

5. If an infant has severe hypoxemia and/or decreased tissue perfusion, anaerobic metabolism will cause metabolic acidosis. This should be treated by improving the underlying problem, rather than by administering additional base.

II. Oxygen Content of Blood

A. Oxygen is carried in the blood in two ways:
   1. Dissolved in plasma. In the normal infant (or adult), the amount of oxygen dissolved in plasma is trivial compared with the amount of oxygen that is bound to hemoglobin. Approximately 0.3 mL O_2 is dissolved in 100 mL plasma per 100 torr O_2 partial pressure.
   2. Bound to hemoglobin. The amount of O_2 that is carried in the blood bound to hemoglobin is dependent on both the hemoglobin level and the hemoglobin saturation (% S_aO_2). In the normal infant with a hemoglobin level of 15 g/100 mL and S_aO_2 of 100%, approximately 20 mL O_2 is bound to the hemoglobin in 100 mL blood.

B. Significantly increasing PaO_2, beyond that which is needed to fully saturate (Hb), will slightly increase the amount of O_2 dissolved in plasma, but will not increase the amount of O_2 bound to Hb.

C. The PaO_2 that is required to fully saturate Hb is dependent on the oxygen-hemoglobin dissociation curve. This curve is dependent on many factors, including the relative amount of fetal Hb in the blood (fetal Hb is fully saturated at a lower PaO_2 than is adult Hb). For this reason, arterial saturation (S_aO_2) is a better indicator of the amount of oxygen in the blood than is PaO_2.

III. Oxygen Delivery and Mixed Venous Oxygen Saturation

A. The amount of oxygen delivered to the tissues depends on the amount of oxygen in the blood (C_aO_2) and cardiac output (CO).
   1. Assume an average infant has a C_aO_2 of 20 mL O_2/100 mL blood and a CO of 120 mL/kg/min.
   2. Therefore, the amount of oxygen available for delivery to the body can be calculated as the product of C_aO_2 and CO.
   3. (20 mL O_2/100 mL blood)(120 mL/kg/min) = 24 mL O_2/kg/min available for delivery to tissues

B. Under stable conditions, oxygen consumption for the average infant is approximately 6 mL O_2/kg/min.

C. If an infant is delivering oxygen to the systemic circulation at a rate of 24 mL/kg/min and is utilizing O_2 at a rate of 6 mL/kg/min, then 25% of the oxygen in the blood is utilized by tissues. 75% of the oxygen (18 mL/kg/min) is not utilized by the tissues, so the blood returning to the right atrium from the systemic circulation is 75% saturated.
   1. Mixed venous saturation (S_vO_2) is the saturation of blood as it enters the pulmonary artery. This can be measured directly with a pulmo-

nary artery catheter in older patients, and can be approximated by a sample of blood from the right atrium.

2. S_vO_2 is an important measurement in patients with questionable CO. A low S_vO_2 (<75%) means that the amount of oxygen delivered to the tissues is less than normal.

3. Causes of low S_vO_2 include inadequate oxygenation of the blood, anemia, or low CO. The combination of low S_vO_2 with normal S_aO_2 and normal Hb is diagnostic of inadequate CO.

4. S_vO_2 is typically used to monitor the adequacy of tissue perfusion in patients receiving extracorporeal membrane oxygenation (ECMO) and can be useful in any patient where adequacy of CO is uncertain.

IV. Errors in Blood Gas Measurements

A. An air bubble in a blood gas sample will cause the blood to equilibrate with room air.

1. PCO_2 will be artificially lowered.

2. PO_2 will move closer to the partial pressure of O_2 in room air (approximately 140 torr or 18.7 kPa, depending on altitude and humidity).

B. Dilution of a blood gas sample with IV fluid of any sort will cause both CO_2 and O_2 to diffuse from the blood into the diluting fluid.

1. PO_2 will be artificially lowered.

2. PCO_2 will be artificially lowered.

3. Because of the buffering capability of the blood, pH will not change as much as will PCO_2. The combination of relatively normal pH and decreased PCO_2 will appear to be a respiratory alkalosis with metabolic acidosis.

C. If a blood gas sample is left for a long period at room temperature, the blood cells will continue to metabolize oxygen and produce CO_2.

D. Most blood gas machines calculate S_aO_2 from P_aO_2, assuming that all of the Hb is adult Hb. In an infant with a significant amount of fetal Hb, this calculated value will be much lower than the actual measured S_aO_2.

E. Capillary blood gas values are frequently assumed to approximate arterial blood gas values. However, there is marked variation in the correlation of capillary and arterial values. Capillary blood gases should be interpreted with caution.

F. Blood gases obtained by arterial puncture or capillary stick are painful and disturb the infant, frequently causing agitation, desaturation, or hyperventilation. They should be interpreted with caution.

V. Clinical Interpretation of Blood Gases (Table 15)

Blood gas values, by themselves, convey relatively little information; they must be interpreted in a clinical context. When interpreting blood gas results, a number of other factors must be assessed simultaneously.

Table 15
Target Ranges for Blood Gases and pH

	pH	PCO_2 torr	PCO_2 kPa	PO_2 torr	PO_2 kPa	HCO_3^- mEq/L	% O_2 Saturation
Arterial	7.30–7.45	35–45	4.7–6.0	50–70	6.7–9.3	20–24	92–95
Venous	7.25–7.35	40–50	5.3–6.7	35–45	4.7–6.0	18–24	70–75
Capillary	7.25–7.35	40–50	5.3–6.7	35–50	4.7–6.7	18–24	70–75

A. How hard is the infant working to breathe?
   1. A normal blood gas in an infant who is clearly struggling to breathe is not necessarily reassuring.
   2. An elevated PCO_2 in an infant with chronic lung disease who is comfortable is not necessarily concerning.
B. Does a recent change in blood gas values represent a change in the patient, or is it an artifact?
C. If a blood gas is used to make decisions about ventilator strategy, how much of the total respiratory work is being done by the patient, and how much is being done by the ventilator?
D. Where is the patient in the course of the disease? A PCO_2 of 65 torr (8.7 kPa) may be very concerning in an infant in the first few hours of life, but perfectly acceptable in an infant with chronic lung disease.
E. When deciding whether to obtain a blood gas sample, ask yourself whether you will learn anything from it that you cannot learn from clinical examination of the patient.

Suggested Reading

Clark JS, Votteri B, Ariagno RL, et al: Noninvasive assessment of blood gases. Am Rev Respir Dis 1992; 145:220-232.

Courtney SE, Weber KR, Breakie LA, et al: Capillary blood gases in the neonate: a reassessment and review of the literature. Am J Dis Child 1990; 144:168-172.

Dennis RC, Ng R, Yeston NS, Statland B: Effect of sample dilutions on arterial blood gas determinations. Crit Care Med 1985; 13:1067-1068.

Dudell G, Cornish JD, Bartlett RH: What constitutes adequate oxygenation? Pediatrics 1990; 85:39-41.

Kim EH, Cohen RS, Ramachandran P: Effect of vascular puncture on blood gases in the newborn. Pediatr Pulmonol 1991; 10:287-290.

Chapter 8

Neonatal Graphic Monitoring

Joanne J. Nicks

I. **Indications**
 A. Optimizing mechanical ventilation parameters including:
   1. Peak inspiratory pressure (PIP)
   2. Positive end-expiratory pressure (PEEP)
   3. Inspiratory and expiratory tidal volume (V_{TI} or V_{TE})
   4. Inspiratory time (T_I)
   5. Expiratory time (T_E)
   6. Flow rate
   7. Synchronization
 B. Evaluation of infant's spontaneous effort:
   1. Spontaneous V_T compared to mechanical V_T
   2. Minute ventilation (MV)
   3. Respiratory pattern
   4. Readiness to extubate
 C. Therapeutic response to pharmacologic agents
   1. Surfactant delivery
   2. Bronchodilators
   3. Diuretics
   4. Steroids
 D. Evaluation of respiratory waveforms, loops, and mechanics
   1. Waveforms
     a. Pressure
     b. Flow
     c. Volume
   2. Loops
     a. Pressure-volume loop
     b. Flow-volume loop
   3. Mechanics
     a. Dynamic compliance (C_D) or static compliance (C_{ST})

        b. Resistance (R_I, inspiratory; R_E, expiratory)

        c. Time constants

    E. Disease evaluation

        1. Restrictive

        2. Obstructive

        3. Severity

        4. Recovery

II. Ventilator Monitoring Devices

Ventilator graphic monitoring devices are capable of providing continuous, real-time feedback regarding the interaction between the patient and the ventilator. They are reliable, accurate, and moderately priced, and are excellent teaching tools.

    A. Sensors

        1. Heated wire anemometer: measures the amount of current required to keep a heated wire at a constant temperature as gas flows past the wire and heat is convected.

        2. Differential pressure pneumotachometer: as gas flows through the sensor across an element, a differential pressure is created between the upstream and downstream sensing ports. The change in pressure across an element is proportional to flow.

    B. Monitors

        1. VIP BIRD/BIRD® Graphic Monitor (Bird Products Corp., Palm Springs, CA, USA)
Variable orifice differential pressure transducer flow sensor monitors at the proximal airway

            a. Waveforms

            b. Loops

            c. Trends

            d. Reference cursor/reference loops

            e. C_D, C_{ST}, resistance (peak expiratory or static), C_{20}/C_D

            f. Patient monitor ventilator settings screen

        2. Bear Cub 750 PSV® with Ventilator Graphics Monitor (Bear Medical, Riverside, CA, USA)
Heated wire flow sensor monitors at the proximal airway

            a. Waveforms

            b. Loops

            c. C_D, peak expiratory resistance

        3. Dräger Babylog 8000 Plus® (Dräger, Lübeck, Germany)
Heated wire flow sensor monitors at the proximal airway

            a. Integrated data

                (1) Single pressure or flow waveform

                (2) Display screens of monitored and set values

(3) Trends of main ventilation parameters

(4) Lung function monitoring of C_D, resistance (linear regression, C_{20}/C_D, and time constant)

b. Babylink® (requires computer interface)

(1) Displays all waveforms

(2) Loops

(3) Overlapping reference function

(4) Trending option (Evitaview®)

(5) Display of all set and measured parameters

4. Nellcor Puritan Bennett Star Series/Star Track® (Nellcor Puritan Bennett, Pleasanton, CA, USA)

Heated wire flow sensor monitors at the proximal airway

a. Waveforms

b. Loops

c. Dynamic compliance

5. Siemens Servo 390® Graphics Screen (Siemens-Elema AB, Solna, Sweden)

Pneumotachometer monitors values back at the ventilator

a. Waveforms

b. Loops

c. Trends

d. C_D, C_{ST}, R_E, and R_I

e. CO_2 analyzer for dead space/tidal ratios (C_D/V_T)

f. Numeric display of data

g. Clinical help file

III. Graphic Waveforms

A. Pressure

1. Pressure waveform (Figure 21)

a. The upsweep of the waveform represents inspiration and the downsweep represents expiration.

b. PIP is the maximum pressure point on the curve (A).

c. PEEP is the baseline pressure level (B).

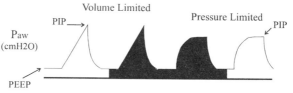

Figure 21. Pressure waveform for both volume- and pressure-limited breaths.

      d. The area within the curve represents the mean airway pressure (Paw) (shaded).

      e. The shape of the curve represents the breath type, e.g., volume (triangular) or pressure (square).

      f. Presence of a plateau at peak pressure is caused by an inflation hold or prolonged inspiratory time. This may improve distribution of ventilation but is not usually desirable in infants because it may disrupt synchrony and results in a higher mean airway pressure (Figure 22).

B. Flow waveform (Figure 23)

    1. Horizontal line is the zero flow point (A). Upsweep of the flow waveform above the zero reference is inspiration (B), and downsweep is expiration (C).

    2. Greatest deflection above reference equals peak inspiratory flow.

    3. Greatest deflection below reference equals peak expiratory flow.

    4. Shape of the flow waveform is typically square or constant flow waveform seen in volume ventilation, or a decelerating flow seen in pressure ventilation.

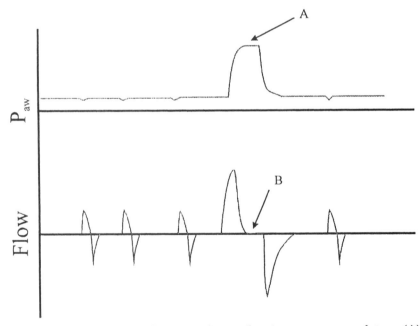

Figure 22. Pressure and flow waveforms showing a pressure plateau **(A)** caused by an inspiratory hold; note the delay **(B)** before expiratory flow is seen.

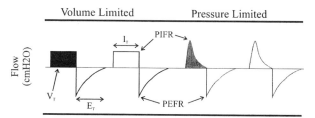

Figure 23. Flow waveforms for both volume- and pressure-limited breath types. Inspiratory flow is above the baseline, expiratory flow is below. Peak inspiratory (PIFR) and peak expiratory (PEFR) flow rates are shown.

5. Inspiratory time is measured from the initial flow delivery (A) until expiratory flow begins (C).
6. Inflation time of the lung is measured from initial inspiratory flow delivery (A) to the point when flow returns to zero (B). When ventilating newborns, clinicians should evaluate this time interval to set an appropriate inspiratory time.
7. Termination sensitivity® and flow cycling allow a mechanical breath to be triggered into expiration by a specific algorithm (usually 5–25% of peak flow). These breath types are available on the

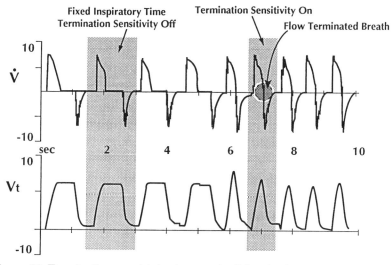

Figure 24. Termination sensitivity is turned off for the first four breaths, then activated. Note that the breath then ends by a decrease in inspiratory flow rather than the preset inspiratory time. (From Nicks JJ: *Graphics Monitoring in the Neonatal Intensive Care Unit.* Palm Springs, CA, Bird Products Corp., 1995, with permission.)

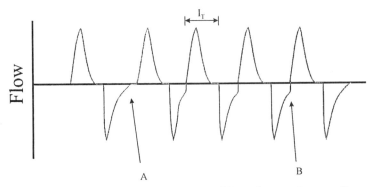

Figure 25. Demonstration of gas trapping. Note that expiratory flow completely returns to baseline in breath A (zero flow state is achieved), whereas in breath B, there is insufficient expiratory time, and onset of next breath occurs before zero flow state is ever achieved.

       VIP BIRD, Bear Cub 750 PSV, and with ventilators having pressure support (Figure 24).

8. Expiratory time is the point where expiratory flow begins (D) until the next inspiration begins (F).
9. When expiratory flow returns to zero, lung deflation is complete. This is represented on a waveform from the point where expiration begins (D) to where expiratory flow returns to zero (E).
10. If flow has not reached zero before the next breath is delivered, gas trapping may occur (Figure 25).
11. Gas trapping is more likely to occur in airways with increased resistance showing slow emptying time (Figure 26).

C. Volume waveform (Figure 27)
1. Inspiration is represented as the waveform sweeps upward and expiration as the waveform sweeps downward.
2. The dashed line represents delivered inspiratory tidal volume.
3. An endotracheal tube leak is observed when the expiratory portion of the waveform fails to return to the zero baseline.
4. The relationship between mechanical volumes vs. spontaneous volumes in synchronized intermittent mandatory ventilation (SIMV) may be helpful in determining readiness to wean (Figure 28).
5. Asynchronous ventilation may be observed with the volume waveform. In intermittent mandatory ventilation (IMV), the mechanical breaths delivered are ineffective; however, with SIMV, ventilation is much more effective (Figure 29).

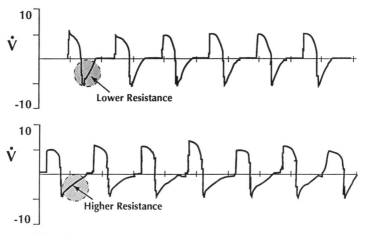

Figure 26. The shape of a specific waveform can help to identify airway and pulmonary abnormalities. In the lower example, higher airway resistance causes flow to return to baseline more slowly on expiration compared to the upper example, where resistance is lower. (From Nicks JJ: *Graphics Monitoring in the Neonatal Intensive Care Unit.* Palm Springs, CA, Bird Products Corp., 1995, with permission.)

IV. Graphic Loops

    A. Pressure-volume (P–V) loop (Figure 30)

        1. A P–V loop compares the relationship of pressure to volume (compliance).

        2. Pressure is displayed along the horizontal axis and volume is displayed on the vertical axis.

        3. Inspiration is represented by the upsweep from the baseline (PEEP) terminating at PIP and V_{TI}. Expiration is the downsweep from PIP and V_{TI} back to baseline.

        4. A line drawn from each endpoint represents compliance ($\Delta V / \Delta P$).

        5. A P-V loop that lies flat indicates poor compliance, and one that

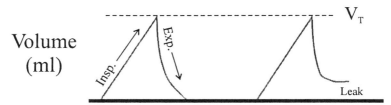

Figure 27. Volume waveform. Inspiration (Insp.) is represented by the upsweep of the waveform, and expiration (Exp.) is the downward sweep.

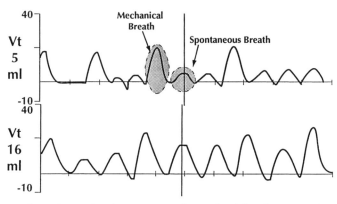

Figure 28. The relationship between mechanical tidal volumes and spontaneous tidal volumes in SIMV may be helpful in determining readiness to wean. (From Nicks JJ: *Graphics Monitoring in the Neonatal Intensive Care Unit.* Palm Springs, CA, Bird Products Corp., 1995, with permission.)

stands upright shows improved compliance. Recovery from respiratory distress syndrome or response to surfactant therapy demonstrates improvement in compliance (Figure 31).

6. Graphic monitoring is useful in identifying appropriateness of pressure delivery. A "beaking" of the P-V loop often indicates overdistension. This occurs when pressure continues to rise with

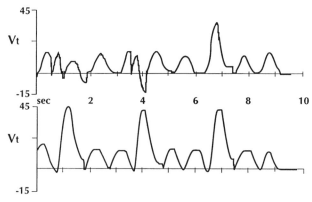

Figure 29. Waveforms may be helpful to assess patient-ventilator interaction (synchrony). In IMV **(top)**, the infant may "fight" the ventilator, resulting in inconsistent tidal volume delivery. In SIMV **(bottom)**, the synchronized interaction between patient and ventilator results in a more consistent tidal volume delivery. (From Nicks JJ: *Graphics Monitoring in the Neonatal Intensive Care Unit.* Palm Springs, CA, Bird Products Corp., 1995, with permission.)

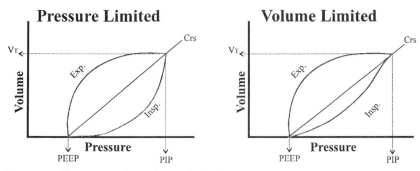

Figure 30. Pressure-volume loops for both pressure-limited **(left)** and volume-limited **(right)** breath types. Note the inspiratory (Insp.) and expiratory (Exp.) limbs, origin positive end-expiratory pressure (PEEP), peak inspiratory pressure (PIP), tidal volume (V_T), and compliance line (C_{rs}), drawn by connecting the origin with the point of PIP.

minimal change in volume (Figure 32). Note that the compliance of the last 20% of the P-V loop is lower than the C_D of the entire loop. This relationship is often expressed as a mechanics calculation (C_{20}/C_D ratio). A ratio of less than one usually indicates overdistension. When this is seen, it is appropriate to evaluate the PIP or V_T and attempt to reduce either of these.

7. P–V loops can help evaluate whether flow delivery from the ventilator is adequate to meet the needs of the patient. Inadequate flow is represented by cusping of the inspiratory portion of the curve (Figure 33). Severe flow limitation may appear as a figure of eight. This indicates that volume is increasing more rapidly than pressure (i.e., inadequate flow).

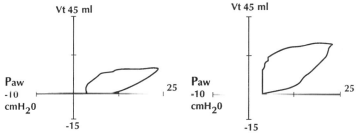

Figure 31. Compliance is the relationship between volume and pressure. On a pressure-volume loop, pressure is on the horizontal axis, volume is on the vertical axis. A flattened loop **(left)** indicates poor compliance. A more upright loop **(right)** indicates improved compliance. This change is typically seen after administration of surfactant to an infant with respiratory distress syndrome. (From Nicks JJ: *Graphics Monitoring in the Neonatal Intensive Care Unit.* Palm Springs, CA, Bird Products Corp., 1995, with permission.)

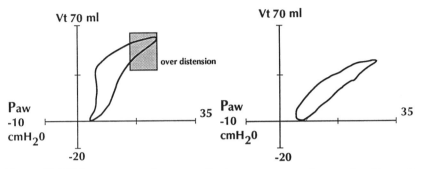

Figure 32. With pressure-volume monitoring, a pressure change should result in a linear change in volume, as seen on the right. On the loop on the left, however, the last third of the curve is flattened, indicating that pressure continues to be delivered with only a minimal increase in volume. This is a sign of overdistension. (From Nicks JJ: *Graphics Monitoring in the Neonatal Intensive Care Unit.* Palm Springs, CA, Bird Products Corp., 1995, with permission.)

    B. Flow-volume (F–V) loop (Figure 34)

        1. An F–V loop displays the relationship between volume and flow. Volume is plotted on the horizontal axis and flow is plotted on the vertical axis.

        2. In this example of a F-V loop (may vary with monitor type), the breath starts at the zero axis and moves downward and to the left

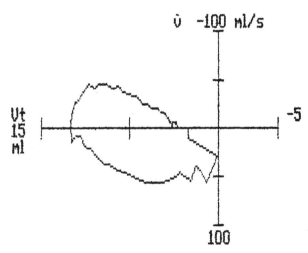

Figure 33. Flow-volume loop displaying inadequate flow in which there is cusping of the inspiratory portion of the loop.

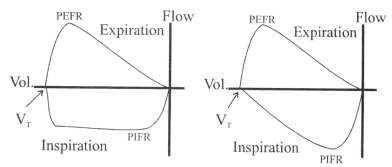

Figure 34. Flow-volume loops. **Left.** Inspiratory flow limitation is demonstrated by flattening of the loop. Peak flow (PIFR) is lower for a given volume. **Right.** Decreasing the resistance (such as by using a bronchodilator) results in improved PIFR and a more normal appearance to the inspiratory flow-volume loop.

on inspiration, terminating at the delivered inspiratory volume and upward, to the right, back to zero on expiration. Note the constant flow delivered with a volume breath type (square inspiratory flow on left loop) vs. decelerating inspiratory flow (right loop) with a pressure breath type.

3. The F-V loop is useful in evaluating airway dynamics. During conditions of high airway resistance, (Raw) peak flow is lower for a given volume. Typically, expiratory resistance is higher with airway collapse or bronchospasm.

4. Conditions in the newborn that often result in increased expiratory resistance from airway obstruction include meconium aspiration syndrome (MAS) and bronchopulmonary dysplasia (BPD).

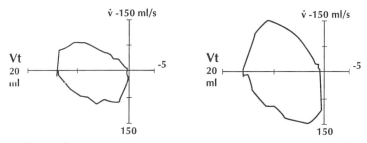

Figure 35. Another example of evaluating a treatment by using pulmonary graphics. **On the left** is a flow-volume loop before administration of a bronchodilator, and **on the right** is the loop following treatment. Note the marked improvement in both inspiratory and expiratory flows in this patient. (From Nicks JJ: *Graphics Monitoring in the Neonatal Intensive Care Unit.* Palm Springs, CA, Bird Products Corp., 1995, with permission.)

71

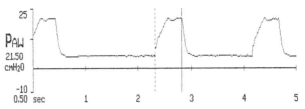

Figure 36. A static pressure waveform caused by an inspiratory hold maneuver.

    5. The F-V loop is useful for evaluating the effectiveness of bronchodilators in treating airway reactivity. In Figure 35, increased expiratory flow is seen in the loop on the right compared to the loop on the left.

V. Dynamics Measurements/Calculations

    A. Tidal volume is measured on inspiration and expiration. Normal delivered V_T is 4–8 mL/kg.

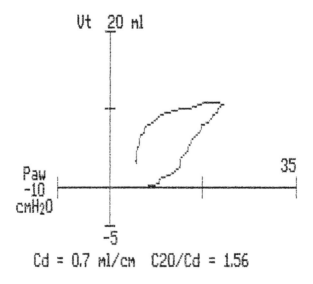

Figure 37. A pressure-volume loop showing a dynamic compliance measurement.

B. Minute ventilation (MV) is the product of V_T and respiratory rate. The normal range is 240–360 mL/kg/min.

C. Pressure may be measured as PIP or static pressure. Static pressure is obtained by doing an inspiratory hold maneuver, which measures pressure obtained by closing the exhalation valve and stopping flow delivery during a mechanical breath (Figure 36).

D. Compliance is the relationship between a change in volume and a change in pressure.

    1. Dynamic compliance (C_D) is the measurement of compliance based on peak pressure (Figure 37).

$$C_D = \frac{V_{TI}}{PIP - PEEP}$$

    2. Static compliance (C_{ST}) is the measurement based on static pressure

$$C_{ST} = \frac{V_{TI}}{P_{ST} - PEEP}$$

    3. C_{20}/C_D is the ratio of compliance of the last 20% to the entire curve. With overdistension this ratio will be <1.

E. Resistance is the relationship of pressure to flow. The pressure may be

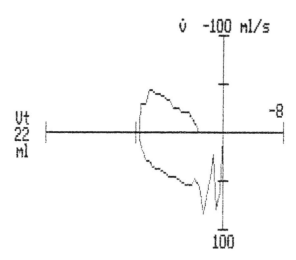

Rpk = 750   Pk Exh Flow = 43 ml/sec

Figure 38. A flow-volume loop showing peak expiratory flow and peak expiratory resistance measurement.

dynamic or static, and flow measurements are taken from various measurements (Figure 38).

1. Peak flow is the maximum flow on either inspiration or expiration.
2. Average flow is based on multiple point linear regression.
3. Mid-volume flow is based on the flow measured at a point of mid-volume delivery.
4.

$$R_{AW}(cmH_2O/L/sec) = \frac{PIP - PEEP}{Flow}$$

Suggested Reading

Cunningham MD, Wood BR: Monitoring of pulmonary function. In Goldsmith JP, Karotkin EH (Eds.): *Assisted Ventilation of the Neonate, 3rd Edition.* Philadelphia, PA, W.B. Saunders Co., 1996, pp. 273-289.

Donn SM (Ed.): *Neonatal and Pediatric Pulmonary Graphics: Principles and Clinical Applications.* Armonk, NY, Futura Publishing Co., 1998.

Nicks JJ: *Grahics Monitoring in the Neonatal Intensive Care Unit: Maximizing the Effectiveness of Mechanical Ventilation.* Palm Springs, CA, Bird Products Corp., 1995.

Sinha SK, Nicks JJ, Donn SM: Graphic analysis of pulmonary mechanics in neonates receiving assisted ventilation. *Arch Dis Child* 1996; 75:F213-F218.

Wilson BF, Cheifetz IM, Meliones JN: *Mechanical Ventilation in Infants and Children with the Use of Airway Graphics.* Palm Springs, CA, Bird Products Corp., 1995.

Chapter 9

Continuous Monitoring Techniques

Christian F. Poets, David P. Southall

I. **Transcutaneous Oxygen ($TcPO_2$) Monitoring**

  A. Principle of operation

    1. Electrodes consist of a platinum cathode and silver reference anode, encased in an electrolyte solution and separated from the skin by an O_2-permeable membrane.

    2. Electrodes are heated to improve oxygen diffusion and to arterialize the capillary blood.

    3. Oxygen is reduced at the cathode, generating an electric current proportional to the O_2 concentration in the capillary bed underneath the sensor.

    4. Sensors require a 10–15 minute warm-up period after application and have to be calibrated q4–8h.

  B. Factors influencing measurements

    1. Sensor temperature

      a. Good agreement with PaO_2 only at 44°C, but then frequent (q2–4h) repositioning is necessary.

      b. At lower sensor temperatures, the PaO_2-$TcPO_2$ difference increases with increasing PaO_2.

    2. Probe placement

      a. $TcPO_2$ will underread PaO_2 if sensor is placed on a bony surface, if pressure is applied on sensor, or if too much contact gel is used.

      b. With patent ductus arteriosus and right-to-left shunt, $TcPO_2$ will be higher on upper than on lower half of thorax.

    3. Peripheral perfusion

      a. $TcPO_2$ is dependent upon skin perfusion.

      b. If the latter is reduced, e.g., hypotension, anemia, acidosis (pH <7.05), hypothermia, or marked skin edema, $TcPO_2$ will be falsely low.

      c. If underreading of PaO_2 occurs, check patient for these conditions.

    4. Skin thickness. Close agreement with PaO_2 only in newborns; beyond 8 weeks of age, $TcPO_2$ will only be in the region of 80% of PaO_2.

    5. Response times. *In vivo* response time to a sudden fall in PaO_2 is 16–20 seconds.

C. Detection of hypoxemia and hyperoxemia. Sensitivity to these conditions (at 44°C sensor temperature) is approximately 85%.

II. Pulse Oximetry (SpO₂)

A. Principle of operation

    1. The ratio of the absorbance of red and infrared light sent through a tissue correlates with the proportion of oxygenated to deoxygenated hemoglobin in the tissue.

    2. The arterial component within this absorbance is determined by identifying the peaks and troughs in the absorbance over time, thereby obtaining a "pulse-added" absorbance that is independent of the absorbance characteristics of the nonpulsating parts of the tissue.

    3. These pulse-added light absorbances are then associated algorithmically with empirically determined arterial oxygen saturation (SaO_2) values.

B. Factors influencing measurements

    1. Probe placement

        a. Light receiving diode must be placed exactly opposite emitting diode; both must be shielded against ambient light and not be applied with too much pressure.

        b. Light bypassing the tissue can cause both falsely high and falsely low values.

        c. Sensor site must be checked q6–8h.

        d. Highly flexible sensors provide better skin contact and thus better signal-to-noise ratio.

    2. Peripheral perfusion. Most oximeters require a pulse pressure above 20 mm Hg or a systolic blood pressure above 30 mm Hg to operate reliably.

    3. Response times

        a. Depend on the averaging time used

        b. Longer averaging times may reduce alarm rates but will increase response time and will hide true severity of short-lived hypoxemic episodes.

    4. Movement artifact

        a. Most frequent cause of false alarms

        b. May be reduced with some newly developed instruments, but potentially at the expense of an unreliable detection of true alarms

     c. Can be identified from analysis of the pulse waveform signal displayed by some instruments or by comparing pulse rate with heart rate

  5. Other hemoglobins and pigments

     a. Methemoglobin (MetHb) will cause SpO_2 readings to tend towards 85%, independent of SaO_2.

     b. Carboxyhemoglobin (COHb) will cause overestimation of SaO_2 by 1% for each percent COHb in the blood.

     c. Fetal hemoglobin (HbF) and bilirubin do not affect pulse oximeters, but may lead to an underestimation of SaO_2 by co-oximeters.

     d. In patients with dark skin, SpO_2 values may be falsely high, particularly during hypoxemia.

  6. Algorithms

     a. These may vary between brands and even between different software versions from the same manufacturer.

     b. Some instruments assume *a priori* the typical levels of COHb, MetHb, etc., in healthy nonsmoking adults from their measurements, and will thus display SpO_2 values that are 2–3% lower than those displayed by other instruments.

  7. Detection of hypoxemia and hyperoxemia

     a. In the absence of movement, pulse oximeters have a high sensitivity for the detection of hypoxemia.

     b. Because of the shape of the O_2 dissociation curve, they are less well suited for detecting hyperoxemia.

       (1) The upper alarm limits at which hyperoxemia can be reliably avoided with different instruments range from 88–95%.

       (2) For a reliable detection of PaO_2 values >80 torr (10.7 kPa), $TcPO_2$ should also be monitored.

III. Transcutaneous Carbon Dioxide ($TcPCO_2$) Monitoring

  A. Principle of operation

     1. $TcPCO_2$ sensor consists of a pH-sensing glass electrode and a silver-silver chloride reference electrode, covered by a hydrophobic CO_2-permeable membrane from which they are separated by a sodium bicarbonate-electrolyte solution.

     2. As CO_2 diffuses across the membrane, there is a pH change of the electrolyte solution ($CO_2 + H_2O/HCO_3^- + H^+$), which is sensed by the glass electrode.

     3. All instruments have built-in correction factors, since their uncorrected measurements will be 50% higher than arterial PCO_2. They must also be calibrated at regular intervals and require a 10–15 min. equilibration time following repositioning.

B. Factors influencing measurements

    1. Sensor temperature. Optimal sensor temperature is 42°C, but if sensors are used in combination with a $TcPO_2$ sensor, a temperature of 44°C can be used without jeopardizing the precision of the $TcPCO_2$ measurement.

    2. Sensor placement and skin thickness. $TcPCO_2$ measurements are relatively independent of sensor site or skin thickness, but $TcPCO_2$ may be falsely high if pressure is applied to the sensor.

    3. Peripheral perfusion

        a. $TcPCO_2$ may be falsely high in severe shock.

        b. Precision may already be affected if $PaCO_2$ is >45 torr (6 kPa) and/or arterial pH is <7.30, but there is no systematic over- or underestimation of $PaCO_2$ under these conditions.

    4. Response times. 90% response time to a sudden change in $PaCO_2$ is between 30 and 50 seconds.

    5. Detection of hypocarbia and hypercarbia. Sensitivity to both hypocarbia and hypercarbia is 80–90%.

IV. End-tidal Carbon Dioxide ($ETCO_2$) Monitoring (Capnometry)

  A. Principle of operation. An infrared beam is directed through a gas sample and the amount of light absorbed by the CO_2 molecules in the sample measured; this is proportional to the CO_2 concentration in the sample.

  B. Factors influence measurements

    1. Gas sampling technique

        a. With mainstream capnometers

            (1) The CO_2 analyzer is built into an adapter, which is placed in the breathing circuit.

            (2) Advantage: fast response time (10 msec), therefore reliable even at high respiratory rates

            (3) Disadvantages: 1–10 mL extra dead space; risk of tube kinking

        b. Sidestream capnometers

            (1) Aspirate the expired air via a sample flow

            (2) Advantages: no extra dead space; can be used in nonintubated patients

            (3) Disadvantages: risk of dilution of expired gas by entrainment of ambient air at the sampling tube-patient interface; longer response time; falsely low values at high respiratory rates (>60/min)

    2. Influence of ventilation/perfusion ($\dot{V}/\dot{Q}$) mismatch

        a. $ETCO_2$ will only approximate $PaCO_2$ if:

            (1) CO_2 equilibrium is achieved between end-capillary blood and alveolar gas,

(2) $ETCO_2$ approximates the average alveolar CO_2 during a respiratory cycle, and

(3) V/Q relationships are uniform within the lung

    b. These conditions are rarely achieved in patients with respiratory disorders.

    c. The reliability of an $ETCO_2$ measurement can be assessed from the expiratory signal: this must have a steep rise, a clear end-expiratory plateau, and no detectable CO_2 during inspiration.

V. **Chest Wall Movements**

    A. Impedance plethysmography

        1. Changes in the ratio of air-to-fluid in the thorax, occurring during the respiratory cycle, create changes in transthoracic impedance.

        2. Cannot be used to quantify respiration

        3. May be heavily influenced by cardiac and movement artifacts

    B. Inductance plethysmography

        1. Changes in the volume of the thoracic and abdominal compartment create changes in inductance, which are registered via abdominal and thoracic bands.

        2. The sum of these changes is proportional to tidal volume, and several methods have been developed to calibrate the systems so that tidal volume can be quantified.

        3. This only works as long as the patient does not shift position.

    C. Strain gauges (usually mercury in silicon rubber) sense respiratory efforts by measuring changes in electrical resistance in response to stretching. These measurements, however, are not reproducible enough to quantitate tidal volume.

    D. Pressure (or volume expansion) capsules

        1. Detect movements of an infant's diaphragm by means of an air-filled capsule that is taped to the abdomen and connected to a pressure transducer via a narrow air-filled tube

        2. The outward movement of the abdomen during inspiration compresses the capsule to produce a positive pressure pulse that is interpreted as a breath.

        3. The technique is predominantly used in apnea monitors and trigger devices for infant ventilators and is not suitable for quantifying tidal volume.

VI. **Electrocardiography (ECG)**

    A. The ECG records electrical depolarization of the myocardium.

    B. During continuous single lead monitoring, only heart rate can be determined with sufficient precision; any analysis of P and T waves, axis, rhythm or QT times requires a printout and/or a 12-lead ECG.

VII. **Continuous Blood Gas Monitoring Using a Multiparameter Intra-arterial Sensor**
  A. Method
    1. Indwelling fiberoptic catheter measures blood gases spectrophotometrically.
    2. Provides continuous readings for pH, PaO_2, and $PaCO_2$
  B. Advantages
    1. Reduces iatrogenic blood loss from repetitive sampling
    2. Provides continuous information
    3. Enables earlier intervention if patient deteriorates
  C. Disadvantages
    1. Presently expensive
    2. Can only be used through umbilical artery
    3. Requires further clinical investigation to establish reliability, accuracy, and cost/benefit analysis.

Suggested Reading

Morgan C, Newell SJ, Ducker DA, et al: Continuous neonatal blood gas monitoring using a multiparameter intra-arterial sensor. Arch Dis Child 1999; 80:F93-F98.

Poets CF, Southall DP: Non-invasive monitoring of oxygenation in infants and children: practical considerations and areas of concern. Pediatrics 1994; 3:737-746.

Poets CF, Martin R: Noninvasive determination of blood gases. In Stocks J, Sly PD, Tepper RS, Morgan WJ (Eds.): *Infant Respiratory Function Testing*. New York, AJ Wiley & Sons, 1996, pp. 411-444.

Poets CF: Polygraphic sleep studies in infants and children. In Carlsen KH, Sennhauser F, Warner JO, Zach MS (Eds.): *New Diagnostic Techniques in Paediatric Respiratory Medicine*. Eur Respir Mono, 1997; 2:179-213.

Sackner MA, Krieger BP. Noninvasive respiratory monitoring. In Scharf SM, Cassidy SS, (Eds.): *Heart-Lung Interactions in Health and Disease*. New York, Marcel Dekker, 1989, pp. 663-805.

Chapter 10

Echocardiography

Jonathan P. Wyllie

I. **Background**

Until the advent of echocardiography, cardiac function in the ventilated baby was monitored by clinical assessment and invasive monitoring, which is limited by the size of the patient. Ideally the parameter of interest is tissue perfusion, which depends upon peripheral resistance and cardiac output. Previously, heart rate and blood pressure have been utilized as indicators of these parameters. Echocardiography now offers a number of different modalities which can be used to assess cardiac function in the ventilated infant.

II. **Influences on Newborn Cardiovascular Adaptation**

    A. Preterm delivery

    B. Surfactant deficiency

    C. Ventilation

    D. Hypoxia

    E. Acidosis

III. **Effects of Prematurity and Respiratory Disease on Cardiovascular Adaptation**

    A. Delayed fall in pulmonary vascular resistance

    B. Myocardial dysfunction

    C. Ductal patency

    D. Ventilation and diminished venous return

    E. Hypovolemia

IV. **Ideal Cardiac Assessment**

    A. Cardiac output

    B. Cardiac function

    C. Pulmonary resistance

    D. Tissue perfusion

    E. Systemic vascular resistance

V. **Echocardiographic assessment**

    A. Echocardiographic principles

        1. Cross-sectional echocardiography is used to assess anatomy, allow accurate positioning of an M-mode, continuous wave Doppler, or pulsed wave Doppler beam, and to give a subjective impression of function.

        2. Views used include:

            a. Long axis parasternal (Figure 39)

            b. Short axis parasternal mitral (Figure 40)

            c. Short axis parasternal pulmonary (Figure 41)

            d. Apical four chamber (Figure 42)

            e. Subcostal

            f. Suprasternal view of aortic arch or ductal arch

    B. M-mode obtains detailed echocardiographic information along a thin beam. It is simplest to first position using a cross-sectional image (Figure 39) and then switch to M-mode. It is used to obtain views of the left ventricle at the level of the mitral leaflets (Figure 43), in assessment of left ventricular function and measurement of left ventricular dimensions. It is also used in measurement of the left atrium and aorta (Figure 44).

    C. Pulsed wave Doppler uses Doppler shift of sound waves from moving red cells to assess flow velocity. It can sample the velocity at a point specified on a cross-sectional image (range gated), but is only useful for relatively low velocities. It is useful for velocity measure-

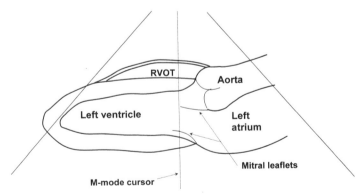

Figure 39. Long axis parasternal view. Positioning of M-mode cursor for left ventricular measurements is shown. RVOT = right ventricular outflow tract.

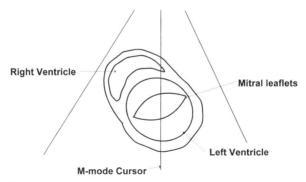

Figure 40. Short axis parasternal view. Positioning of M-mode cursor for left ventricular measurements is shown.

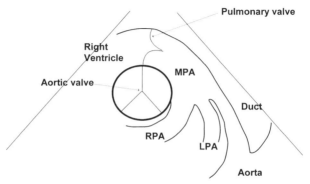

Figure 41. Short axis parasternal view. MPA = main pulmonary artery; RPA = right pulmonary artery; LPA = left pulmonary artery.

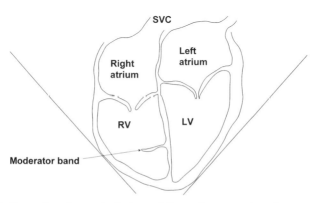

Figure 42. Four chamber apical view. Offset of tricuspid and mitral valves is seen. SVC = superior vena cava; RV = right ventricle; LV = left ventricle.

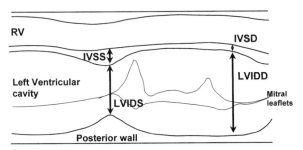

Figure 43. M-view of left ventricle showing measurements. (See text for definition of abbreviations.)

ment in the pulmonary artery, ductus arteriosus (Figure 45), and foramen ovale.

D. Continuous wave Doppler also uses Doppler shift of sound waves from moving red cells to assess flow velocity but is not range gated and samples velocities along the cursor line (Figure 46). It can be used in line with cross-sectional views or with a stand-alone "pencil" probe. Both continuous and pulsed wave Doppler beams must be within 15° of the direction of flow to be accurate.

E. Color Doppler simplifies accurate diagnosis and delineation of ductal patency. It also enables identification of tricuspid regurgitation and patency of the foramen ovale as well as the direction of flow. Flow velocity measurement is possible when used in conjunction with continuous or pulsed wave Doppler.

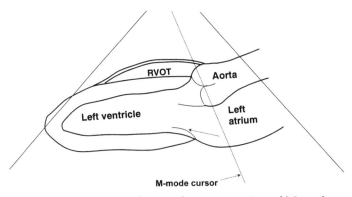

Figure 44. Long axis parasternal view showing position of M-mode cursor in measuring the aorta and left atrium.

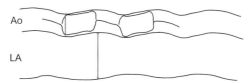

Figure 45. M-mode of aorta and left atrium at the level of the valve leaflets. Measurements are shown.

VI.   Indications for Echocardiographic Assessment
A. Suspected congenital heart disease
B. Suspected persistent pulmonary hypertension
C. Suspected patent ductus arteriosus
D. Hypotension or shock
E. Asphyxia
F. Suspected cardiac dysfunction
G. Use of high PEEP
H. High-frequency oscillatory ventilation

VII. Cardiac Function
Depressed ventricular function may occur in neonatal disease processes such as hypoxia, sepsis, hemolytic disease, hyaline membrane disease (RDS), persistent pulmonary hypertension, and transient tachypnea. A dysfunctional heart may be tachycardic, bradycardic, or have a normal rate. In hypotensive newborns, cardiac function may be depressed, normal, or even hyperdynamic.

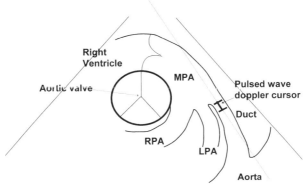

Figure 46. Short axis parasternal view showing the position of the pulsed wave Doppler cursor for sampling ductal flow velocity.

VIII. Left Ventricular Assessment

A. Cross-sectional and M-mode assessment

B. Cross-sectional echocardiography permits accurate positioning of the M-mode beam just at the mitral leaflet tips in the long axis (parasternal, Figure 39) or centered in the short axis parasternal views (Figure 40) of the left ventricle. Measurements must be taken from standard and reproducible positions, otherwise increased variability will obscure the results.

C. On the M-mode picture (Figure 43), the interventricular septal (IVS), left ventricular internal diameter (LVID), and posterior wall dimensions are measured at end-systole (S) and end-diastole (D). From these measurements several parameters of ventricular function can be calculated.

1. Fractional shortening characterizes left ventricular contractility, although it is also affected by preload and afterload.

$$\text{Fractional shortening (\%)} = \frac{\text{LVIDD} - \text{LVIDS}}{\text{LVIDD}} \times 100\%$$

   Normal ranges: 25-45% adults
   25-41% term babies
   23-40% preterm babies
   Errors in fractional shortening estimation may occur in early preterm life from distortion of the left ventricle and abnormal wall motion.

2. Circumferential fiber shortening
   Mean velocity of circumferential fiber shortening (VCF) has been suggested as a simple alternative measurement of left ventricular contractility. It is less sensitive to minor dimensional discrepancies and involves no assumptions about ventricular shape, offering a reproducible measurement of neonatal ventricular contractility.

3. LVIDD and LVIDS are measured as above, but ejection time is measured from the time of mitral valve closure to the onset of mitral valve opening.

$$\text{VCF} = \frac{\text{LVIDD} - \text{LVIDS}}{\text{LVIDD} \times \text{ejection time}}$$

   The units are circumferences per second.

4. Stroke volume
   a. Stroke volume (SV) measurement assumes an ellipsoidal ventricle. Using measurements of left ventricular internal diameter in diastole (LVIDD) and systole (LVIDS), the stroke volume can be calculated:

$$\text{SV} = \text{LVIDD}^3 - \text{LVIDS}^3$$

b. Similarly, a proportion of ventricular contents or ejection fraction (EF) can be calculated :

$$EF = \frac{SV}{\text{end-diastolic volume}} = \frac{LVIDD^3 - LVIDS^3}{LVIDD^3}$$

5. Volume load assessment

    a. M-mode assessment of the left ventricle and atrial size provides information about changes in ventricular preload. The ratio of these chambers to the aorta is used to assess the effect of shunts upon the heart, especially the ductus arteriosus.

    b. Normal left atrial to aortic ratio is 0.84–1.39 in preterm infants and 0.95–1.38 in term infants.

    c. Left atrial: aortic ratio >1.5 suggests volume loading

IX. Doppler Assessment of Cardiac Function

    A. Stroke volume (SV). Calculated from the product of the integral of the Doppler velocity-time curve (VTI, also known as stroke distance) and the cross-sectional area of the aorta derived from the M-mode diameter.

$$SV = VTI \times \pi(\text{aortic diameter}/2)^2$$

    B. Cardiac output. Multiplying SV by the heart rate (HR) produces the left ventricular output (CO)

$$CO = VTI \times \pi(\text{aortic diameter}/2)^2 \times HR$$

Note: Minute distance (MD = VTI × HR) is directly related to cardiac output but removes the aortic diameter from the calculation, which is the major source of error. This can be used to assess changes in therapy.

X. Right Ventricular Assessment

The normal shape of the right ventricle is more complex than the left. It consists of inflow, outflow, and apical segments and is wrapped around the left ventricle. This makes quantitative evaluation by M-mode difficult at any age and not useful in the newborn. However, qualitative information about right ventricular systolic function can be obtained by the experienced operator from cross-sectional views. Paradoxical movement of the intraventricular septum is seen in right ventricular dysfunction.

XI. Doppler Assessment of Systolic Function

    A. One of the most important determinants of right ventricular systolic function in newborns is pulmonary arterial pressure. This can be estimated in several ways.

    B. Tricuspid regurgitation. If present, the most accurate assessment of right ventricular (and therefore pulmonary) pressure is obtained by measuring the velocity of the regurgitant jet (V). Then, assuming right atrial pressure is low,

$$\text{Pulmonary pressure} = 4V^2$$

   C. Pre-ejection period-to-right ventricular ejection time is inversely related to pulmonary pressure and requires ECG monitoring while echoing the subject. It is useful for assessment of babies with chronic lung disease but difficult to interpret acutely.
   D. Ductal flow. If the ductus arteriosus is patent, the direction of flow (as well as the pattern) gives an indication of pulmonary pressure (i.e., right-to-left = pulmonary > systemic). However, the velocity of flow cannot accurately predict pulmonary pressure.
   E. Foramen ovale. Right-to-left flow is suggestive of high right-sided pressures or dysfunction. It is seen best in the subcostal view.
   F. Diastolic function. Few studies of diastolic function have been carried out in children or infants. Right ventricular filling is modified by positive pressure ventilation and especially by high positive end-expiratory pressure and oscillatory ventilation.

XII. **Assessment of the Patent Ductus Arteriosus (see Chapter 50)**
   A. The ductus arteriosus is best seen in the parasternal short axis view (Figure 41), although the suprasternal and subcostal approaches may be needed in babies with overdistended lungs. Color Doppler simplifies identification and allows subjective assessment of flow and velocity. Doppler interrogation of the ductus arteriosus (Figure 45) demonstrates the pattern of flow and the velocity profile. Velocity depends upon both the size of the vessel and the pressure difference between aorta and pulmonary artery. The size can be estimated in cross-sectional view in relation to the branch pulmonary arteries or aorta.
   B. Measurement of the left atrium:aortic ratio (see above) gives some indication of flow but may not be accurate if the left atrium decompresses through the foramen ovale.
   C. Echocardiographic evidence of a significant ductus arteriosus precedes clinical evidence. On day 3 of life it can predict significance with 100% sensitivity and 85% specificity.

XIII. **Accuracy and Reproducibility**
   A. M-mode measurements have been made using both leading and trailing edges. In measurements of the left ventricle both leading and trailing edges are used. Intraobserver variability for these measurements range from 5% for distances to 10% for calculated volumes. Interobserver variability is greater, ranging from 7% to 25% for volume measurements.

B. Measurement of the aorta and left atrium by M-mode is more reproducible in newborns if it is made from trailing-to-leading echo edge (i.e., the internal aortic diameter). Accuracy is vital, as a 1 mm error in the measurement of a 10 mm aorta will produce a 17% error in cardiac output.

C. The main sources of error in Doppler measurement are from the site of sampling and the angle of incidence of the Doppler wave. If the angle is <15°, the error will be <3%. A further source of error in calculating cardiac output is coronary artery flow, which may cause a 10–15% underestimate in flow.

Suggested Reading

Evans N, Kluckow M: Early determinants of right and left ventricular output in ventilated preterm infants. Arch Dis Child 1996; 74:F88-F94.

Gill AB, Weinding AM: Echocardiographic assessment of cardiac function in shocked very low birthweight infants. Arch Dis Child 1993; 68:17-21.

Hudson I, Houston A, Aitchison T, et al: Reproducibility of measurements of cardiac output in newborn infants by Doppler ultrasound. Arch Dis Child 1990; 65:15-19.

Skinner JR, Boys RJ, Hunter S, Hey EN: Pulmonary and systemic arterial pressure in hyaline membrane disease. Arch Dis Child 1992; 67:366-373.

SECTION III

Neonatal Respiratory Failure

Chapter 11

Indications for Mechanical Ventilation

Anne Greenough, Anthony D. Milner

I. Absolute Indications

A. In the delivery room

1. Failure to establish adequate spontaneous respiration immediately after delivery despite adequate face mask ventilation
2. Persistent bradycardia unresponsive to face mask ventilation
3. A large diaphragmatic hernia. Affected infants should be ventilated and paralyzed from birth to stop them from swallowing, which increases the dimensions of the bowel and worsens respiratory failure.

B. In the neonatal intensive care unit (NICU)

1. Sudden collapse with apnea and bradycardia with failure to establish satisfactory ventilation after a short period of face mask ventilation
2. Massive pulmonary hemorrhage. Such infants should be intubated, preferably paralyzed, and ventilated with high levels of positive end-expiratory pressure (PEEP).

II. Relative Indications

A. In the delivery room

1. Infants <28 weeks of gestational age are frequently electively intubated unless vigorous at birth.
2. Infants <32 weeks of gestational age may be electively intubated to receive prophylactic surfactant therapy.

B. In the NICU

1. Worsening respiratory failure – the criteria will depend on the gestational age of the infant

   a. 28 weeks gestation – arterial carbon dioxide tension ($PaCO_2$) >50–55 torr (6.7–7.3 kPa), the lower limit if associated with a pH <7.25 and/or arterial oxygen tension (PaO_2) <50–60 torr (6.7–8 kPa) in a fractional inspired oxygen (FiO_2) of >0.40, although if the infant only has poor oxygenation, nasal continuous positive airway pressure (CPAP) may be tried first

   b. 28–34 weeks gestation – $PaCO_2$ >50–55 torr (6.7–7.0 kPa), the lower limit being used if the pH is <7.25 and/or PaO_2 <50–60 torr (6.7–8 kPa) in an FiO_2 of >0.6, if nasal CPAP has failed to improve blood gas tensions.

   c. 35 weeks gestation – if the $PaCO_2$ exceeds 60 torr (8 kPa) with a pH below 7.25 and/or PaO_2 <45 torr (6 kPa) in an FiO_2 of >0.80. CPAP is usually poorly tolerated in mature infants.

2. Stabilization of infants at risk for sudden collapse

   a. Small preterm infants with recurrent apnea unresponsive to nasal CPAP and administration of methylxanthines

   b. Severe sepsis

   c. Need to maintain airway patency

3. To maintain control of carbon dioxide tension

   a. Persistent pulmonary hypertension

   b. Following severe asphyxia

Suggested Reading

Greenough A, Milner AD, Roberton NRC (Eds.): *Neonatal Respiratory Disorders.* London, Edward Arnold, 1996.

Chapter 12

Mechanisms of Respiratory Failure

Anne Greenough, Anthony D. Milner

I. **Definition**

   A. Respiratory failure is present when there is a major abnormality of gas exchange.

      1. In an adult, the limits of normality are a PaO_2 of >60 torr (8 kPa).

      2. In the newborn, the oxygen tension needed to maintain the arterial saturation above 90% varies between 40 and 60 torr (5.3–8 kPa), depending on the proportion of hemoglobin that is fetal, and the arterial pH (a drop in pH of 0.2 eliminates the left shift produced by 70% of the hemoglobin being fetal). Thus, in the newborn period, respiratory failure is best defined in terms of oxygen saturation. There are, however, no agreed upon criteria (see below).

      3. Hypoxia may be associated with hypercarbia ($PaCO_2$ >55 torr [6.7 kPa])

$$PaCO_2 = \frac{CO_2 \text{ production}}{\text{alveolar ventilation}}$$

Alveolar ventilation = (tidal volume − dead space × frequency)

   B. Respiratory failure associated with hypercarbia will occur, therefore, in situations associated with reduction in tidal volume and/or frequency.

      1. Respiratory failure in the neonatal period may be defined as: PaO_2 <50 torr (6.7 kPa) in an inspired oxygen of at least 50% with/ without $PaCO_2$ >50 torr (6.7 kPa)

      2. Hypoxemia in the neonatal period can result from multiple causes

         a. Ventilation/perfusion mismatch

            (1) Distinguished by a good response to supplementary oxygen (intrapulmonary shunting)

            (2) Increased physiologic dead space

            (3) Found in the following conditions:

(a) Respiratory distress syndrome (RDS)

(b) Pneumonia

(c) Meconium aspiration syndrome (MAS)

(d) Bronchopulmonary dysplasia (BPD)

b. Extrapulmonary (right-to-left) shunts are distinguished by relatively little improvement with supplementary oxygen and are found in:

(1) Pulmonary hypertension

(2) Cyanotic congenital heart disease*

c. Methemoglobinemia*

d. Inadequate inspired oxygen*

*Note – although these situations produce cyanosis, this is not from respiratory failure. Cyanosis appears when the reduced hemoglobin concentration of the blood in the capillaries is more than 5 g/dL. Cyanosis, therefore, does not occur in severe anemic hypoxia (hypoxia is oxygen deficiency at the tissue level).

e. Hypoventilation (reduced alveolar ventilation, reduction in tidal volume and/or frequency)

(1) Distinguished by a high $PaCO_2$ in association with hypoxemia

(a) Reduced respiratory compliance

(b) Found in the following conditions:

(i) RDS

(ii) Pneumonia

(2) Reduced lung volume

(a) RDS

(b) Pulmonary hypoplasia

(3) Compressed lung, found in:

(a) Pneumothorax

(b) Pleural effusion

(c) Lobar emphysema

(d) Cystic adenomatoid malformation

(e) Asphyxiating thoracic dystrophy

(4) Ventilatory pump failure

(a) Reduced central drive, found in:

(i) Maternal opiate treatment (high levels of sedation)

(ii) Cerebral ischemia

(iii) Intracerebral hemorrhage

(iv) Apnea of prematurity

(v) Central alveolar hypoventilation syndrome

(b) Impaired ventilatory muscle function

(c) Miscellaneous conditions

     (i) Drugs (corticosteroids, paralytics – synergism with aminoglycosides)

     (ii) Disuse atrophy (first signs occur after 1–2 days of mechanical ventilation)

     (iii) Protein calorie malnutrition

     (iv) Disadvantageous tension-length relationship (e.g., hyperinflation – diaphragm must contract with a much higher than normal tension. When completely flat, contraction of the diaphragm draws in the lower rib cage, producing an expiratory rather than inspiratory action.

     (v) Neuromuscular disorders (Werdnig-Hoffmann disease, myotonic dystrophy)

     (vi) Diaphragmatic problems (e.g., hernia, eventration)

     (vii) Phrenic nerve palsy (birth trauma – with Erb's palsy)

  (d) Increased respiratory muscle workload, found in

     (i) "Obesity," chest wall edema (hydrops)

     (ii) Upper airway obstruction/endotracheal tube with insufficient compensatory ventilatory support

     (iii) Pulmonary edema, pneumonia

     (iv) Intrinsic (inadvertent) positive end-expiratory pressure (PEEP)

(5) Disorders affecting the alveolar-capillary interface, distinguished, if incomplete, by a good response to increased supplementary oxygen

  (a) Diffusion abnormalities (interstitial lung disease) e.g., pulmonary lymphangiectasia (Noonan's syndrome)

  (b) Anemia

  (c) Alveolar-capillary dysplasia

Suggested Reading

Aldrich TK, Prezant DJ: Indications for mechanical ventilation. In Tobin MJ (Ed.): *Principles and Practice of Mechanical Ventilation.* New York, McGraw-Hill, Inc., 1994, pp. 155–189.

Roussos C, Macklem PT: The respiratory muscles. N Engl J Med 1982; 307: 786–797.

Chapter 13

Tissue Hypoxia

Anne Greenough, Anthony D. Milner

I. **Definition**

   A. Tissue hypoxia occurs when oxygen transport is reduced below a critical level (i.e., below the metabolic demand), at which point either metabolism must be maintained anaerobically or tissue metabolic rate must be reduced.

   B. Under experimental conditions, if demands are kept constant, there is a biphasic response in oxygen consumption as oxygen transport is progressively reduced.

   1. Initially, oxygen consumption is independent of oxygen transport.

   2. Subsequently, oxygen consumption becomes dependent on oxygen transport and declines in proportion (physiologic supply dependency).

II. **Evaluating Tissue Oxygenation**

   A. There is no very good method.

   B. Mixed venous saturation identifies global tissue hypoxia, but tissue hypoxia can exist with a normal mixed venous saturation.

   C. Blood lactate levels – elevation can be present in the absence of tissue hypoxia, particularly in patients with sepsis.

III. **Oxygen Transport**

   A. Determinants

   1. Tissue blood flow (cardiac output)

   2. Hemoglobin concentration

   3. To a lesser extent, hemoglobin saturation

   B. Oxygen-hemoglobin dissociation curve
   The quaternary structure of hemoglobin determines its affinity for oxygen. By shifting the relationship of its four component polypeptide chains, and hence a change in the position of the heme moieties, it can assume:

1. A relaxed (R) state, which favors O_2 binding
2. A tense (T) state, which decreases O_2 binding

When hemoglobin takes up a small amount of the oxygen, the R state is favored and additional O_2 uptake is facilitated. The oxygen-hemoglobin dissociation curve (which relates percentage oxygen saturation of hemoglobin to PaO_2) has a sigmoid shape.

C. Factors affecting the affinity of hemoglobin for oxygen:
   1. Temperature
   2. pH
   3. 2,3-diphosphoglycerate (2,3-DPG)

   A rise in temperature, a fall in pH (Bohr effect, elevated $PaCO_2$), or an increase in 2,3-DPG all shift the curve to the right, liberating more oxygen. The P_{50} is the PaO_2 at which the hemoglobin is half saturated with O_2; the higher the P_{50} the lower the affinity of hemoglobin for oxygen. A right shift of the curve means a higher P_{50} (i.e., a higher PaO_2 is required for hemoglobin to bind a given amount of O_2).

D. 2,3-DPG
   1. Formed from 3-phosphoglyceride, a product of glycolysis
   2. It is a high charged anion, which binds to the β chains of deoxygenated hemoglobin, but not those of oxyhemoglobin.
   3. 2,3-DPG concentration
      a. Increased by:
         1. Thyroid hormones
         2. Growth hormones
         3. Androgens
         4. Exercise
         5. Ascent to high altitude (secondary to alkalosis)
      b. Decreased by:
         1. Acidosis (which inhibits red blood cell glycolysis)
         2. Fetal hemoglobin (HbF) has a greater affinity for O_2 than adult hemoglobin (HbA); this is caused by the poor binding of 2,3-DPG to the δ chains of HbF. Increasing concentrations of 2,3-DPG have much less effect on altering the P_{50} if there is HbF rather than HbA.

IV. **Response to Reduced Oxygen Transport**
   A. From low cardiac output
      If chronic, 2,3-DPG increases unless there is systemic acidemia.
   B. From anemia
      1. Cardiac output and oxygen extraction increase.
      2. If chronic, the HbO_2 (hemoglobin, oxygenated) dissociation curve shifts to the right.

    C. From alveolar hypoxemia
       1. Increased cardiac output and oxygen extraction
       2. Increased hemoglobin

V. Oxygen extraction increases progressively as oxygen transport is reduced if oxygen consumption remains constant.

    A. Alterations in vascular resistance with adjustments to the microcirculation – opening of previously closed capillaries. This has three positive effects:

       1. The increase in capillary density decreases the distance for diffusion between the blood and site of oxygen utilization.

       2. It increases the lateral surface area for diffusion.

       3. The increase in cross-sectional area of the capillaries reduces the blood linear velocity and increases the transit time for diffusion.

    B. Changes in hemoglobin-oxygen affinity

       1. Increase in hydrogen (H^+) concentration results in a right shift of the dissociation curve.

       2. Changes in the 2,3-DPG concentration

       3. The concentration of 2,3-DPG is regulated by red blood cell H^+ concentration (as the rate-limiting enzyme is pH sensitive) – a high pH stimulates 2,3-DPG synthesis.

       4. Deoxyhemoglobin provides better buffering than oxyhemoglobin and thereby raises red cell pH; thus low venous oxygen promotes DPG synthesis.
       Note: this adaptive mechanism is less prominent in young infants with high levels of HbF, as HbF binds 2,3-DPG poorly and its synthesis is inhibited by unbound DPG.

VI. Consequences of Tissue Hypoxia

    A. Reduced oxidative phosphorylation

    B. Electron transport chain slows

    C. Reduced phosphorylation of adenosine-5'-diphosphate (ADP) to adenosine-5'-triphosphate (ATP)

    D. Increased adenosine-5'-monophosphate (AMP), which is rapidly catabolized to inosine and hypoxanthine during hypoxia

    E. Creatinine phosphate acts as a "supplementary" energy reservoir if creatinine kinase is available, but becomes rapidly depleted.

    F. ADP can be phosphorylated anaerobically, but this is much less efficient than aerobic metabolism. During aerobic glycolysis, production of ATP is 19 times greater than it is under anerobic conditions (i.e, production of 38 vs. 2 mmol of ATP). Lactic acid accumulates.

G. Adverse effect on immune function and inflammation
   1. Increased neutrophil sequestration
   2. Increased vascular permeability
   3. Decreased cellular immune function

Suggested Reading

Lister G: Oxygen transport and consumption. In Gluckman PD, Heymann MA (Eds.): *Pediatrics and Perinatology: The Scientific Basis, 2nd Edition.* London, Edward Arnold, 1996, pp. 778–790.

Chapter 14

Neonatal Resuscitation

Janet M. Rennie

"Time is of the utmost importance. *Delay* is damaging to the infant. *Act* promptly, accurately and gently." *Virginia Apgar*

I. **Anticipating Resuscitation**
Some form of resuscitation is required in about 2% of all deliveries; advanced resuscitation is required in as few as 2 per 1,000 deliveries. An individual with resuscitation skills should be present at the following types of deliveries:
   A. Preterm delivery
   B. Multiple deliveries
   C. Breech delivery
   D. Instrumental delivery
   E. Meconium staining
   F. Fetal distress (whether cesarean section or vaginal delivery)

II. **Normal Postnatal Transition**
Most babies establish independent breathing and circulation quickly after birth, crying lustily and becoming pink within a few minutes. During the period of time the infant normally:
   A. Clears lung liquid from the trachea and alveoli
   B. Establishes a functional residual volume with the aid of surfactant
   C. Reduces pulmonary vascular resistance (oxygenation, nitric oxide, prostaglandins)
   D. Increases pulmonary blood flow

III. **Equipment Needed for Resuscitation**
In order that resuscitation can take place quickly and effectively, appropriate facilities and equipment must be available. The following are essential:
   A. A warm, well-lit area in which resuscitation can take place

101

B. A heater

C. Towels, gloves, hat for baby

D. Immediate access to a telephone

E. An assured oxygen supply with a suitable pressure valve to limit the pressure

F. A supply of medical gases

G. A suction device with a range of catheter sizes

H. Laryngoscopes with back-up bulbs and batteries, assorted blades

I. Endotracheal tubes varying from 2.5–4.5 mm

J. A mask resuscitation system

K. All systems capable of providing respiratory support should have protective "blow-off devices." However, in case high pressures are needed on an individual basis, the resuscitator should be able to override such a device.

L. Equipment for placing a peripheral and/or umbilical venous line

M. Scissors

N. Stethoscope

O. A timing device

P. Fluids and drugs (sodium bicarbonate, naloxone, adrenaline, dextrose, saline)

IV. **Assessing the Infant after Birth**

A. Start the clock.

B. Receive the baby, remove any wet wraps, and dry the baby with a warm towel.

C. Place the infant on the resuscitation surface, cover with a warm towel, and make an assessment of breathing, heart rate, and color.

D. Babies fall into one of three categories at this point:

1. Pink, breathing spontaneously and regularly; heart rate >100; active tone

2. Cyanosed, breathing irregularly, with a heart rate >100; some tone

3. White, floppy, not breathing, heart rate <100

V. **The Apgar Score (Table 16)**

The Apgar score can be helpful in categorizing infants at this stage. A score <3 means that advanced resuscitation is required immediately and is an indication to call for help.

VI. **Initiating Resuscitation**

Babies who are pink, breathing, and have a good heart rate should be returned to their mothers as soon as possible, without any further intervention. If the baby falls into one of the other two categories above

Table 16
The Apgar Score

Score	0	1	2
A Appearance	Pale or blue	Body pink, but extremities blue	Pink
P Pulse rate	Absent	<100	>100
G Grimace	Nil	Some	Cry
A Activity (muscle tone)	Limp	Some flexion	Well flexed
R Respiratory effort	Absent	Hypoventilation	Good

where respiration is not established, resuscitation should be started. Babies who are blue but with a good heart rate usually respond to simple resuscitation. Babies who are white, floppy, and not breathing will most likely need full resuscitation with intubation and chest compression following the A, B, C, D approach outlined below. Optimally, two people should be dedicated to the resuscitation of the infant. Call for help immediately if this has not been established.

The A, B, C, D approach to resuscitation is:

A. Airway

   1. Make sure the airway is clear.

   2. Position the baby supine with the jaw drawn forward.

   3. Gently suction the mouth, then the nose if secretions are present. Many babies will resuscitate themselves once the airway is clear.

   4. Do not insert the suction catheter too far into the oropharynx or it will initiate a vagal response with bradycardia and apnea.

   5. Do not suction for more than 5 seconds at a time.

   6. Suction is particularly important for babies born through meconium.

B. Breathing

   1. If resuscitation does not commence rapidly, try gentle stimulation – rubbing the soles of the feet, drying the body with the towel.

   2. If respirations do not commence within 20 seconds, or remain irregular, the baby will require artificial lung inflation.

   3. Choose a face mask that fits over the baby's mouth and nose but does not overhang the chin or cover the eyes.

   4. Hold the mask over the face making a tight seal.

   5. Begin to inflate the lungs with the Y piece (easier and better – can give sustained inflation) or self-inflating bag.

   6. Ventilate at 30–40 breaths per minute, giving the first few breaths a long (2 sec) inflation time.

     a. The first few breaths need to overcome surface tension.

     b. The pressure given should be enough to move the chest wall; about 20 cm H_2O water, although the first few breaths may need to be 30-40 cm H_2O water pressure.

    c. Watch to see that the chest moves and listen to the heart rate, which should rapidly rise.

    d. If the heart rate remains low, or falls in spite of adequate ventilation, the baby will need intubation and external chest compression.

C. Circulation

    1. When the heart rate is <60 bpm, circulatory support is required.

    2. The best method for external chest compression in babies is to encircle the chest with both hands at the level of the lower third of the sternum, and to compress the sternum with the thumbs.

    3. Press down about 2–3 cm in a term baby at a rate of about 80 per minute.

    4. Inflate the lungs after every few compressions, in a ratio of 3:1.

D. Drugs

Rarely, there is still no response even after intubation with effective ventilation and chest movement and chest compression. The baby remains white, not breathing, and with a heart rate ≤60 bpm. In this situation drugs can sometimes achieve a "jump start" of the system. The ideal route is via the umbilicus.

    1. Adrenaline 0.1–0.3 mL/kg 1:10,000 by IV or endotracheal tube

    2. Sodium bicarbonate 2 mL/kg IV (4.2%), if ventilating

    3. Dextrose 2 mL/kg, 10% solution

    4. Naloxone is of use if the mother was given opiate analgesia <6 hours before delivery. Use 100 μg/kg. The dose may need to be repeated. *Do not* give if there is a history or suspicion of maternal drug abuse as it may initiate neonatal withdrawal.

    5. Calcium – there is no evidence that calcium is useful in resuscitation

VII. Monitoring the Response to Resuscitation

    A. Resuscitation does not end with the baby achieving a good heart rate and spontaneous breathing.

    B. Observations should continue and a decision made as to whether it is safe for the baby to remain with the mother or whether he/she should be admitted to the nursery for observation.

    C. Any baby who has required resuscitation should have early glucose screening until stable.

VIII. Reasons for Failure to Respond to Resuscitation

    A. There is a leak in the system delivering oxygen or air to the baby.

    B. The endotracheal tube is in the esophagus.

    C. Hemorrhagic shock – consider blood transfusion.

    D. Sepsis, including pneumonia

    E. Pneumothorax

    F. Pleural effusion

    G. Pulmonary hypoplasia – may respond to high ventilatory pressures

    H. Laryngeal abnormality; choanal atresia; Pierre-Robin sequence

    I. Congenital diaphragmatic hernia

    J. Congenital heart disease

    K. Spinal cord injury

IX. **Abandoning Resuscitation**

    A. This decision should only be made by a senior neonatologist.

    B. If there has been no cardiac output after 20 minutes of resuscitation, attempts should be abandoned.

    C. If the baby has a heart beat but is not making respiratory effort, artificial ventilation should continue while further information is sought.

X. **Record Keeping – Good Records are Vital**

    A. Condition at birth, color/tone/respiration

    B. Time to first gasp, time to regular respiration, cry

    C. Heart rate at the start and at intervals: time when heart rate rose above 100 bpm

    D. Apgar scores at 5-minute intervals to supplement the above (but not to replace these observations)

    E. Time commencing bag and mask ventilation, duration

    F. Time at tracheal intubation, duration of intubation

    G. Umbilical cord pH (specify whether arterial or venous)

    H. Drugs given, dose, route, and time

    I. Names and designations of personnel; time of their arrival

    J. Reasons for any delay

    K. Information given to the parents

Suggested Reading

Bloom RS, Cropley C: *Textbook of Neonatal Resuscitation.* Dallas, American Heart Association/American Academy of Pediatrics, 1987.

Royal College of Paediatrics and Child Health, Royal College of Obstetricians and Gynaecologists: *Resuscitation of Babies at Birth.* London, England, BMJ Publishing Group, 1997.

SECTION IV

Mechanical Ventilation

Chapter 15

Basic Principles of Mechanical Ventilation

Waldemar A. Carlo, Namasivayam Ambalavanan, Robert L. Chatburn

The ventilatory needs of a patient depend largely on the mechanical properties of the respiratory system and the derangement of gas exchange.

I. **Pulmonary Mechanics**
   A. The mechanical properties of the lungs determine the interaction between the ventilator and the infant.
   B. A pressure gradient between the airway opening and alveoli drives the flow of gases.
   C. The pressure gradient is largely determined by the compliance and resistance.

II. **Compliance**
   A. Compliance describes the elasticity or distensibility of the lungs or respiratory system (lungs plus the chest wall).
   B. It is calculated as follows:

$$\text{Compliance} = \frac{\Delta \text{volume}}{\Delta \text{pressure}}$$

   C. Compliance in infants with normal lungs ranges from 3–5 mL/cm H_2O/kg.
   D. Compliance in infants with respiratory distress syndrome (RDS) ranges from 0.1–1 mL/cm H_2O/kg.

III. **Resistance**
   A. Resistance describes the ability of the gas conducting parts of the lungs or respiratory system (lungs plus chest wall) to resist airflow.

B. It is calculated as follows:

$$\text{Resistance} = \frac{\Delta\text{pressure}}{\Delta\text{flow}}$$

C. Resistance in infants with normal lungs ranges from 25–50 cm H_2O/ L/sec. Resistance is not markedly altered in infants with RDS or other acute pulmonary disorders, but can be increased to 100 cm H_2O/L/sec or more by small endotracheal tubes.

IV. Time Constant

A. The time constant is a measure of the time (expressed in seconds) necessary for the alveolar pressure (or volume) to reach 63% of a change in airway pressure (or volume) (Figure 47).

B. It is calculated as follows:

$$\text{Time constant} = \text{compliance} \times \text{resistance}$$

For example, if an infant has lung compliance of 3 mL/cm H_2O (0.003 L/cm H_2O) and a resistance of 40 cm H_2O/L/sec, time constant is calculated as follows:

$$\text{Time constant} = 0.003 \text{ L/cm } H_2O \times 40 \text{ cm } H_2O/\text{L/sec}$$

$$\text{Time constant} = 0.120 \text{ sec}$$

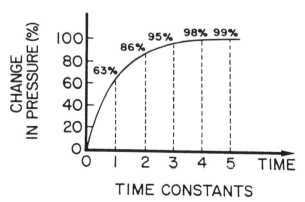

TIME CONSTANTS

Figure 47. Percentage change in pressure in relation to the time (in time constants) allowed for equilibration. As a longer time is allowed for equilibration, a higher percentage change in pressure will occur. The same rules govern the equilibrium for step changes in volume. Changes in pressure during inspiration and expiration are illustrated. (Modified from Carlo WA, Chatburn RL: Assisted ventilation of the newborn. In Carlo WA, Chatburn RL [Eds.]: *Neonatal Respiratory Care, 2nd Edition.* Chicago, Year Book Medical Publishers, 1988, p. 323, with permission.)

Note that in the calculation of the time constant, compliance is not corrected for unit of weight.

C. A duration of inspiration or expiration equivalent to 3–5 time constants is required for a relatively complete inspiration or expiration, respectively. Thus, in the infant described above, inspiratory and expiratory duration should be around 360–600 msec each (or 0.36–0.6 sec).

D. The time constant will be shorter if compliance is decreased (e.g., in patients with RDS) or if resistance is decreased. The time constant will be longer if compliance is high (e.g., large infants with normal lungs) or if resistance is high (e.g., infants with chronic lung disease).

E. Patients with a short time constant ventilate well with short inspiratory and expiratory times and high ventilatory frequency, while patients with a long time constant require longer inspiratory and expiratory times and lower rates.

F. If inspiratory time is too short (i.e., a duration shorter than approximately 3–5 time constants), there will be a decrease in tidal volume delivery and mean airway pressure (Figure 48).

G. If expiratory time is too short (i.e., a duration shorter than approximately 3–5 time constants), there will be gas trapping and inadvertent positive end-expiratory pressure (PEEP) (Figure 49).

H. While the respiratory system is often modeled as being composed of a single compliance and a single resistance, it is known that the mechanical properties vary with changes in the lung volume, even within a breath. Furthermore, the mechanical characteristics of the respiratory system change somewhat between inspiration and expiration. In addition, lung disease can be heterogeneous, and thus, different areas of the lungs can have varying mechanical characteristics.

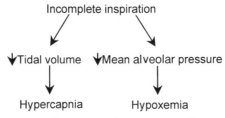

Figure 48. Effect of incomplete inspiration on gas exchange. (From Carlo WA, Greenough A, Chatburn RL: Advances in mechanical ventilation. In Boynton BR, Carlo WA, Jobe AH [Eds.]: *New Therapies for Neonatal Respiratory Failure: A Physiologic Approach*. Cambridge, Cambridge University Press, 1994, p. 137, with permission.)

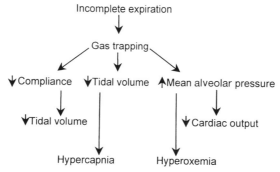

Figure 49. Effect of incomplete expiration on gas exchange. (From Carlo WA, Greenough A, Chatburn RL: Advances in mechanical ventilation. In Boynton BR, Carlo WA, Jobe AH [Eds.]: *New Therapies for Neonatal Respiratory Failure: A Physiologic Approach.* Cambridge, Cambridge University Press, 1994, p. 137, with permission.)

V. **Equation of Motion**

    A. The pressure necessary to drive the respiratory system is the sum of the elastic, resistive, and inertial components and can be calculated as follows:

$$P = \frac{1}{C}V + R\dot{V} + I\ddot{V}$$

        Where P is pressure
            C is compliance
            V is volume
            R is resistance
            $\dot{V}$ is flow
            $\ddot{V}$ is the rate of change in flow
            I is inertance

    B. Because the inertial component is small at physiologic flows, the last component ($I\ddot{V}$) can be neglected

    C. The equation of motion can be used to derive estimates of compliance and resistance. For example, between points of $\dot{V} = 0$ (points of no flow) the pressure gradient results from compliance.

VI. **Gas Exchange**

    A. Hypercapnia and/or hypoxemia occur during respiratory failure. Although impairment in CO_2 elimination and oxygen uptake and delivery may coexist, some conditions may affect gas exchange differentially.

VII. Gas Exchange During Transition to Extrauterine Life

A. Hemodynamic changes during transition to extrauterine life:
   1. Systemic vascular resistance increases.
   2. Pulmonary vascular resistance decreases.
   3. Pulmonary blood flow increases.

B. Blood gas values in the perinatal period

	At birth	*10 min of age*
PaO_2 (mm Hg)	15–20	46–57
$PaCO_2$ (mm Hg)	49–76	40–47

VIII. Determinants of Pulmonary Gas Exchange

A. Composition and volume of alveolar gas
B. Composition and volume of mixed venous blood
C. Mechanisms of gas exchange

IX. Composition of Inspired and Alveolar Gases

A. Partial pressure of oxygen in dry air
Partial pressure of O_2 = fractional content x total gas pressure
If barometric pressure = 760 mm Hg, then

$$PO_2 = 0.21(760 \text{ mm Hg})$$

$$PO_2 = 160 \text{ mm Hg}$$

B. Partial pressure of oxygen in humidified air
Partial pressure O_2 = fractional content $\times$ (total gas pressure − water vapor pressure)

$$PiO_2 = 0.21(760 - 47 \text{ mm Hg})$$

$$PiO_2 = 149 \text{ mm Hg}$$

C. Partial pressure of oxygen in humidified alveolar gas

$$\text{Partial pressure of alveolar } O_2 = PiO_2 - PACO_2$$
$$\times (FiO_2 + [1 - FiO_2]/R)$$

where $PACO_2$ is alveolar PCO_2 and R is the respiratory quotient. Because CO_2 diffuses so well through the alveoli, $PACO_2 \approx PaCO_2$.

If barometric pressure = 760 mm Hg and water vapor pressure is 47 mm Hg, then

$$PiO_2 = 713$$

If FiO_2 is 1.00, $(FiO_2 + [1 - FiO_2]/R) = 1.0$, then

$$PaO_2 = 713 - 40 = 673 \text{ mm Hg}$$

If FiO_2 is 0.21, then

$$PaO_2 = 149 - 40(0.21 + [1 - 0.21]/0.8) = 100 \text{ mm Hg}$$

X. **Composition of Mixed Venous Blood**
    A. Mixed venous PO_2 (PvO_2) depends on arterial O_2 content, cardiac output, and metabolic rate.
    B. Oxygen content of blood per 100 mL of blood

    $$\text{Dissolved } O_2 = 0.003 \text{ mL } O_2/PaO_2$$

    Hemoglobin bound O_2 = O_2 sat × 1.34/gm hemoglobin
    × hemoglobin concentration

    For example, 1 kg infant (blood volume ≈ 100 mL) with PaO_2 = 100 mm Hg (O_2 sat = 100%, or 1.0), and hemoglobin = 17 mg/dL

    $$O_2 \text{ content} = \text{hemoglobin bound } O_2 + \text{dissolved } O_2$$

    $$O_2 \text{ content} = 1.00 \times 1.34 \times 17 + 0.003 \times 100$$

    $$O_2 \text{ content} = 22.78 + 0.3 \text{ mL } O_2$$

    $$O_2 \text{ content} = 23.08 \text{ mL } O_2$$

    C. CO_2 content of blood
        CO_2 is carried in three forms:
        1. Dissolved in plasma and red cells
        2. As bicarbonate
        3. Bound to hemoglobin

XI. **Hypoxemia**
    The pathophysiologic mechanisms responsible for hypoxemia are ventilation/perfusion ($\dot{V}/\dot{Q}$) mismatch, shunt, hypoventilation, and diffusion limitation (Figures 50, 51, 52):

    A. $\dot{V}/\dot{Q}$ mismatch. $\dot{V}/\dot{Q}$ mismatch is an important cause of hypoxemia in newborns. Supplemental oxygen can largely overcome the hypoxemia resulting from $\dot{V}/\dot{Q}$ mismatch.
    B. Shunt
        Shunt is a common cause of hypoxemia in newborns. A shunt may be

V_AQ Relationships

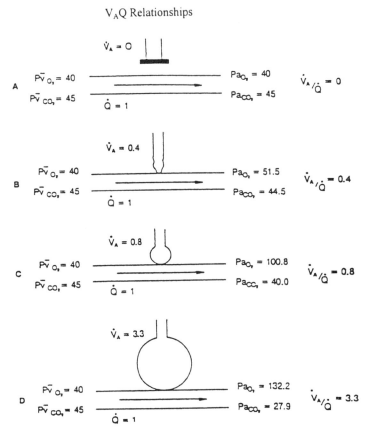

Figure 50. Effects of various ventilation/perfusion ratios on blood gas tensions. **A.** Direct venoarterial shunting ($\dot{V}_A/\dot{Q} = 0$). **B.** Alveolus with a low $\dot{V}_A/\dot{Q}$ ratio. **C.** Normal alveolus. **D.** Underperfused alveolus with high $\dot{V}_A/\dot{Q}$ ratio. (From Krauss AN: Ventilation-perfusion relationships in neonates. In Thibeault DW, Gregory GA [Eds.]: *Neonatal Pulmonary Care, 2nd Edition*. Norwalk, CT, Appleton-Century-Crofts, 1986, p. 127, with permission.)

physiologic, intracardiac (e.g., persistent pulmonary hypertension of the newborn, congenital cyanotic heart disease), or pulmonary (e.g., atelectasis). It can be thought of as a $\dot{V}/\dot{Q} = 0$ and supplemental O_2 cannot reverse the hypoxemia.

C. Hypoventilation
Hypoventilation results from a decrease in tidal volume or respiratory rate. During hypoventilation, the rate of oxygen uptake from the alveoli exceeds its replenishment. Thus, alveolar PO_2 falls and PaO_2 decreases. It can be thought of as low $\dot{V}/\dot{Q}$ and supplemental O_2 can

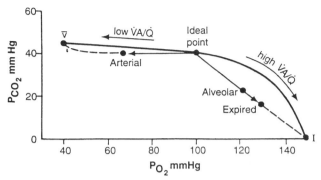

Figure 51. O_2-CO_2 diagram showing the arterial, ideal, alveolar, and expired points. The curved line indicates the PO_2 and PCO_2 of all lung units having different ventilation/perfusion ratios. (From West JB: Gas exchange. In West JB [Ed.]: *Pulmonary Pathophysiology: The Essentials.* Baltimore, Williams & Wilkins, 1977, p. 27, with permission.)

overcome the hypoxemia easily. Causes of hypoventilation include: depression of respiratory drive, weakness of the respiratory muscles, restrictive lung disease, and airway obstruction.

D. Diffusion limitation

Diffusion limitation is an uncommon cause of hypoxemia, even in the presence of lung disease. Diffusion limitation occurs when mixed venous blood does not equilibrate with alveolar gas. Supplemental O_2 can overcome hypoxemia secondary to diffusion limitation.

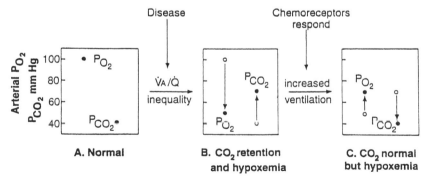

Figure 52. PO_2 and PCO_2 in different stages of ventilation/perfusion inequality. Initially, there must be both a fall in oxygen and a rise in carbon dioxide tensions. However, when the ventilation to the alveoli is increased, the PCO_2 returns to normal, but the PO_2 remains abnormally low. (From West JB: Gas exchange. In West JB [Ed.]: *Pulmonary Pathophysiology: The Essentials.* Baltimore, Williams & Wilkins, 1977, p. 30, with permission.)

XII. Oxygenation During Assisted Ventilation

A. Oxygenation may be largely dependent on lung volume, which in turn depends on mean airway pressure (Figure 53).

B. On a pressure ventilator, any of the following will increase mean airway pressure: increasing inspiratory flow, increasing peak inspiratory pressure (PIP), increasing the inspiratory-to-expiratory (I:E) ratio, or increasing PEEP.

C. Mean airway pressure maybe calculated as follows:

$$\text{Mean airway pressure} = K(PIP - PEEP)[T_I/(T_I + T_E)] + PEEP$$

where K is a constant that depends on the shape of the early inspiratory part of the airway pressure curve (K ranges from approximately 0.8 to 0.9 during pressure-limited ventilation); T_I is inspiratory time; T_E is expiratory time.

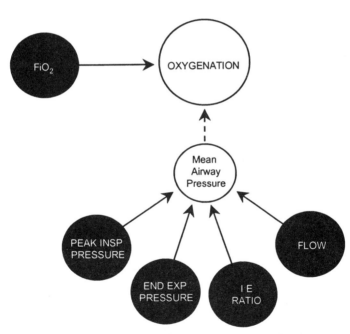

Figure 53. Determinants of oxygenation during pressure-limited, time-cycled ventilation. Shaded circles represent ventilator-controlled variables. Solid lines represent the simple mathematical relationships that determine mean airway pressure and oxygenation, whereas dashed lines represent relationships that cannot be quantified. (From Carlo WA, Greenough A, Chatburn RL: Advances in mechanical ventilation. In Boynton BR, Carlo WA, Jobe AH [Eds.]: *New Therapies for Neonatal Respiratory Failure: A Physiologic Approach*. Cambridge, Cambridge University Press, 1994, p. 134, with permission.)

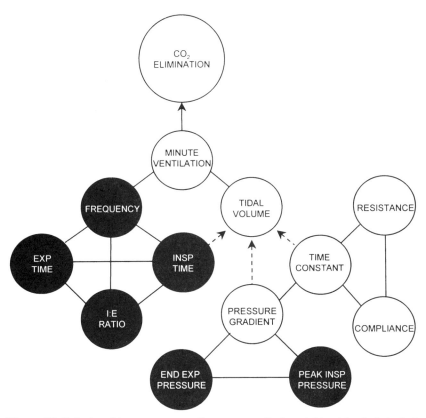

Figure 54. Relationships among ventilator-controlled variables (shaded circles) and pulmonary mechanics (unshaded circles) that determine minute ventilation during time-cycled, pressure-limited ventilation. Relationships between circles joined by solid lines are mathematically derived. The dashed lines represent relationships which cannot be precisely calculated without considering other variables such as pulmonary mechanics. Alveolar ventilation can be calculated from the product of tidal volume and frequency when dead space is subtracted from the former. (From Carlo WA, Greenough A, Chathurn RL: Advances in mechanical ventilation. In Boynton BR, Carlo WA, Jobe AH [Eds.]: *New Therapies for Neonatal Respiratory Failure: A Physiologic Approach.* Cambridge, Cambridge University Press, 1994, p. 133, with permission.)

For the same change in mean air way pressure, increases in PIP and PEEP increase oxygenation more. A very high mean airway pressure transmitted to the intrathoracic structures may impair cardiac output and thus decrease oxygen transport despite an adequate PaO_2.

Table 17
Blood Gas Classifications*

Classification	pH	PaCO$_2$	HCO$_3$$^-$	BE
Respiratory disorder				
Uncompensated acidosis	↓	↑	N	N
Partly compensated acidosis	↓	↑	↑	↑
Compensated acidosis	N	↑	↑	↑
Uncompensated alkalosis	↑	↓	N	N
Partly compensated alkalosis	↑	↓	↓	↓
Compensated alkalosis	N	↓	↓	↓
Metabolic disorder				
Uncompensated acidosis	↓	N	↓	↓
Partly compensated acidosis	↓	↓	↓	↓
Uncompensated alkalosis	↑	N	↑	↑
Partly compensated alkalosis	↑	↑	↑	↑
Compensated alkalosis	N	↑	↑	↑

* Arrows = elevated or depressed values; N = normal; BE = base excess.
(From Carlo WA, Chatburn RL: Assessment of neonatal gas exchange. In Carlo WA, Chatburn RL [Eds.]: *Neonatal Respiratory Care, 2nd Edition.* Chicago, Year Book Medical Publishers, 1988, p. 51, with permission.)

XIII. Hypercapnia

The pathophysiologic mechanisms responsible for hypercapnia are severe $\dot{V}/\dot{Q}$ mismatch, shunt, hypoventilation, and increased physiologic dead space. The physiologic dead space results in part from areas of inefficient gas exchange because of low perfusion (wasted ventilation). Physiologic dead space includes ventilation to conducting airways and alveolar spaces not perfused (i.e., anatomic dead space).

XIV. CO$_2$ Elimination During Assisted Ventilation

A. CO$_2$ diffuses easily into the alveoli and its elimination depends largely on the total amount of gas that comes in contact with the alveoli (alveolar ventilation). Minute alveolar ventilation is calculated from the product of the frequency (per minute) and the alveolar tidal volume (tidal volume minus dead space).

Minute alveolar ventilation = frequency $\times$ (tidal volume − dead space)

B. On a volume-cycled ventilator the tidal volume is preset. On a pressure-controlled ventilator, the tidal volume depends on the pressure gradient between the airway opening and the alveoli; this is PIP minus the PEEP, or amplitude (ΔP).

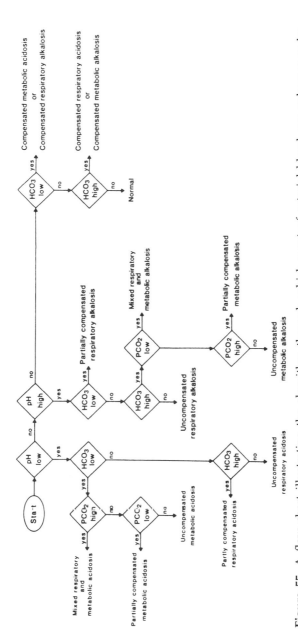

Figure 55. A flow chart illustrating the algorithm through which a set of arterial blood gas values may be interpreted. (From Chatburn RL, Carlo WA: Assessment of neonatal gas exchange. In Carlo WA, Chatburn RL [Eds.]: *Neonatal Respiratory Care, 2nd Edition.* Chicago, Year Book Medical Publishers, 1988, p. 56, with permission.)

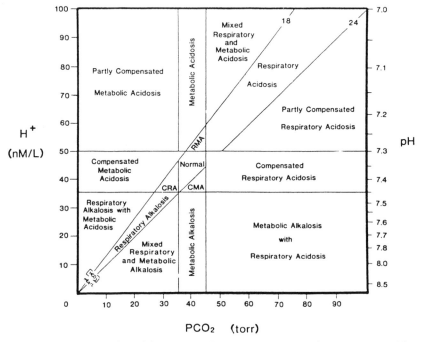

Figure 56. A neonatal acid-base map. CRA = compensated respiratory acidosis; CMA = compensated metabolic acidosis; RMA = mixed respiratory and metabolic acidosis. (From Chatburn RL, Carlo WA: Assessment of neonatal gas exchange. In Carlo WA, Chatburn RL [Eds.]: *Neonatal Respiratory Care, 2nd Edition.* Chicago, Year Book Medical Publishers, 1988, p. 58, with permission.)

    C. Depending on the time constant of the respiratory system (and the ventilator), a very short T_I may reduce the tidal volume, and a very short T_E may cause gas trapping and inadvertent PEEP, and consequently may also reduce tidal volume (see above).

    D. Figure 54 illustrates the relationships among ventilator controls, pulmonary mechanics, and minute ventilation. Ventilator controls are shown in shaded circles.

XV. Blood Gas Analysis
    A careful interpretation is essential for appropriate respiratory care (Table 17, Figures 55, 56; see also Chapter 7).

    A. Respiratory acidosis (low pH, high $PaCO_2$, normal HCO_3^-)
        1. From $\dot{V}/\dot{Q}$ mismatch, shunt and/or hypoventilation
        2. Secondary renal compensation
            a. Reduction in bicarbonate excretion
            b. Increased hydrogen ion excretion

B. Respiratory alkalosis (high pH, low $PaCO_2$, normal HCO_3^-)
  1. From hyperventilation
  2. Secondary renal compensation
     a. Increased bicarbonate excretion
     b. Retention of chloride
     c. Reduced excretion of acid salts and ammonia
C. Metabolic acidosis (low pH, normal $PaCO_2$, low HCO_3^-)
  1. From increased acid production or impaired acid elimination
  2. Secondary pulmonary compensation – hyperventilation with decreased $PaCO_2$
D. Metabolic alkalosis (high pH, normal $PaCO_2$, high HCO_3^-)
  1. From excessive $NaHCO_3$ administration, diuretic therapy, and loss of gastric secretions
  2. Secondary pulmonary compensation – hypoventilation

Suggested Reading

Carlo WA, Chatburn RL: Assisted ventilation of the newborn. In Carlo WA, Chatburn RL (Eds.): *Neonatal Respiratory Care, 2nd Edition.* Chicago, Year Book Medical Publishers, 1988, pp. 320–346.

Carlo WA, Greenough A, Chatburn RL: Advances in conventional mechanical ventilation. In Boynton BR, Carlo WA, Jobe AH (Eds.): *New Therapies for Neonatal Respiratory Failure: A Physiologic Approach.* Cambridge, England, Cambridge University Press, 1994, pp. 131–151.

Donn SM (Ed.): *Neonatal and Pediatric Pulmonary Graphics: Principles and Clinical Applications.* Armonk, NY, Futura Publishing Co., 1997.

Greenough A: Respiratory support. In Greenough A, Roberton NRC, Milner AD (Eds.): *Neonatal Respiratory Disorders.* New York, Oxford University Press, 1996, pp. 115–151.

Krauss AN: Ventilation-perfusion relationship in neonates. In Thibeault DW, Gregory GA (Eds.): *Neonatal Pulmonary Care, 2nd Edition.* Norwalk, CT, Appleton-Century-Crofts, 1986, p. 127.

Mariani GL, Carlo WA: Ventilatory management in neonates: Science or art? Clin Perinatol 1998; 25:33–48.

Spitzer AR, Fox WW: Positive-pressure ventilation: pressure-limited and time-cycled ventilators. In Goldsmith JP, Karotkin EH (Eds.): *Assisted Ventilation of the Neonate, 3rd Edition.* Philadelphia, W.B. Saunders Co., 1996, pp. 167–186.

West JB: Gas exchange. In West JB (Ed.): *Pulmonary Pathophysiology: The Essentials.* Baltimore, Williams & Wilkins, 1977, p. 32.

Chapter 16

Classification of Mechanical Ventilation Devices

Waldemar A. Carlo, Namasivayam Ambalavanan, Robert L. Chatburn

I. **Introduction**
   Ventilators can be classified by the variables that are controlled (e.g., pressure or volume), as well as those that start (or trigger), sustain (or limit), and end (cycle) inspiration and those that maintain the expiratory support (or baseline pressure).

II. **Control Variables**
   A ventilator can be classified as a pressure, volume, or flow controller (Figure 57). Ventilators control more than one variable at different times.

   A. Pressure controller. This type of ventilator controls either:
      1. Airway pressure, making it rise above the body surface pressure (i.e., positive pressure ventilator); or
      2. Body surface pressure, making it fall below the airway pressure (i.e., negative pressure ventilator).

   B. Volume controller
      This type of ventilator controls and measures the tidal volume generated by the ventilator despite changes in loads. In the past, the usefulness of this type of ventilator in newborns has been limited because the control variable was regulated near the ventilator and not near the patient, resulting in a tidal volume lower than the set one.

   C. Flow controller
      This type of ventilator controls the tidal volume but does not measure it directly. A ventilator is a flow controller if the gas delivery is limited by flow.

   D. Time controller
      This type of ventilator controls the timing of the ventilatory cycle but not the pressure or volume. Most high-frequency ventilators are time controllers.

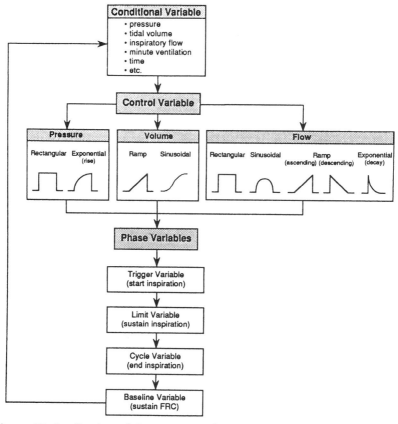

Figure 57. Application of the equation of motion for the respiratory system. Common waveform for each control variable is shown. Pressure, volume, flow, and time are also used as phase variables that determine the characteristics of each ventilatory cycle (e.g., trigger sensitivity, inspiratory time, baseline pressure). This emphasizes that each breath may have a different set of control and phase variables, depending on the mode of ventilation desired. (From Chathurn RL: Classification of mechanical ventilators. In Branson RD, Huess DR, Chatburn RL [Eds.]: *Respiratory Care Equipment.* Philadelphia, J.B. Lippincott, 1995, p. 280, with permission.)

III. Phase Variables

The ventilatory cycle has four phases: 1) the change from expiration to inspiration (trigger); 2) inspiration (limit); 3) the change from inspiration to expiration (cycle); and 4) expiration (baseline pressure) (Figure 58).

A. Trigger

One or more variables in the equation of motion (i.e., pressure, volume,

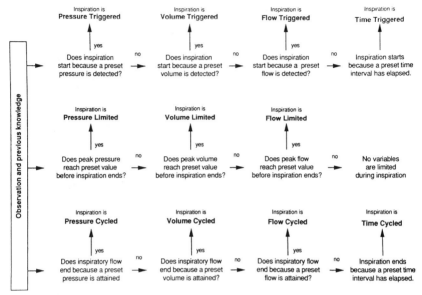

Figure 58. Criteria for determining the phase variables during a ventilator-supported breath. (From Chatburn RL: Classification of mechanical ventilators. In Branson RD, Huess DR, Chatburn RL [Eds.]: *Respiratory Care Equipment.* Philadelphia, J.B. Lippincott, 1995, p. 280, with permission.)

flow, and time) is measured by the ventilator and used to trigger (or start) inspiration. Inspiration begins when one of these variables reaches a preset value. The most common trigger variables are time (i.e., after a predefined time, the ventilator is triggered to start inspiration as in intermittent mandatory ventilation) and pressure (i.e., when an inspiratory effort is detected as a change in the end-expiratory pressure, the ventilator is triggered to start inspiration as in patient-triggered ventilation).

B. Limit
Pressure, volume, and flow increase during inspiration. A limit variable restricts the inspiratory increase to a preset value but does not limit the duration. Many neonatal ventilators are pressure-limited.

C. Cycle
The cycle variable is used to end inspiration. Many neonatal ventilators, including high-frequency ventilators, are time-cycled.

D. Baseline
The baseline variable maintains expiratory pressure and expiratory lung volume (e.g., positive end-expiratory pressure).

IV. Ventilatory Modes
This classification of mechanical ventilation devices can be applied to the various ventilatory modes (Table 18).

Table 18
Ventilatory Modes

Mode	Mandatory				Spontaneous			
	Control	Trigger[a]	Limit	Cycle	Control	Trigger	Limit	Cycle
Control	Flow[b]	Time	Volume Flow	Volume Time	NA[c]	NA	NA	NA
A/C or CMV	Flow	Pressure Volume Time	Volume Flow	Volume Time	NA	NA	NA	NA
IMV (continuous flow)	Pressure Flow	Time	Volume Flow	Volume Time	—[d]	—	—	—
SIMV (continuous flow)	Pressure Flow	Pressure Volume Flow Time	Pressure Volume Flow Time	Volume Time	—	—	—	—
SIMV (demand flow)	Pressure Flow	Pressure Volume Flow Time	Pressure Volume Flow Time	Volume Time	Pressure Flow	Pressure	Pressure	Pressure
PS	—	—	—	—	Pressure	Pressure	Pressure	Flow

(continued)

125

Table 18 (continued)

Mode	Mandatory				Spontaneous			
	Control	Trigger[a]	Limit	Cycle	Control	Trigger	Limit	Cycle
PS + SIMV	Pressure Flow	Pressure Volume Flow Time	Pressure Volume Flow Time	Time	Pressure	Pressure Flow	Pressure	Flow
CAP or CPAP (continuous flow)	—	—	—	—	Pressure	—	Pressure	—
CAP or CPAP (demand flow)	—	—	—	—	Pressure	Pressure Flow	Pressure	—
PC	Pressure	Time	Pressure	Time	NA	NA	NA	—

[a] Whether or not a breath is patient-triggered depends on the sensitivity setting and the magnitude of the patient's inspiratory effort.

[b] For the purposes of this table, flow control is equivalent to volume control. Baseline PEEP is assumed to be available for all modes.

[c] NA, not applicable.

[d] Ventilator does not respond.

A/C = assist/control; CMV = conventional mandatory ventilation; IMV = intermittent mandatory ventilation; PS = pressure support; SIMV = synchronized mandatory ventilation; CAP = constant airway pressure; CPAP = continuous positive airway pressure; PC = pressure control.

(From Carlo WA, Greenough A, Chatburn RL: Advances in conventional mechanical ventilation. *New Therapies for Neonatal Respiratory Failure: A Physiologic Approach.* Cambridge, Cambridge University Press, 1994, p. 144, with permission.)

Suggested Reading

Carlo WA, Greenough A, Chatburn RL: Advances in conventional mechanical ventilation. In Boynton BR, Carlo WA, Jobe AH (Eds.): *New Therapies for Neonatal Respiratory Failure: A Physiologic Approach.* Cambridge, England, Cambridge University Press, 1994, pp. 131–151.

Chatburn RL: Classification of mechanical ventilators. In Branson RD, Hess DR, Chatburn RL (Eds.): *Respiratory Care Equipment.* Philadelphia, J.B. Lippincott Company, 1995, pp. 264–293.

Chapter 17

Ventilator Parameters

Waldemar A. Carlo, Namasivayam Ambalavanan, Robert L. Chatburn

I. **Peak Inspiratory Pressure (PIP)**

   A. Physiological effects

   PIP, in part, determines the pressure gradient between the onset and end of inspiration, and thus, affects the tidal volume and minute ventilation. Note: During volume ventilation an increase in tidal volume corresponds to an increase in PIP during pressure ventilation. If tidal volume is not measured, initial PIP can be selected based on observation of the chest wall movement and magnitude of the breath sounds.

   B. Gas exchange effects

   An increase in PIP will increase tidal volume, increase CO_2 elimination, and decrease $PaCO_2$. An increase in PIP will increase mean airway pressure, and thus improve oxygenation.

   C. Side effects

   An elevated PIP may increase the risk of barotrauma, volutrauma, and bronchopulmonary dysplasia/chronic lung disease. There is increasing evidence that lung injury is primarily caused by large tidal volume delivery and lung overdistention. Thus, it is important to adjust PIP based on lung compliance, and ventilate with relatively small tidal volumes. (e.g., 4–6 mL/kg).

II. **Positive End-Expiratory Pressure (PEEP)**

   A. Physiological effects

   PEEP in part determines lung volume during the expiratory phase, improves ventilation/perfusion mismatch, and prevents alveolar collapse. PEEP contributes to the pressure gradient between the onset and end of inspiration, and thus affects the tidal volume and minute ventilation. A minimum "physiological" PEEP of 2–3 cm H_2O should be used in most newborns.

   B. Gas exchange effects

   An increase in PEEP increases expiratory lung volume (functional residual capacity) during the expiratory phase, and thus improves ventilation/perfusion matching and oxygenation in patients whose disease state reduces expiratory lung volume. An increase in PEEP will increase mean airway pressure, and thus improve oxygenation. An increase in PEEP will also reduce the pressure gradient during inspiration, and thus reduce tidal volume, reduce CO_2 elimination, and increase $PaCO_2$.

C. Side effects

An elevated PEEP may overdistend the lungs and lead to decreased lung compliance, decreased tidal volume, less CO_2 elimination, and an increase in $PaCO_2$. While use of low-to-moderate PEEP may improve lung volume, a very high PEEP may cause overdistention and impaired CO_2 elimination secondary to decreased compliance and gas trapping. Furthermore, a very high PEEP may decrease cardiac output and oxygen transport.

III. **Frequency**

A. Physiological effects

The ventilator frequency (or rate) in part determines minute ventilation, and thus, CO_2 elimination. Ventilation at high rates ($\geq 60/$min) frequently facilitates synchronization of the ventilator with spontaneous breaths. Spontaneous breathing rates are inversely related to gestational age and the time constant of the respiratory system. Thus, infants with smaller and less compliant lungs tend to breathe faster.

B. Gas exchange effects

When very high frequencies are used, the problem of insufficient inspiratory time (T_I) or insufficient expiratory time (T_E) may occur (see below).

C. Side effects

Use of very high ventilator frequencies may lead to insufficient T_I and decreased tidal volume or insufficient T_E and gas trapping.

IV. **Inspiratory Time, Expiratory Time , and Inspiratory-to-Expiratory Ratio (I:E Ratio)**

A. Physiological effects

The effects of the T_I and T_E are strongly influenced by the relationship of those times to the T_I and T_E constants. A T_I as long as 3–5 time constants allows relatively complete inspiration. T_I of 0.2–0.5 seconds are usually adequate for newborns with respiratory distress syndrome (RDS). Use of a longer T_I generally does not improve ventilation or gas exchange. A very prolonged T_I may lead to ventilator asynchrony. A very short T_I will lead to decreased tidal volume. However, infants with a long time constant (e.g., chronic lung disease) may benefit from a longer T_I (up to approximately 0.6–0.8 sec).

B. Gas exchange effects

Changes in T_I, T_E, and I:E ratio generally have modest effects on gas exchange. A sufficient T_I is necessary for adequate tidal volume delivery and CO_2 elimination. Use of relatively long T_I or high I:E ratio improves oxygenation slightly.

C. Side effects
Very short T_I or T_E can lead to insufficient times and decrease tidal volume and increase gas trapping, respectively.

V. Inspired Oxygen Concentration (FiO$_2$)

A. Physiological effects
Changes in FiO$_2$ alter alveolar oxygen pressure, and thus, oxygenation. Because both FiO$_2$ and mean airway pressure determine oxygenation, the most effective and less adverse approach should be used to optimize oxygenation. When FiO$_2$ is above 0.6–0.7, increases in mean airway pressure are generally warranted. When FiO$_2$ is below 0.3–0.4, decreases in mean airway pressure are generally preferred.

B. Gas exchange effects
FiO$_2$ directly determines alveolar PO$_2$ and thus PaO$_2$.

C. Side effects
A very high FiO$_2$ can damage the lung tissue, but the absolute level of FiO$_2$ that is toxic has not been determined.

VI. Flow
Changes in flow rate have not been well studied in infants, but they probably impact arterial blood gases minimally as long as a sufficient flow is used (which is generally the case with most ventilators).

VII. In summary, depending on the desired change in blood gases, the corresponding ventilator parameter changes shown in (Table 19) can be performed.

VIII. Algorithm for Changes in Ventilator Parameters
Based on the principles addressed above, an algorithm for ventilatory management of infants with RDS is suggested (Figure 59 and Table 20).

Table 19
Desired Blood Gas Goal and Corresponding Ventilator Parameter Changes

Desired Goal	Ventilator Parameter Change				
	PIP	*PEEP*	*Frequency*	*I:E Ratio*	*Flow*
Decrease PaCO$_2$	↑	↓	↑	—	± ↑
Increase PaCO$_2$	↓	↑	↓	—	± ↑
Decrease PaO$_2$	↓	↓	—	↓	± ↑
Increase PaO$_2$	↑	↑	—	↑	± ↑

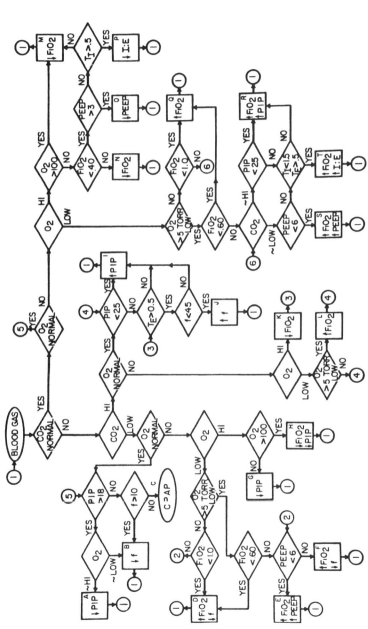

Figure 59. Simplified flow chart illustrating an algorithm used to optimize pressure-limited mechanical ventilation of infants with RDS. Diamond-shaped symbols call for decisions, while squares indicate types and directions of ventilator setting changes. Algorithm is entered at top, where "blood gas" appears in an oval. Flow chart is followed until a square is reached. If a number other than 1 is reached, reenter the algorithm as appropriate. See Table 20 for explanation of abbreviations. (From Chatburn RL, Carlo WA, Lough MD: Clinical algorithm for pressure-limited ventilation of neonates with respiratory distress syndrome. Respir Care 1983; 28:1579, with permission.)

Table 20
Abbreviations and Symbols Used in the Flowchart in Figure 59

CO_2	Arterial carbon dioxide tension (mm Hg)
O_2	Arterial oxygen tension (mm Hg)
FiO_2	Fraction of inspired oxygen
PIP	Peak inspiratory pressure (cm H_2O)
Pāw	Mean airway pressure (cm H_2O)
PEEP	Positive end-expiratory pressure (cm H_2O)
CPAP	Continuous positive airway pressure without mechanical ventilation (cm H_2O)
I:E	Ratio of inspiratory to expiratory time
f	Ventilator frequency (breaths/min). Unless otherwise specified, a change in frequency should be accompanied by a change in I:E to maintain the same T_I, so that tidal volume remains constant
T_I	Inspiratory time (sec)
T_E	Expiratory time (sec)
HI	The variable in the decision symbol is above normal range
LOW	The variable in the decision symbol is below normal range
≈HI	The variable in the decision symbol is at the high end of normal
≈LOW	The variable in the decision symbol is at the low end of normal
↑	Increase
↓	Decrease
>	Greater than
<	Less than
Torr	Unit of pressure; 1 torr − 1 mm Hg

From Carlo WA, Chatburn RL: Assisted ventilation of the newborn. In Carlo WA, Chatburn RL (Eds.): *Neonatal Respiratory Care, 2nd Edition.* Chicago, Year Book Medical Publishers, 1988 p. 339, with permission.

Suggested Reading

Donn SM (Ed.): *Neonatal and Pediatric Pulmonary Graphics: Principles and Clinical Applications.* Armonk, NY, Futura Publishing Co., 1997.

Greenough A: Respiratory support. In Greenough A, Roberton NRC, Milner AD (Eds.): *Neonatal Respiratory Disorders.* New York, Oxford University Press, 1996, pp. 115–151.

Mariani GL, Carlo WA: Ventilatory management in neonates: Science or art Clin Perinatol 1998; 25:33–48.

Spitzer AR, Fox WW: Positive-pressure ventilation: pressure-limited and time-cycled ventilators. In Goldsmith JP, Karotkin EH (Eds.): *Assisted Ventilation of the Neonate, 3rd Edition.* Philadelphia, W.B. Saunders Co., 1996, pp. 167–186.

SECTION V

Conventional Ventilation

Chapter 18

Continuous Positive Airway Pressure

Colin J. Morley

I. **Definition**

   A. Continuous positive airway pressure (CPAP) is a positive pressure applied to the airways of a spontaneously breathing baby throughout the respiratory cycle.

   B. Positive end-expiratory pressure (PEEP) is a pressure applied to the airways during the expiratory phase of ventilation.

   C. CPAP and PEEP are used to treat babies with acute respiratory difficulty, mainly premature infants with respiratory distress syndrome (RDS). CPAP is also used to treat premature infants with apnea or airway obstruction.

II. **CPAP and PEEP are Needed to Avoid Alveolar Collapse to Below Functional Residual Capacity.**

   A. The newborn with a low lung volume may grunt to maintain functional residual capacity (FRC). During this process, the baby inspires, closes the larynx, contracts the abdominal muscles to increase intrathoracic pressure, and prevent the alveoli and airway from collapsing. The newborn then exhales through a narrowed larynx with the gas under pressure to maintain alveolar distention. If the baby tires, or cannot maintain laryngeal tone, or the larynx is bypassed, he/she may rapidly loose lung volume.

   B. In term neonates, the lung fluid leaves the air spaces soon after birth. Inflation of the lungs moves the liquid from the lung lumen into distensible perivascular spaces, distant from the sites of gas exchange. Large positive pressures are generated with the first few breaths to open the lung. The postnatal clearance of lung liquid is much slower after premature birth. The premature lung may even continue to secrete fluid into the alveoli adding to the problem of maintaining alveolar patency. Elevated left atrial pressure and low plasma protein concentrations also slow the rate at which lung liquid is removed from potential air spaces.

C. The newborn lung has an FRC that is close to airway closing volume. Babies may have to maintain lung volume by shortening their expiratory time so that the lung has not completely emptied.

D. The upper airway in the term infant is supported by a fat laden superficial fascia and also actively held open by the pharyngeal muscles. In the premature infant it is not so well stabilized and is much more likely to collapse. Pharyngeal closure or narrowing can occur with relatively small changes in airway pressure. If the infant has large negative pharyngeal pressures during inspiration, this may collapse the extrathoracic airway. Infants with periodic breathing easily develop obstruction of the pharynx, which is reversible by CPAP.

E. The premature infant has an immature lung structure with a relatively undeveloped internal architecture to maintain lung volume so that it is not held open by internal support. The immature lung also has thicker and fewer alveolar septa. This reduces gas exchange.

F. The newborn's chest wall is very compliant – probably five times more than the normal lung tissue. The chest wall of the premature baby is so soft and flexible that it is incapable of holding the lung open during excessive inspiratory efforts and the pull of the diaphragm and negative pressure generated distorts the chest wall and reduces the tidal volume.

G. The round shape of the premature infant's chest wall with horizontal ribs also reduces the potential for lung expansion. The diaphragm of the preterm infant is relatively flat and potentially less effective. During rapid eye movememt (REM) sleep there is loss of intercostal muscle activity. This destabilizes the chest wall so that rib cage and abdominal respiratory movements are out of phase. This results in a further loss of end-expiratory lung volume. Atelectasis and airway closure develop easily especially considering the relative paucity of collateral ventilation channels in the newborn.

H. Premature babies often have a patent ductus arteriosus with a shunt from the aorta to the pulmonary arteries. This increases the fluid in the lungs and predisposes to pulmonary edema.

I. Surfactant in normal lungs has two important functions:
  1. It lowers the surface tension and facilitates lung expansion at birth, and
  2. It "solidifies" and splints the lung open during expiration.
    Premature lungs lack adequate surfactant so they tend to have low lung volume or airway collapse during expiration. This results in loss of surfactant from the alveolar surface by squeeze-out.

J. The epithelium of the collapsing lung is easily damaged and plasma proteins exude onto the surface. These compound the problem of inadequate surfactant by inhibiting its function.

K. A decrease in lung volume is associated with a persistently elevated alveolar-arterial oxygen gradient and ventilation/perfusion mismatch with increased arterial CO_2 levels. Oxygenation is related to the surface area. If this is reduced, then oxygenation is compromised.

135

CO_2 elimination is related to the minute volume. This can also be compromised by low lung volume and atelectasis.

L. Reduced arterial oxygen availability impairs the respiratory pump including the diaphragm.

III. How CPAP or PEEP Helps

A. It abolishes upper airway occlusion and decreases upper airway resistance by mechanical splinting. It increases the pharyngeal cross-sectional area and decreases genioglossus activity.

B. It increases diaphragmatic activity.

C. It improves lung compliance and decreases airway resistance in the infant with unstable lung mechanics. This allows a greater tidal volume for a given pressure with subsequent reduction in the work of breathing and stabilization of the minute ventilation.

D. It increases the tidal volume if the lung is stiff and the FRC is low.

E. It increases the mean airway pressure, and the associated increase in FRC should improve ventilation/perfusion and potentially reduce oxygen requirements.

F. It conserves surfactant on the alveolar surface.

G. It diminishes alveolar edema and prevents alveolar flooding.

H. It helps overcome the resistance of the endotracheal tube.

I. Successful extubation may be more likely to succeed if the baby is treated with nasal CPAP.

IV. Indication for CPAP or Increasing PEEP

A. Increased work of breathing indicated by:
1. Increased respiratory rate
2. Retractions, grunting, nasal flaring
3. The need for increased inspired oxygen

B. Poorly expanded or infiltrated lung fields on chest radiograph

C. Pulmonary edema

D. Atelectasis

E. Apnea of prematurity

F. Recent extubation

G. Tracheomalacia or other abnormalities of the airways predisposing to airway collapse

V. How CPAP Can Be Given

A. The American Association for Respiratory Care has published some useful advice about how to administer CPAP. The following devices have been used:

1. Face mask. This can provide positive pressure but has several drawbacks. It is difficult to get a good seal without excessive pressure on the baby's face. The mask has to be removed and the pressure is lost when the mouth and nose are cleared by suction. It is difficult to place a nasogastric or orogastric tube because of the difficulty with the seal.

2. Head box with a seal. The original method devised by Gregory et al. was a special head box that sealed around the neck and had a blow-off relief valve to control the pressure. It had a number of problems. It was difficult to get a good seal. There was poor access to the baby's face, and any attention to the baby's face caused a loss of pressure. There was a high flow of gas cooling the baby's head. It was very noisy.

3. Negative pressure box. This is a small cuirass that encircles the chest and abdomen and maintains a negative pressure outside the lung to help keep it open. Although effective, it has many practical problems. It is difficult to get a good seal. There is poor access to the baby's body. Any attention to the baby's body causes a loss of pressure. There is a high flow of gas cooling the baby.

4. Nose piece. This can be effective but is difficult to attach to the baby and get a good seal without undue pressure.

5. Endotracheal tube. Whenever a baby has an endotracheal tube and the larynx is bypassed, PEEP should be applied to prevent loss of lung volume. However, an endotracheal tube should not be used solely for the purpose of delivering CPAP because the resistance of the endotracheal tube makes it difficult for the baby to breathe effectively for more than a short time. Endotracheal CPAP can be used for a short while just before extubation to ensure that the baby does not become apneic when intermittent inflation is not present.

6. Nasal prongs. This is the most satisfactory (or least unsatisfactory) method of delivering CPAP. For the most part, newborns are obligatory nose breathers; therefore nasal CPAP is easily facilitated. This is accomplished by inserting nasopharyngeal tubes or nasal prongs.

    a. One or two prongs are inserted into one or two nostrils and attached to a ventilator or a device for delivering CPAP. Although there are proponents for double prongs, they have not been shown to be more effective in delivering CPAP than a single prong appropriately used. A newer fluidic device is said to reduce the work of breathing but there are few clinical data to substantiate any superiority over other devices. The prong can be short, inserted into the nostril about 1.5 cm, or deep into the pharynx. Long nasal prongs have not been shown to be superior to short prongs and they have the added difficulty of higher resistance for the baby to breathe through and are more likely to become blocked by secretions.

    b. A pacifier in the baby's mouth has been shown to help maintain the pharyngeal pressure. The biggest problems with nasal

CPAP are that the tubes become displaced and pressure is lost, the tubes become blocked and pressure is not delivered, the baby cries and pressure is lost, and they make the nose sore.

VI. **What Levels of CPAP or PEEP Can Be Used?**

A. As each baby's respiratory problems are unique, the level of CPAP/PEEP required needs to be individualized and should be altered to suit the baby's problems as they change. The level therefore needs to be adjusted for each baby at each use.

1. Providing the infant has stiff lungs or low lung volumes, increasing CPAP/PEEP improves oxygenation up to about 8 cm H_2O. Some babies with very stiff lungs may need a higher pressure. However, if the pressure is too high, overdistension occurs and the oxygenation may be compromised.

2. Increasing CPAP/PEEP tends to increase CO_2 retention, so there may be a trade-off between improving the oxygenation and a rise in the CO_2 levels. Conversely, if a baby is being treated with CPAP/PEEP and the CO_2 levels are high, then reducing the pressure may improve the CO_2 exchange.

B. The way to determine the appropriate level of CPAP or PEEP for a baby is:

1. Look at the chest radiograph. Do the lungs look collapsed or edematous or are they well expanded? High or low pressures may be required depending on the problem.

2. If oxygenation is the main problem, increase the pressure.

3. If CO_2 retention is the main problem reduce the pressure.

4. Start at 4–5 cm H_2O and gradually increase up to 10 cm H_2O to stabilize the oxygenation while maintaining a pH >7.25 and $PaCO_2$ <60 torr (8.0 kPa).

5. For PEEP applied through an endotracheal tube, pulmonary mechanics measurements or graphics may help to determine the optimal PEEP.

VII. **Use of CPAP After a Baby Has Been Extubated**

Several studies have shown that babies breathe and oxygenate better and are less likely to need reintubation, particularly if they were ventilated for RDS, if they are treated with nasal CPAP immediately after extubation. This may be because the larynx has been stretched and is edematous and not functioning properly during the few hours after extubation. Alternatively, CPAP helps to maintain alveolar distention and lower the work of breathing.

VIII. **Contraindications to CPAP**

A. The need for intubation or ventilation because of ventilatory failure – inability to maintain oxygenation and the $PaCO_2$ >60 torr (8 kPa) and pH <7.25

    B. Upper airway abnormalities (cleft palate, choanal atresia, tracheo-esophageal fistula, and diaphragmatic hernia)

    C. Severe cardiovascular instability

    D. Unstable respiratory drive with frequent apnea and or bradycardia

XI. **Hazards/Complications of CPAP or PEEP**

    A. Obstruction of the nasal tubes so the baby mouth breathes and gets less oxygen and pressure than expected

    B. It may cause overdistension of the lung and reduce the tidal volume if the lung is very compliant and the pressure is relatively high within the lung leading to:

       1. Air leaks

       2. CO_2 retention

       3. Increased work of breathing

       4. Impedance of pulmonary blood flow with subsequent increased pulmonary vascular resistance and decreased cardiac output

       5. Gastric insufflation and distension

       6. Nasal irritation, damage to the septum and mucosal damage

       7. Skin irritation and necrosis from the fixation devices

       8. Failure of the disconnect alarms because of the increased resistance in the tube or obstruction in the tubes continuing to measure a high pressure

       9. Inadvertent decannulation

X. **Inadvertent PEEP**

The development of inadvertent PEEP has been considered a problem in ventilated babies where it is thought that fast rate ventilation may have an expiratory time that is so short that there is inadequate time for full expiration. This can be a problem and care has to be taken with babies who have "normal" lungs (i.e., babies undergoing surgery), or babies ventilated with low inspired oxygen or low peak pressures (i.e., <16 cm H_2O), or with normally expanded lungs on the chest radiograph. Clinically, this can be recognized because oxygenation deteriorates as the pressure is increased. Except in babies with chronic lung disease, an expiratory time of 0.5 seconds will usually be sufficient. It must be recognized that babies frequently shorten their own expiratory time by increasing the respiratory rate in order to create intrinsic PEEP.

XI. **Weaning Babies from CPAP**

Nasal CPAP is very useful after babies are extubated from intermittent positive pressure ventilation (IPPV). Once on CPAP, the level of pressure required and the length of time it is used has to be determined by clinical experience. A baby who is not having apneic or bradycardic episodes and who requires a low inspired oxygen concentration can be tried without CPAP. It is a matter of trial and error to see how they manage. Conversely, a baby who requires a high level of inspired oxygen and is clinically unstable will probably benefit from CPAP.

Suggested Reading

AARC Clinical Practice Guideline: Application of continuous positive airway pressure to neonates via nasal prongs or nasopharyngeal tube. Respir Care 1994; 39:817–823.

Alex CG, Aronson RM, Onal E, Lopata M: Effects of continuous positive airway pressure on upper airway and respiratory muscle activity. J Appl Physiol 1987; 62:2026–2030.

Bartholomew KM, Brownlee KG, Snowden S, Dear PRF: To PEEP or not to PEEP. Arch Dis Child 1994; 70:F209–F212.

Da Silva WJ, Abbasi S, Pereira G, Bhutani VK: Role of positive end-expiratory pressure changes on functional residual capacity in surfactant treated preterm infants. Pediatr Pulmonol 1994; 18:89–92.

Gregory GA, Kitterman JA, Phibbs RH, et al: Treatment of the idiopathic respiratory distress syndrome with continuous positive airway pressure. N Engl J Med 1971; 284:1333–1340.

Klausner JF, Lee AY, Hutchinson AA: Decreased imposed work with a new nasal continuous positive airway pressure device. Pediatr Pulmonol 1996; 22:188–194.

Kosch PC, Stark AR: Dynamic maintenance of end-expiratory lung volume in full term infants. J Appl Physiol: Respirat Environ Exercise Physiol 1984; 57:1126–1133.

Robertson NJ, McCarthy LS, Hamilton PA, Moss ALH: Nasal deformities resulting from flow driver continuous positive airway pressure. Arch Dis Child 1996; 75:F209–F212.

So B, Tamura M, Mishina J, et al: Application of nasal continuous positive airway pressure to early extubation in very low birthweight infants. Arch Dis Child 1995; 72:F191–F193.

Verder H, Robertson B, Greisen G, et al: Surfactant therapy and nasal continuous positive airway pressure for newborns with respiratory distress syndrome. N Engl J Med 1994; 331:1051–1055.

Vilstrup CT, Bjorklund LJ, Larsson A, et al: Functional residual capacity and ventilation homogeneity in mechanically ventilated small neonates. J Appl Physiol 1992; 73:276–283

Chapter 19

Intermittent Mandatory Ventilation

Cheryll K. Hagus

I. **Description**

A. Definition

Intermittent mandatory ventilation (IMV) is a mode which combines a fixed amount of mechanical ventilation, predetermined by the clinician, with the patient's own spontaneous breathing. This mode may be utilized in the acute care phase (i.e., higher preset breath rates) or the weaning phase (i.e., lower preset rates). This mode has been historically called time-cycled, pressure-limited ventilation (TCPLV).

B. Characteristics

1. Mandatory breaths occur at fixed intervals determined by the preset breath rate (BR) divided by 60 sec/min (termed total cycle time [TCT]).

2. The mandatory tidal volume (V_T) breath-to-breath is determined by the preset pressure limit (PL), flow, and inspiratory time (T_I), as well as the patient's compliance (C_L) and airway resistance (R_{AW}).

3. V_T may not be stable breath-to-breath, particularly if the patient is breathing asynchronously with the ventilator.

4. The patient may breath spontaneously between mandatory breaths from a flow of gas, with a preset oxygen fraction (FiO_2), provided from the ventilator (continuous and/or demand flow).

5. The spontaneous BR, V_T, peak flow, and T_I are determined by the patient.

6. The baseline pressure (positive end-expiratory pressure, PEEP) may be increased to a preset level to enhance the patient's oxygenation status.

C. Indications

1. Hypoxemic respiratory failure – PaO_2 <50 torr (6.7 kPa) while receiving FiO_2 ≥0.5

2. Hypercapnic respiratory failure – $PaCO_2$ >60 torr (8 kPa)

3. Unstable cardiovascular status (bradycardia, hypotension)

4. Impaired respiratory drive (apnea, neurologic impairment)

5. Excessive work of breathing (impaired pulmonary function, airway obstruction)

D. Management of potential complications

    1. Overdistension/barotrauma/volutrauma

        a. If possible, avoid PL settings above 35 cm H_2O. Wean pressure aggressively.

        b. The risk of barotrauma increases when the patient is breathing asynchronously with the ventilator. Consider use of sedation and/or paralytics.

    2. Intraventricular hemorrhage risk increases when the patient is breathing asynchronously. Consider use of sedation and/or paralytics.

    3. Cardiovascular compromise

        a. The risk increases at mean airway pressures >15 cm H_2O. Avoid excessive ventilator settings whenever possible.

        b. Medical management of hypotension and/or hypovolemia may be required.

    4. Airway complications including upper airway trauma, endotracheal tube malpositioning, tube obstruction (plugging/kinking).

        a. Endotracheal tubes and ventilator circuits should be firmly secured to avoid excessive movement.

        b. Lavage and suction should be performed when the physical assessment indicates the need to do so.

    5. Oxygen toxicity

        a. Utilize optimum mean airway pressure and PEEP to improve oxygenation status.

        b. Wean oxygen as quickly as possible.

    6. Ventilator-acquired infection

        a. Infection control policies and procedures should be strictly followed.

        b. Prophylactic use of antibiotics is a common practice, although of unproven efficacy and potentially risky.

II. Controls, Monitors, and Alarms

    A. Controls

        1. Breath rate (BR)

            a. BR adjusts the number of mandatory (i.e., ventilator-controlled breaths) delivered each minute.

            b. Conventional ventilators typically have a range from zero (CPAP) to 150 BPM.

            c. Initial BR will generally be between 30–40 BPM; however, rates ≥60 BPM may be necessary.

        2. Pressure limit (PL)

            a. PL adjusts the peak inspiratory pressure (PIP) applied to the airway during the inspiratory phase. It is the primary determinant of the delivered V_T (i.e., the depth of inspiration).

  b. Typically the adjustable range will be from 3–80 cm H_2O.

  c. The PL is usually started at a low level (e.g., 15–20 cm H_2O) and adjusted upward in 1–2 cm H_2O increments.

  d. If the ventilator system in use has a V_T monitor, PL may be set to achieve a desired V_T based on weight. General rules are 4–6 mL/kg for very low birthweight (VLBW), 6–8 mL/kg for low birthweight (LBW), and ≥ 8 mL/kg for term infants.

3. Inspiratory time (T_I)

  a. T_I adjusts the length of time pressure is applied to the airway during inspiration (i.e., the length of the inspiratory phase).

  b. The adjustable range is typically 0.1–3.0 seconds.

  c. Initial T_I generally ranges from 0.3–0.5 seconds. A shorter T_I may be required with BR >60 BPM.

4. Flow rate

  a. This control generally has a dual purpose. First, it adjusts the magnitude of flow directed to the airway during the inspiratory phase of each breath. It also determines the flow available for spontaneous breathing between mandatory breaths. Some ventilators automatically adjust the flow available for spontaneous breathing to a value lower than the preset inspiratory flow to reduce expiratory resistance.

  b. The range of flow varies from ventilator to ventilator. The low end is usually 2–3 liters per minute (LPM) with the high end 20–30 LPM, and in some cases, up to 40 LPM.

  c. To avoid excessive expiratory resistance the flow rate should be set to the lowest value which will generate the desired inspiratory pressure and pressure waveform. This will typically be 5–8 LPM in VLBW and LBW infants and up 12 LPM for larger infants.

5. PEEP

  a. PEEP enhances lung volume (FRC) by discouraging the collapse of alveoli at end-expiration. Increases in PEEP increase mean airway pressure, which correlates with improvement in oxygenation.

  b. The range of PEEP available on most ventilators is 1.0–20-25 cm H_2O.

  c. PEEP should be started at low levels (3-5 cm H_2O) and increased in 1 cm H_2O increments until the desired effect is achieved. In newborns, PEEP levels higher than 10 cm H_2O are rarely utilized.

6. Fraction of inspired oxygen (FiO_2)
Raises the fractional concentration of inspired oxygen above room air (0.21). It is adjustable from 0.21–1.0.

B. Monitors and alarms

1. The PIP monitor reflects the highest pressure recorded during the inspiratory phase of mandatory breaths. It reflects the PL control setting and, therefore, it usually does not vary breath-to-breath. Ventilators also have an airway pressure gauge which reflects the dynamic increase and decrease in pressure between the PL and PEEP (ΔP or amplitude).

   a. The high pressure alarm, which is set 5–10 cm H_2O above the PL setting, audibly and visually alerts an increase in airway pressure. Potential causes are an occluded/kinked patient circuit or patient coughing.

   b. The low pressure alarm, which is set 5–10 cm H_2O below the peak pressure, audibly alerts a patient circuit leak or disconnect.

   c. The low PEEP alarm is set 2–3 cm H_2O below the PEEP setting and also alerts a patient circuit leak or disconnect.

2. The mean airway pressure monitor reflects the average pressure applied over time (i.e., a moving average). This monitor responds to changes in the PL, BR, T_I, flow, and PEEP settings.

3. In IMV, the BR and T_I monitors reflect the control settings for these parameters. The expiratory time (T_E) and I:E ratio monitors reflect calculated values based on the T_I and BR settings. I:E ratio and T_E are valuable in evaluating the risk of air trapping and (inadvertent) auto-PEEP. The apnea alarm reflects decreases in respiratory rate. Often the apnea alarm is factory preset at 20 seconds but may be adjustable from 10 seconds to 2 minutes on some ventilators.

4. Most neonatal ventilators do not include an oxygen analyzer that displays the FiO_2. However, a stand-alone monitor is often added externally. Most monitors include a high and low FiO_2 alarm which are usually set 0.05 above and below the preset level.

5. Some third generation ventilators include V_T and minute volume monitors, either built-in or as external options. Inspiratory/Expiratory V_T is the volume in milliliters which is inspired or expired per breath. When both are provided, the degree of airway leak can be assessed. Minute volume is the volume exhaled during a 1-minute time frame.

   a. The V_T monitor is a valuable tool for titrating the PL setting to achieve an optimal V_T based on patient weight (see above).

   b. The low minute volume alarm can alert a significant drop in V_T, BR, or a leak/disconnect in the patient circuit. It may be set 20–25% below the prevailing minute volume.

6. An early sign of failure to wean from mechanical ventilation may be tachypnea. Some ventilator monitoring systems may include a high breath rate alarm or a high minute volume alarm to alert this situation.

7. Most ventilators include alarms for loss of air and/or oxygen gas pressure, loss of electrical power, and ventilator inoperative conditions. These alarm conditions should be addressed immediately as patient compromise is highly likely.

III. Patient Management
A. Ventilation
   1. The primary controls which adjust the level of ventilation are the PL and BR.
   2. PL should be adjusted to achieve adequate lung inflation and discourage atelectasis. Assessment of bilateral breath sounds, chest excursion, exhaled V_T, and chest radiography can guide subsequent adjustments.
   3. Once adequate lung inflation has been achieved, BR should be adjusted for $PaCO_2$ and pH within the target ranges.
   4. In general, $PaCO_2$ of 40–60 torr (5.3–8 kPa) and pH of 7.35–7.45 are acceptable. However, certain diagnosis may warrant a $PaCO_2$ >60 torr (8 kPa) with a pH of >7.25, or $PaCO_2$ <40 torr (5.3 kPa) with a pH <7.35.
B. Oxygenation
   1. The primary parameters that adjust oxygenation are FiO_2 and $P\bar{a}w$.
   2. In general, PaO_2 of 50–80 torr (6.7–10.7 kPa) with an oxygen saturation of >92% are acceptable.
   3. FiO_2 should be maintained below 0.6, if possible, to avoid increased risk of oxygen toxicity.
   4. Excessive PEEP levels should be avoided to reduce the risk of cardiovascular compromise.
   5. Mean airway pressure correlates with oxygenation. Increases in T_I may improve oxygenation, without changes in FiO_2 or PEEP, and without significantly changing the patient's ventilation status.
C. Weaning
   1. As the patient's compliance increases, delivered V_T will increase. To avoid overinflation, the PL should be decreased in 1–2 cm H_2O decrements for minor adjustments, and 3–5 cm H_2O decrements for moderate adjustments, to a minimum of 12–15 cm H_2O.
   2. BR should be decreased in 3–5 BPM decrements for slight adjustments in $PaCO_2$, and 5–10 BPM decrements for moderate adjustments, to a minimum of 5–10 BPM.
   3. PEEP should be weaned in 1–2 cm H_2O decrements to a minimum of 2 cm H_2O.
   4. FiO_2 should be weaned aggressively to <0.4.
   5. Once ventilator parameters have been weaned to minimum values, readiness for extubation may be assessed. Evaluation of respiratory parameters, chest radiography, airway clearance, and hemodynamics can aid the decision process.

Suggested Reading

Aloan CA, Hill TV: *Respiratory Care of the Newborn, 2nd Edition.* Philadelphia, Lippincott, 1997.

Barnhart SL, Czervinske MP: *Perinatal and Pediatric Respiratory Care.* Philadelphia, W.B. Saunders Co., 1995.

Donn SM (Ed.): *Neonatal and Pediatric Pulmonary Graphics: Principles and Clinical Applications.* Armonk, NY, Futura Publishing Co., Inc., 1998.

Goldsmith JP, Karatokin EH (Eds.): *Assisted Ventilation of the Neonate, 3rd Edition.* Philadelphia, W.B. Saunders Co., 1996.

Koff PB, Eitzman D, Neu J: *Neonatal and Pediatric Respiratory Care.* St. Louis, Mosby, 1993.

Whitaker KB: *Comprehensive Perinatal and Pediatric Respiratory Care.* Albany, NY, Delmar Publishers, Inc., 1992.

Chapter 20

Assist/Control Ventilation

Steven M. Donn, Sunil K. Sinha

I. **Description**
  A. Ventilatory mode in which mechanical breaths are either patient (assist) or ventilator (control) initiated.
  B. Also referred to as patient-triggered ventilation (PTV)

II. **Cycling Mechanisms**
  A. Time
  B. Flow
  C. Volume

III. **Trigger Mechanisms**
  A. Airway flow
    1. Differential pressure transducer
    2. Heated wire anemometer
  B. Airway pressure
  C. Thoracic impedance
  D. Abdominal impedance

IV. **Assist Breath**
  A. If patient effort exceeds trigger threshold, mechanical breath is initiated
    1. Trigger delay is the time from signal detection to rise in proximal airway pressure.
    2. Long trigger delay increases work of breathing as patient may complete own inspiratory cycle before receiving mechanical breath.
  B. Patient-controlled variables
    1. Respiratory rate

    2. Inspiratory time (if flow-cycled)

C. Clinician-controlled variables

    1. Peak inspiratory pressure (if pressure-limited)

    2. Tidal volume delivery (if volume-cycled)

    3. Inspiratory time (if time-cycled)

    4. Flow

    5. Control rate

D. Flow-cycling

    1. Inspiration is terminated at a percentage of peak flow rather than time.

    2. Fully synchronizes patient and ventilator

    3. Prevents inversion of inspiratory:expiratory ratio and minimizes gas trapping

    4. May result in insufficient inspiratory time and tidal volume delivery

V. Control Breath

A. Essentially a back-up intermittent mandatory ventilation (IMV) in case of insufficient patient effort or apnea

B. Provides a minimal minute ventilation if baby is unable to trigger the ventilator or fails to breathe

C. If rate set too high, patient may "ride" the ventilator and not breathe spontaneously.

D. If patient is consistently breathing above the control rate, lowering it has no effect on the mechanical ventilatory rate.

VI. Patient Management

A. Indications

    1. Works well for virtually all patients

    2. Flow-triggering especially useful in extremely low birth weight infants

    3. Provides full ventilatory support

    4. Synchrony can decrease need for sedatives/paralytics.

B. Initiation

    1. Use minimal assist sensitivity.

    2. Set control rate at reasonable level until patient demonstrates reliable respiratory drive.

    3. For flow-cycling, termination at 5% of peak flow generally works best but check to see that patient is receiving adequate tidal volume.

    4. Other parameters set as for IMV

C. Weaning
   1. Since reduction in ventilator rate will have no impact on minute ventilation if patient breathes above control rate, primary weaning parameter is peak inspiratory pressure.
   2. If P_aCO_2 is too low, it is most likely the result of overventilation (too high a peak inspiratory pressure), as the infant is unlikely to spontaneously hyperventilate. Lower the pressure.
   3. As soon as patient demonstrates reliable respiratory drive, lower the control rate (20–30 BPM).
   4. Can extubate directly from assist/control or switch to synchronized intermittent mandatory ventilation (SIMV)
   5. Can also wean by increasing assist sensitivity, thus increasing patient work to increase tolerance

VII. Problems
   A. Auto-cycling and false triggering
      1. Leaks anywhere in the system (around endotracheal tube, in circuit, etc.) can cause flow and pressure-triggered devices to misread this as patient effort resulting in delivery of a mechanical breath.
      2. Thoracic impedance triggering may result in mechanical breaths secondary to cardiac impulses rather than respiratory motion
      3. Abdominal impedance device may trigger from artifactual motion
   B. Failure to trigger
      1. Assist sensitivity too high
      2. Patient unable to reach trigger threshold
      3. Patient fatigue
      4. Sedative drugs
   C. Inadequate inspiratory time (flow-cycling) results in inadequate tidal volume delivery. Patient may compensate by breathing rapidly.

Suggested Reading

Donn SM, Nicks JJ, Becker MA: Flow-synchronized ventilation of preterm infants with respiratory distress syndrome. J Perinatol 1994; 14:90–94.

Donn SM, Sinha SK: Controversies in patient-triggered ventilation. Clin Perinatol 1998; 25:49–62.

Donn SM, Nicks JJ: Special ventilator techniques and modalities I: patient-triggered ventilation. In Goldsmith JP, Karotkin EH (Eds.): *Assisted Ventilation of the Neonate, 3rd Edition.* Orlando, FL, W.B. Saunders Co., 1996, pp. 215–228.

Sinha SK, Donn SM: Advances in neonatal conventional ventilation. Arch Dis Child 1996; 75:F135–F140.

Chapter 21

Synchronized Intermittent Mandatory Ventilation

Steven M. Donn, Sunil K. Sinha

I. **Description**

   A. Ventilatory mode in which mechanical breaths are synchronized to the onset of a spontaneous patient breath (if trigger threshold is met), or delivered at a fixed rate if patient effort is inadequate or absent. Spontaneous patient breaths between mechanically assisted breaths are supported by baseline pressure only.

   B. A form of patient-triggered ventilation (PTV)

II. **Cycling Mechanisms**

   A. Time

   B. Flow

   C. Volume

III. **Trigger Mechanisms**

   A. Airway flow
      1. Differential pressure transducer
      2. Heated wire anemometer
   B. Airway pressure
   C. Abdominal impedance

IV. **Synchronized Intermittent Mandatory Ventilation (SIMV) Breath**

   A. In SIMV, breathing time is divided into "breath periods" or "assist windows" based on the selected ventilatory rate.

   B. The first time a patient attempts to initiate a breath during an assist window (which begins immediately after a mechanically delivered breath), the ventilator delivers an assisted breath, provided that patient effort exceeds trigger threshold.

    C. Further attempts to breathe during the same assist window result only in spontaneous breaths, supported only by the baseline pressure.

    D. Mechanical breaths are only delivered if there is insufficient patient effort or apnea during the preceding assist window.

    E. Patient-controlled variables

       1. Respiratory rate

       2. Inspiratory time (if flow-cycled)

    F. Clinician-controlled variables

       1. Peak inspiratory pressure (if pressure-limited)

       2. Tidal volume delivery (if volume-cycled)

       3. Inspiratory time (if time-cycled)

       4. Flow

       5. SIMV rate

    G. Flow-cycling

       1. Inspiration is terminated at a percentage of peak flow rather than time.

       2. Synchronizes expiratory as well as inspiratory phase, and thus total patient/ventilator synchrony can be achieved for assisted breaths.

V. Spontaneous Breath

    A. Supported by baseline pressure (positive end-expiratory pressure) only

    B. Work of breathing higher than for assist/control or pressure support ventilation

    C. Observation of spontaneous tidal volume is a useful indicator of suitability to wean.

VI. Patient Management

    A. Indications

       1. Works best as a weaning mode, although many clinicians prefer it to assist/control as a primary management mode

       2. Flow-triggering especially useful in extremely low birthweight infants

       3. Provides partial ventilatory support

       4. Synchrony can decrease need for sedatives/paralytics

    B. Initiation

       1. Use minimal assist sensitivity

       2. Set SIMV rate at reasonable level to maintain adequate minute ventilation.

       3. For flow-cycling, termination at 5% of peak flow generally works best but must check to see that patient is receiving adequate tidal volume

       4. Other parameters set as for IMV

C. Weaning
1. Primary weaning parameters include SIMV rate, peak inspiratory pressure (for time- or flow-cycling), and tidal volume (for volume-cycling).
2. If P_aCO_2 is too low, it is most likely the result of overventilation. Lower rate, pressure, or volume depending on lung mechanics.
3. As patient status improves, spontaneous tidal volumes will increase, enabling lowering of SIMV rate.
4. Can extubate directly from SIMV, or add or switch to pressure support ventilation
5. Can also wean by increasing assist sensitivity, thus increasing patient work to increase tolerance

VII. Problems

A. Auto-cycling and false triggering
1. Leaks anywhere in the system (around the endotracheal tube, in circuit, etc.) can cause flow- and pressure-triggered devices to misread this as patient effort, resulting in delivery of a mechanical breath.
2. Abdominal impedance device may trigger from artifactual motion.

B. Failure to trigger
1. Assist sensitivity too high
2. Patient unable to reach trigger threshold
3. Patient fatigue

C. Inadequate inspiratory time (flow-cycling) results in inadequate tidal volume delivery. Patient may compensate by breathing rapidly.

Suggested Reading

Donn SM, Nicks JJ, Becker MA: Flow-synchronized ventilation of preterm infants with respiratory distress syndrome. J Perinatol 1994; 14:90–94.

Donn SM, Sinha SK: Controversies in patient-triggered ventilation. Clin Perinatol 1998; 25:49–62.

Donn SM, Nicks JJ: Special ventilator techniques and modalities I: patient-triggered ventilation. In Goldsmith JP, Karotkin EH (Eds.): *Assisted Ventilation of the Neonate, 3rd Edition.* Orlando, FL, W.B. Saunders Co., 1996, pp. 215–228.

Sinha SK, Donn SM: Advances in neonatal conventional ventilation. Arch Dis Child 1996; 75:F135–F140.

Chapter 22

Volume-Controlled Ventilation

Steven M. Donn, Kenneth P. Bandy

I. **Description**
   A. Form of mechanical ventilation where inspiratory phase ends when a preset volume of gas has been delivered
   B. Tidal volume may be monitored at the ventilator or (more accurately) at the patient airway.
   C. Because uncuffed endotracheal tubes (ETTs) are used in newborns, there may be a variable loss of delivered gas volume from leaks. It is thus more appropriate to describe this form of ventilation as volume-controlled, rather than volume-cycled, ventilation.

II. **Modes that Utilize Volume-Controlled Ventilation (VCV)**
   A. Intermittent mandatory ventilation (IMV)
   B. Synchronized intermittent mandatory ventilation (SIMV)
      1. Alone
      2. With pressure support (PSV)
   C. Assist/control (A/C)
   D. Pressure-regulated volume control (PRVC)
   E. Volume assured pressure support (VAPS)
   F. Mandatory minute ventilation (MMV)

III. **Characteristics of Volume-Controlled Breaths**
   A. May be patient-triggered or machine-initiated
      1. Pressure or flow trigger
      2. May be at proximal airway or in ventilator
   B. Flow-limited (fixed flow rate)
      1. Determines inspiratory time
      2. Square flow waveform
   C. Dependent variable is pressure
      1. Low compliance will result in higher pressure delivery.

153

2. As compliance improves, pressure will be auto-weaned.

3. May be influenced by inspiratory flow setting

D. Tidal volume is guaranteed.

E. Maximum alveolar distension depends on end alveolar pressure.

IV. **Advantages of Volume-Controlled Ventilation**

A. Consistent tidal volume delivery even in the face of changing compliance

B. Volume-limited breaths; avoidance of volutrauma

C. Combination with other modes to facilitate weaning

1. PSV

2. VAPS

3. MMV

V. **Clinical Limitations**

A. Minimal tidal volume delivery

1. Must know smallest tidal volume the machine is capable of delivering

2. Should not exceed patient's physiologic tidal volume

a. <1,000 g: 4–7 mL/kg

b. >1,000 g: 5–8 mL/kg

3. Ventilator circuit should be of reasonable rigidity (compliance) so as not to cause excessive compressible volume loss in circuit if pulmonary compliance is low.

4. Smaller patients with smaller ETT (2.5–3.0 mm) may have difficulty triggering (especially if pressure-triggered).

5. Flow limitation may result in inadequate inspiratory time in smaller patients.

6. Leaks

a. May cause loss in baseline pressure

b. May result in auto-cycling

VI. **Clinical Indications**

A. Respiratory failure in term or near-term infants (>1,500 g)

1. Persistent pulmonary hypertension of the newborn

2. Meconium aspiration syndrome

3. Sepsis/pneumonia

4. Respiratory distress syndrome

5. Congenital diaphragmatic hernia

      6. Pulmonary hypoplasia

      7. Congenital cystic adenomatoid malformation

  B. Ventilator-dependent cardiac disease with normal lungs

  C. Weaning infants recovering from respiratory illness

  D. Bronchopulmonary dysplasia

VII. Initiating Volume Ventilation

  A. Select desired mode.

      1. SIMV or A/C for acute illness

      2. SIMV and/or PSV for weaning

  B. Select desired delivered tidal volume.

      1. <1,000 g: 4–7 mL/kg

      2. >1,000 g: 5–8 mL/kg

      3. Confirm that patient is receiving appropriate tidal volume.

         a. Volume monitoring

         b. Pulmonary graphics

            (1) Tidal volume waveform

            (2) Pressure-volume loop

  C. Set flow rate to achieve desired inspiratory time.

  D. Set mechanical ventilatory rate.

  E. Set trigger sensitivity if using patient-triggered mode.

      1. Generally use minimal setting unless auto-cycling

      2. Ensure patient is able to trigger ventilator

  F. Some clinicians prefer to set a pressure limit; do not set this too close to peak pressure, or desired tidal volume may not be delivered.

  G. Some ventilators have a leak compensation system. While beneficial in maintaining stable baseline in the presence of a leak, it may increase the work of breathing and possibly expiratory resistance.

  H. Assessment of patient

      1. Adequacy of breath sounds

      2. Adequacy of chest excursions

      3. Patient-ventilator synchrony

      4. Patient comfort

      5. Blood gases

      6. Pulmonary mechanics

VIII. Weaning Infants from Volume-Controlled Ventilation

  A. As pulmonary compliance improves, inspiratory pressure will be automatically decreased to maintain set tidal volume delivery.

B. Adjustments in set tidal volume should be made to maintain desired tidal volume delivery.

C. Adjustment in flow rate may need to be made to maintain same inspiratory time or inspiratory:expiratory (I:E) ratio.

D. If using A/C:
    1. Decrease control rate (allow patient to assume greater percentage of work of breathing).
    2. May also increase assist (trigger) sensitivity

E. If using SIMV:
    1. Decrease SIMV rate, but remember that patient receives no support for spontaneous breaths other than positive end-expiratory pressure.
    2. Consider adding pressure support (see Chapter 23), or even switching to it completely if the baby has consistently reliable respiratory drive.

F. Newer modes (VAPS, MMV) may prove even more beneficial for weaning but have limited clinical experience in the newborn at present.

Suggested Reading

Bandy KP, Nicks JJ, Donn SM: Volume-controlled ventilation for severe neonatal respiratory failure. Neonat Intens Care 1992; 5:70–73.

Donn SM: Alternatives to ECMO. Arch Dis Child 1994; 70:F81–F84.

Donn SM, Becker MA: Baby in control: neonatal pressure support ventilation. Neonat Intens Care 1998; 11:16–20.

Donn SM, Becker MA: Mandatory minute ventilation: a neonatal mode of the future. Neonat Intens Care 1998; 11:22–24.

Nicks JJ, Becker MA, Donn SM: Neonatal respiratory failure: response to volume ventilation. J Perinatol 1993; 13:72–75.

Sinha SK, Donn SM, Gavey J, McCarty M: Randomized trial of volume controlled versus time cycled, pressure limited ventilation in preterm infants with respiratory distress syndrome. Arch Dis Child 1997; 77:F202–F205.

Tsai WC, Bandy KP, Donn SM: Volume controlled ventilation of the newborn. In Donn SM (Ed.): *Neonatal and Pediatric Pulmonary Graphic Analysis: Principles and Clinical Applications.* Armonk, NY, Futura Publishing Co., 1998, pp. 279–300.

Chapter 23

Pressure Support Ventilation

Sunil K. Sinha, Steven M. Donn

I. **Description**

    A. Ventilatory mode in which spontaneous breaths are partially or fully supported by an inspiratory pressure assist above baseline pressure to decrease the imposed work of breathing (endotracheal tube, ventilator circuit, demand valve).

    B. A form of patient-triggered ventilation (PTV); may be used alone in patients with reliable respiratory drive, or in conjunction with volume-controlled synchronized intermittent mandatory ventilation (SIMV).

II. **Cycling Mechanisms**

    A. Time: inspiratory time limit, chosen by clinician

    B. Flow: termination of inspiratory cycle based on a percentage of peak flow. This varies according to both delivered tidal volume and specific algorithm of the ventilator in use.

III. **Trigger Mechanisms**

    A. Airway pressure change (minimum 1.0 cm H_2O)

    B. Airway flow change (minimum 0.2 LPM)

IV. **Pressure Support Breath**

    A. A spontaneous inspiratory effort that exceeds the trigger threshold will initiate delivery of a mechanically generated pressure support breath.

    B. There is a rapid delivery of flow to the patient, which peaks, then decelerates.

    C. The airway pressure will rise to the pressure support level, set by the clinician as a value above baseline (positive end-expiratory pressure [PEEP]).

    D. When flow-cycling criterion is met (decline to the termination level), the breath will end and flow will cease. If this has not occurred by the end of the set inspiratory time limit, the inspiratory phase of the mechanical breath will be stopped.

E. The amount of flow delivered to the patient during inspiration is variable and will be proportional to patient effort.

F. Patient-controlled variables

    1. Respiratory rate

    2. Inspiratory time

    3. Peak inspiratory flow

G. Clinician-controlled variables

    1. Pressure support level

    2. Inspiratory time limit

    3. Baseline flow

    4. Baseline pressure (PEEP)

    5. SIMV rate, flow, inspiratory time, and tidal volume (if SIMV is used)

V. **Patient Management**

  A. Indications

    1. Designed primarily as a weaning mode to enable full or partial unloading of respiratory musculature during mechanical ventilation

    2. Pressure support is fully synchronized with spontaneous breathing and can decrease need for sedatives/paralytics

  B. Initiation

    1. Use minimal assist sensitivity

    2. The pressure support level can be adjusted to provide either full support (PS_{max}), delivering a full tidal volume, or set at a lower level to provide partial support. Remember that the pressure support level is the pressure applied above baseline (i.e., a patient receiving 4 cm H_2O PEEP and 16 cm H_2O pressure support actually gets 20 cm H_2O peak inspiratory pressure).

    3. Set the inspiratory time limit for the pressure support breath.

    4. Set parameters for the (volume-controlled) SIMV breaths if they are to be used.

      a. These can be used analogously to control breaths during assist/control ventilation, providing a "safety net" of background ventilation in the event of inadequate effort (triggering) or apnea.

      b. If the SIMV rate is set too high, and the majority of minute ventilation is provided by SIMV, the patient may have no impetus to breathe, thus defeating the purpose of pressure support.

C. Weaning
1. Weaning may be accomplished in a variety of ways:
   a. Decrease the SIMV rate to as low a level as possible, thus increasing spontaneous effort.
   b. Decrease the pressure support level, thus increasing the percentage of the work of breathing assumed by the patient
   c. Consider the use of pressure support alone in patients with a reliable respiratory drive who have no difficulty triggering.
2. Consider extubation when the pressure support level has been reduced to the point where it delivers about 4 mL/kg tidal volume if the patient appears comfortable and is not tachypneic at this level.

VI. **Problems**
A. Failure to trigger (may occur with small endotracheal tubes and inadequate patient effort)
B. Pressure overshoot
C. Premature termination

VII. **Clinical Applications**
A. Weaning mode for most infants >1,500 g
B. Bronchopulmonary dysplasia (BPD)
1. Infants with BPD exhibit reactive airways with elevated inspiratory resistance.
2. Pulmonary mechanics in most modes display flattened inspiratory flow-volume loop.
3. Variable inspiratory flow during pressure support ventilation enables patient to overcome increased inspiratory resistance and lowers ventilatory work.

VIII. **Advantages of Pressure Support Ventilation**
A. Complete patient-ventilator synchrony
B. Decreased work of breathing compared with other modes
1. Same tidal volume delivered at lower work of breathing
2. Larger tidal volume delivered at same work of breathing
C. Adults treated with pressure support ventilation have described increased comfort and endurance compared with other weaning modes.

IX. **Future Applications**
A. Volume assured pressure support (VAPS)

1. Used primarily in adults, but now available for infant use
2. Combines features of volume-controlled ventilation and pressure support ventilation
3. Clinician determines minimum tidal volume
4. As long as spontaneous patient effort results in delivery of desired tidal volume, breath "behaves" like a pressure support breath.
5. If breath delivers a tidal volume below the desired minimum, it is transitioned to a volume-controlled breath, assuring delivery of desired tidal volume.

B. Mandatory minute ventilation (MMV)
   1. This mode combines pressure support ventilation with SIMV.
   2. Clinician chooses a minute ventilation rate which the patient is to receive by selecting a desired tidal volume and frequency.
   3. As long as spontaneous breathing results in minute ventilation which exceeds the minimum, all breaths are pressure support breaths.
   4. If minute ventilation falls below the set minimum, the ventilator will provide sufficient SIMV breaths to allow the patient to "catch up" to the desired level of minute ventilation. This is based on a moving average.

Suggested Reading

Donn SM, Sinha SK: Controversies in patient-triggered ventilation. Clin Perinatol 1998; 25:49–62.

Donn SM, Nicks JJ: Special ventilator techniques and modalities I: patient-triggered ventilation. In Goldsmith JP, Karotkin EH (Eds.): *Assisted Ventilation of the Neonate, 3rd Edition.* Orlando, FL, W.B. Saunders Co., 1996, pp. 215–228.

Donn SM, Sinha SK: Pressure support ventilation of the newborn. Acta Neonatologica Japonica 1997; 33:472–478.

Donn SM, Becker MA: Baby in control: neonatal pressure support ventilation. Neonat Intens Care 1998; 11:16–20.

Donn SM, Becker MA: Mandatory minute ventilation: a neonatal mode of the future. Neonat Intens Care 1998; 11:20–22.

Nicks JJ, Becker MA, Donn SM: Bronchopulmonary dysplasia: response to pressure support ventilation. J Perinatol 1994; 11:374–376.

Sinha SK, Donn SM: Advances in neonatal conventional ventilation. Arch Dis Child 1996; 75:F135–F140.

Sinha SK, Donn SM: Pressure support ventilation. In Donn SM (Ed.): *Neonatal and Pediatric Pulmonary Graphics: Principles and Clinical Applications.* Armonk, NY, Futura Publishing Co., 1998, pp. 301–312.

Chapter 24

Pressure Control Ventilation and Pressure-Regulated Volume-Controlled Ventilation

Mary K. Dekeon

I. **Pressure Control Ventilation**
  A. Description
    1. Pressure control (PC) ventilation was developed in the early 1980s as a ventilatory mode for the treatment of adult respiratory distress syndrome (ARDS).
    2. This mode delivers a preset pressure and employs a variable flow rate.
    3. The variable flow rate differentiates this mode from traditional time-cycled, pressure-limited ventilation, which incorporates a constant flow rate.
  B. Features
    1. Variable tidal volume
    2. Constant peak inspiratory pressure
    3. A square pressure waveform
    4. Decelerating flow waveform
  C. Clinical indications
    1. Patients with high peak airway pressures who are at risk for barotrauma
      a. Respiratory distress syndrome (RDS)
      b. Bronchopulmonary dysplasia (BPD)
      c. Meconium aspiration syndrome (MAS)
      d. Other
    2. Mode of choice for inverse inspiratory:expiratory (I:E) ratio ventilation
    3. Patients with large endotracheal tube leaks
    4. Patients with airway obstruction
  D. Clinician-set parameters
    1. Peak inspiratory level (above positive end-expiratory pressure, PEEP)
    2. Inspiratory time

3. Ventilatory rate
4. PEEP
5. FiO_2
6. High and low minute ventilation alarms
7. High pressure alarm
8. Trigger sensitivity level
E. Advantages
   1. Peak airway pressures are controlled
   2. Pressure is limited but flow is not; thus, the spontaneously breathing patient is not "flow starved."
   3. Inspiratory time is maintained at the preset peak inspiratory pressure for better distribution of gas within the lung.
F. Disadvantage – tidal volume (V_T) is variable according to lung compliance

II. Pressure-Regulated Volume-Controlled Ventilation

A. Description
   This mode offers the variable flow rate employed in PC but with a targeted V_T. The ventilator, by means of a microprocessor, delivers the first breath with a pressure of 10 cm above PEEP. The pressure is increased until the target V_T is delivered (within three breaths). Maximum pressure is 5 cm H_2O below upper pressure limit control.
   1. V_T is set
   2. Peak pressure is variable
   3. Variable, decelerating flow waveform
   4. Square pressure waveform
B. Indications
   1. Patients with high peak airway pressures at risk for barotrauma (e.g., RDS, BPD, MAS, etc.)
   2. Patients with asthma
   3. Postoperative patients
   4. Patients with large endotracheal tube leaks
   5. Patients with airway obstruction
C. Clinician-set parameters
   1. V_T
   2. Inspiratory time
   3. Ventilator rate
   4. PEEP
   5. FiO_2
   6. High and low minute ventilation alarms
   7. High pressure alarm
   8. Trigger sensitivity level

SECTION VI

Neonatal Ventilators

Chapter 25

VIP BIRD® Infant/Pediatric Ventilator

Michael A. Becker, Steven M. Donn

The VIP BIRD ventilator (Bird Products Corp., Palm Springs, CA, USA) provides both neonatal and pediatric ventilation. The ventilator breaths are synchronized in all modes. Continuous tidal volume and graphic monitoring of waveforms and mechanics are also available.

I. **Monitoring**

    A. Internal

        1. Breath rate

        2. Inspiratory time

        3. Inspiratory:expiratory (I:E) ratio

        4. Peak inspiratory pressure (PIP)

        5. Mean airway pressure

    B. Partner IIi Monitor (Bird Products Corp.)

        1. Proximal inspiratory and expiratory tidal volumes

        2. Proximal expiratory minute ventilation

        3. Proximal inspiratory and expiratory flow

        4. Respiratory rate

    C. Bird Graphic Monitor

        1. Waveforms (2 of the 3 displayed at the same time)

            a. Flow

            b. Volume

            c. Pressure

        2. Mechanics

            a. Pressure-volume loop

            b. Flow-volume loop

        3. Trends (24-hour trend monitoring)

        4. Pulmonary mechanics calculations

            a. Compliance and C_{20}/C ratio

            b. Resistance

II. Alarms
  A. VIP BIRD Ventilator
   1. Low PIP
   2. Low positive end-expiratory pressure (PEEP)
  B. Partner IIi Monitor
   1. High and low respiratory rate
   2. Apnea

III. Modes of Ventilation
  A. Time-cycled, pressure-limited (TCPL) modes
  Continuous flow is present. Mechanical breaths are pressure limited and synchronized to the patient's own respiratory effort. The pressure is constant and the volume is variable with lung compliance changes. The breaths are synchronized by flow changes detected by a proximal flow sensor (pneumotachograph).
   1. TCPL synchronized intermittent mandatory ventilation (SIMV)
   A preset number of SIMV breaths are delivered. Additional spontaneous breaths are generated from the continuous flow in the system with no pressure assistance other than PEEP.
     a. Parameters/initial settings
       (1) Mode: time-cycled/SIMV
       (2) Rate: 40–60 breaths per minute
       (3) Inspiratory time: 0.3–0.5 seconds
       (4) Flow rate: 6-8 liters per minute (LPM)
       (5) PIP
         (a) Adjusted for appropriate tidal volume delivery of 4–8 mL/kg
         (b) Observe chest wall excursion
         (c) Auscultate breath sounds
       (6) PEEP
         (a) Initially set at 3–5 cm H_2O
         (b) May be increased for improved oxygenation, atelectasis, pulmonary edema, or pulmonary hemorrhage
       (7) Assist sensitivity (inspiratory trigger)
       Flow-triggering sensitivity adjustment. Set to make the trigger as sensitive as possible without auto-cycling. Usually 0.2 LPM
       (8) Termination sensitivity (expiratory trigger)
         (a) Termination of inspiration by flow: adjust for an appropriate inspiratory time
         (b) Generally a termination sensitivity of 5–10% will deliver an inspiratory time of 0.2–0.3 seconds (Figure 60).

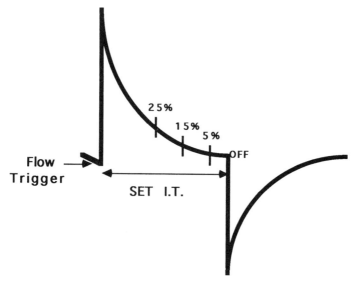

Figure 60. Termination sensitivity®, or expiratory trigger. Inspiration is initiated by a change of flow at the airway. When the lungs have inflated, flow decreases at the proximal airway, which results in the breath being terminated. This point of termination is clinician adjustable, and represents a percentage of peak inspiratory flow. Thus, a 5% termination sensitivity setting means that the breath will be terminated when airway flow has decreased to 5% of peak flow (i.e., there has been a 95% decay of the curve). I.T. = inspiratory time.

  b. Weaning time/flow-cycled SIMV
    (1) Decrease fraction of inspired oxygen (FiO_2) for oxygen saturation >92–94%
    (2) Decrease PEEP to 4 cm H_2O
    (3) Adjust PIP to keep tidal volumes 4–8 mL/kg
    (4) Decrease rate as tolerated
 2. TCPL assist/control
  A preset number of mandatory pressure-limited ventilator breaths are delivered as a back-up (control rate) if the infant makes no ventilatory effort. If the infant triggers the ventilator, it will deliver a pressure-limited (assist) breath with each spontaneous effort.
  a. Parameters/initial settings
    (1) Mode: time-cycled, assist/control
    (2) Rate: 30–40 breaths per minute
    (3) Inspiratory time: 0.3–0.4 seconds
    (4) Flow rate: 5-8 LPM
    (5) PIP

      (a) Adjusted for appropriate tidal volume delivery (4–8 mL/kg)

      (b) Observe chest wall excursion

      (c) Auscultate breath sounds

   (6) PEEP

      (a) Initially set at 3–5 cm H_2O

      (b) May be increased for improved oxygenation, atelectasis, pulmonary edema, pulmonary hemorrhage

   (7) Assist sensitivity (inspiratory trigger)
Flow-triggering sensitivity adjustment. Set to make the trigger as sensitive as possible without auto-cycling. Usually 0.2 LPM

   (8) Termination sensitivity

      (a) Termination of inspiration by flow: adjust for an appropriate inspiratory time

      (b) Generally a termination sensitivity of 5–10% will deliver an inspiratory time of 0.2–0.3 seconds (Figure 60).

  b. Weaning time/flow-cycled, assist/control

   (1) Decrease rate until the infant triggers most, if not all, of the breaths

   (2) Adjust PIP to keep tidal volumes 4–8 mL/kg

   (3) Decrease FiO_2 for oxygen saturations >92–94%

   (4) Decrease PEEP to 4 cm H_2O

  c. Extubation from pressure-limited ventilation evaluation

   (1) Lower ventilator settings with resolving respiratory disease

   (2) Note if effective spontaneous respiratory effort and tidal volumes

   (3) Consider continuous positive airway pressure (CPAP) trial, observe the infant's own spontaneous minute ventilation

B. Volume-controlled (cycled) modes
A preset volume is delivered with each volume ventilated breath. The volume is constant with variable pressure dependent on the patient's lung compliance. The breaths are triggered by a pressure change (which is less sensitive than flow-triggering). The minimum tidal volume leaving the ventilator is 20 mL. Volume ventilation is not recommended for infants <1,500 g. Because cuffed endotracheal tubes are not used in newborns, there is usually some leakage of delivered volume. It is more appropriate to refer to this as volume-controlled or volume-limited ventilation.

  1. Volume assist/control ventilation
A preset volume is delivered at a preset rate. If the infant triggers the ventilator by generating a pressure change, the ventilator will deliver another volume-limited breath. Volume assist/control is not a weaning mode of ventilation and is best used in the acute phase of respiratory disease.

  a. Parameters/initial settings

    (1) Mode: volume assist/control

    (2) Rate: 40–60 breaths per minute

    (3) Tidal volume
  Set at 10 mL/kg to deliver approximately 5–8 mL/kg to the proximal airway. The difference in set tidal volume and the proximal delivered tidal is the volume that is lost from the compliance of the ventilator circuit and compression of gas.

    (4) Inspiratory time: 0.3–0.4 seconds (flow rate and tidal volume determine the inspiratory time)

    (5) Flow rate: adjusted to deliver the desired inspiratory time

    (6) High pressure limit

        (a) Adjusted as a maximum pressure for the system

        (b) If the high pressure limit is achieved the ventilator breath will end, and the ventilator audible and visual alarms will indicate such.

    (7) PEEP

        (a) Initially set at 3–5 cm H_2O

        (b) May be increased for improved oxygenation, atelectasis, pulmonary edema, pulmonary hemorrhage

    (8) Assist sensitivity (inspiratory trigger)
  Pressure-triggering sensitivity adjustment. Set to make the trigger as sensitive as possible without auto-cycling. Usually 1.0 cm H_2O. The VIP BIRD ventilator also has a leak compensation feature that helps to keep a constant PEEP level in the face of a leak around the artificial airway. This feature maybe disabled (turned off) to make the ventilator easier to trigger in the volume ventilation modes.

  b. Weaning volume assist/control

    (1) Wean V_T (which decreases pressure) as patient improves, but maintain 5–8 mL/kg delivery.

    (2) Change mode to volume SIMV/pressure support (see below).

2. Volume SIMV and pressure support ventilation
A preset number of volume ventilator breaths (SIMV) are delivered. The additional spontaneous breaths are supported by pressure-limited breaths. These pressure-limited breaths (pressure support) have variable inspiratory flow (which is proportional to patient effort) which may be more comfortable for some infants. Volume SIMV and pressure support is the weaning mode of volume ventilation.

  a. Parameters/initial settings

    (1) Mode: volume SIMV and pressure support

    (2) Rate: 20–30 breath per minute

(3) Tidal volume

Set at 10 mL/kg to deliver approximately 5–8 mL/kg at the proximal airway. The difference in set tidal volume and the proximal delivered tidal is the volume lost from the tubing compliance and compression of gas.

(4) Inspiratory time: 0.3–0.4 seconds (flow rate and tidal volume determine the inspiratory time)

(5) Flow rate: adjusted to deliver an appropriate inspiratory time (0.3–0.4 seconds)

(6) High pressure limit

(a) Adjusted as a maximum pressure for the system

(b) If the high pressure limit is achieved the ventilator breath will end, and the ventilator audible and visual alarms will indicate such.

(7) PEEP

(a) Initially set at 3–5 cm H_2O

(b) May be increased for improved oxygenation, atelectasis, pulmonary edema, pulmonary hemorrhage

(8) Assist sensitivity (inspiratory trigger)

Pressure-triggering sensitivity adjustment. Set to make the trigger as sensitive as possible without auto-cycling. Usually 1.0 cm H_2O

(9) Pressure support (see Chapter 23)

Spontaneous breaths greater than the SIMV rate are supported with pressure support. Pressure support is pressure above the PEEP level. It should be adjusted to deliver 4–6 mL/kg. The minimal pressure support to overcome the resistance of the endotracheal tube is about 10 cm H_2O.

b. Weaning volume SIMV and pressure support

(1) Decrease the SIMV rate

(2) Do not adjust the tidal volume unless lung compliance improvements cause delivered tidal volumes to be >8 mL/kg.

(3) Adjust the pressure support level to deliver 4–6 mL/kg.

(4) When the SIMV rate is 0 and the pressure support is <10 cm H_2O, consider CPAP trial and extubation.

IV. **VIP Gold/VIP Plus (not yet Food and Drug Administration approved) Will Offer Enhancements to Features of VIP BIRD**

A. Features

1. Flow trigger available in all models

a. Neonatal sensor – at the patient wye (proximal)

b. Pediatric sensor – close to the exhalation valve (distal)

2. Proximal tidal volume measurement with the neonatal sensor; graphic display is provided by the Bird Graphic Monitor.

3. The pediatric sensor provides flow-triggering and distal monitoring.
4. Volume ventilation with a minimum tidal volume of 10 mL.
5. Rise time inspiratory flow rate adjustment in the pressure-limited modes
6. Inspiratory and expiratory holds
7. SIMV/CPAP/pressure support and assist/control are available in all modes
8. Alarms – volume, pressure, rate, pressure support time limit
9. Manual breath

B. Modes
   1. Pressure modes
      a. TCPL
      A pressure-limited breath is delivered with a fixed continuous flow rate that is determined by the clinician.
      b. Pressure support
         (1) A pressure-limited breath that is patient-triggered. The patient has primary control of the inspiratory time and flow.
         (2) The inspiratory flow may be adjusted with rise time, an adjustment that effects the waveform. The setting of 1 is the steepest rise. The breath will be given quickly. The setting of 7 will give the breath more slowly and may be very helpful in the management of infants with high resistance disease or small endotracheal tubes.
      c. Pressure control
      A pressure-limited breath is delivered with a variable flow rate. It accelerates to peak flow and then decelerates. The endotracheal tube resistance and the patient compliance determine the flow rate, which can also be adjusted with rise time.
      d. Volume assured pressure support (VAPS)
      A pressure-limited breath that assures a minimal tidal volume. A volume target is set and if the target is met, the breath will be a pressure support breath. If the volume is not met, the inspiratory time will be extended until the target volume is achieved. This mode will deliver either patient-triggered breaths or a control rate if the patient has not triggered. Flow rate may be adjusted with rise time.
      e. CPAP
      Continuous flow through the system with expiratory resistance to provide the desired PEEP.
   2. Volume modes
      a. Volume control
      A preset volume is delivered from the ventilator. The actual delivered volume to the patient is determined by compliance of the patient and the ventilator circuit. The waveform is adjustable in volume ventilation.

170

3. Combining modes
   a. Combinations are not available in assist/control ventilation. If the patient is in assist/control and triggers the ventilator, another breath of the same mode will be delivered.
   b. Pressure support combination modes
      (1) TCPL with pressure support
      A set number of TCPL breaths; additional breaths are pressure support (TCPL is not available with the pediatric sensor).
      (2) Volume with pressure support
      A set number of volume breaths; additional breaths are pressure support.
      (3) Pressure control with pressure support
      A set number of pressure control breaths, additional breaths are pressure support. The rise time adjustment will effect both the pressure control and pressure support breaths.
      (4) VAPS with pressure support
      A set number of VAPS breaths; additional breaths are pressure support. The rise time adjustment will effect both the VAPS and pressure support breaths.

Suggested Reading

Donn SM, Nicks JJ: Special ventilator techniques and modalities I: Patient-triggered ventilation. In Goldsmith JP, Karotkin EH (Eds.): *Assisted Ventilation of the Neonate, 3rd Edition.* Philadelphia, W.B. Saunders Co., 1996, pp. 215–228.

Donn SM, Nicks JJ, Becker MA: Flow-synchronized ventilation of preterm infants with respiratory distress syndrome. J Perinatol 1994; 14:90–94.

Donn SM, Sinha SK: Controversies in patient-triggered ventilation. Clin Perinatol 1998; 25:49–61.

Sinha SK, Donn SM: Advances in neonatal conventional ventilation. Arch Dis Child 1996; 75:F135–F140.

Sinha SK, Nicks JJ, Donn SM: Graphic analysis of pulmonary mechanics in neonates receiving assisted ventilation. Arch Dis Child 1996; 75:F213–F218.

Chapter 26

Dräger Babylog 8000 Plus® Infant Care Ventilator

Donald M. Null, Jr.

I. **Babylog 8000 Plus Ventilator (Dräger, Lübeck, Germany)**

    A. Time-cycled, expiratory pressure-limited, continuous flow ventilator designed for patients weighing up to 10 kg

    B. Dual microprocessor controlled

        1. Main ventilator functions

        2. Monitor systems

    C. The ventilator front panel consists of dial panel and display/menu key panel.

        1. The lower dial panel contains buttons for main operating modes and dial knobs for oxygen concentration, inspiratory time, inspiratory flow, peak inspiratory pressure, and positive end-expiratory pressure/continuous positive airway pressure (PEEP/CPAP).

        2. The main components of display/menu key panel are the screen and, below this, a number of menu keys with fixed or variable function assignment.

        3. There is an illuminated bar graph above the screen that displays current airway pressure readings.

        4. Also includes alarm silence key, confirm key (for acknowledging alarms or settings), a manual inspiration key, and a calibration configuration key

II. **Technical Data (see Table 21)**

III. **Peak Flow and Volume Measurement**

    A. Parameters are measured with a heated wire anemometer that may be integrated into the wye or into a separate sensor adapter between the wye and the endotracheal tube (ETT). Volume is displayed as expiratory volume. Leak is calculated by the difference between inspiratory and expiratory minute volumes.

Table 21
Technical Data

Parameter	Range	Resolution
Inspiratory time	0.1–2.0 sec	0.1–1.0 sec: 0.01 sec 0.1–2.0 sec: 0.1 sec
Expiratory time	0.7–30 sec	0.2–1.0 sec: 0.01 sec 1.0–10 sec: 0.1 sec 10–30 sec: 1.0 sec
O_2 concentration	21–100%	1%
Inspiratory flow	1–30 LPM	1–10 LPM: 0.1 LPM 10–30 LPM: 1 LPM
Expiratory flow	1–30 LPM	1–10 LPM: 0.1 LPM 10–30 LPM: 1 LPM
Inspiratory pressure	10–80 cm H_2O	1 cm H_2O
PEEP	0–25 cm H_2O	0–1 cm H_2O: 0.1 cm H_2O 0–2 > 10 cm H_2O: 1 cm H_2O
Tidal volume (set)	2–100 mL	2–9.9 mL: 0.1 mL 10–19.5 mL: 0.5 mL 20–100 mL: 1.0 mL

B. Trigger function

1. Spontaneous breathing is detected using a flow measurement. Trigger sensitivity may be set from 1–10 to avoid auto-triggering. At the highest sensitivity setting, V trigger is 0 and inspiratory flow will trigger a breath when it reaches a minimum value of 0.2 LPM.
2. Trigger response time is 40–60 msec.

IV. **Measurement of Lung Mechanics**

A. Dynamic compliance of the respiratory system
B. Airway and ETT resistance
C. Coefficient of correlation
D. Time constant of the respiratory system
E. Lung overdistension index, C_{20}/C
F. Parameters are measured for each respiratory cycle of mechanical breaths and can be displayed using display/menu key panel.

V. **Rate-volume ratio (RVR) is calculated and may be used to assess the effects of weaning. The value is displayed with lung mechanics.**

173

VI. Modes of Ventilation

A. CPAP (0–25 cm H_2O available)

B. Conventional mechanical ventilation/intermittent mandatory ventilation (CMV/IMV)

1. Rate 1–150 BPM
2. Pressure-limited with/without plateau

C. Synchronized intermittent mandatory ventilation (SIMV) and assist/control (A/C)

1. Provided by use of heated wire anemometer
2. Volume measurement triggers the device
3. Sensitivity settings from 1–10 (correspond to 0.2–3.0 mL trigger volume)

D. Pressure support ventilation (PSV)

1. Pressure-limited
2. Patient-triggered
3. Patient-terminated
4. Leak adaption for inspiratory trigger and termination criteria ensures sensitive and exact synchronization with leaks up to 40%.

E. Volume guarantee

1. Uses a preset tidal volume (V_T); each supported breath provides this volume irrespective of patient effort or change in compliance or resistance.
2. Ventilator pattern with plateau is required.
3. Can be used in SIMV, A/C, and PSV

F. Variable inspiratory and variable expiratory flow (VIVE)

1. Allows for independently setting inspiratory and expiratory flows
2. Enables user to set different flow rates for spontaneous and mechanical breaths
3. Using VIVE, inspiratory flow applies to mechanical breaths, and expiratory flow applies to spontaneous breathing and during CPAP.

VII. Monitoring

A. Numerical and graphic displays

B. Set values displayed numerically on one panel

1. Inspiratory time (T_I), expiratory time (T_E), inspiratory:expiratory ratio (I:E)
2. fset (set frequency)
3. O_2 concentration
4. Inspired tidal volume (V_{TI}), expired tidal volume (V_{TE})
5. Pressure limit (PL), PEEP
6. Trigger

C. Measured values, mechanics, and RVR displayed numerically on another panel
   1. Peak inspiratory pressure (PIP), PEEP, mean airway pressure ($\bar{P}w$)
   2. FiO_2 (built-in oxygen sensor)
   3. f_{tot} (total frequency)
   4. Minute volume (expired) (V_E), V_T
   5. Percent spontaneous breathing
   6. Percent leak
D. Graphic displays available
   1. P waveform
   2. V waveform
   3. Trends
E. Outputs for digital or analog interfaces
   1. Analog provides output of measured values, data reports, and communication with patient
   2. Digital data are transmitted using the Dräger Babylink.

Chapter 27

SLE 2000® (HFO) Ventilator

J. Harry Baumer

I. **Ventilator Principles**
    A. Valveless jet ventilator
    B. Designed for use in newborns and infants
    C. Constant gas flow
    D. Pressure-limited
    E. Time-cycled

II. **Modes of Ventilation**
    A. Intermittent mandatory ventilation (IMV)
    B. Assist/control (A/C)
    C. Synchronized intermittent mandatory ventilation (SIMV)
    D. High-frequency oscillatory ventilation (HFOV)
    E. Combined oscillation and IMV

III. **Background**
    A. Prototype valveless jet ventilator, SLE CW200 (Scientific Laboratory Equipment, Ltd., Croydon, England) described in 1988
    B. Resulted in acute improvement in oxygenation in 13 newborn babies with severe respiratory disease who had been ventilated with conventional ventilators
    C. The arrangement of the prototype ventilator is set out schematically in Figure 61. Although the principle is the same, it should be emphasized that this design does not illustrate the SLE 2000.
    D. Introduction in 1991 of SLE 2000
    E. Subsequent development of SIMV and HFOV capabilities (SLE 2000 HFO)

IV. **Design Details**
    A. Gas supply

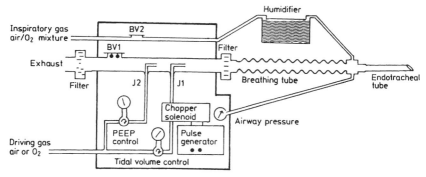

Figure 61. The design of the CW200 prototype. (Reproduced with permission of Scientific Laboratory Equipment, Ltd., Croydon, England.)

1. A continuous flow of warmed, humidified gas at a rate of 5 LPM
2. The humidified gas flow is greater than the minute volume, and the space between the endotracheal tube and the driving jet is greater than the tidal volume.
3. Gas from the driving jet does not reach the infant and does not take part in gas exchange.
4. When gas flow rate is variable, as in conventional ventilator design, increases in gas flow may overcome the capacity of the humidifier, leading to inadequately humidified gas reaching the infant's trachea.
5. The fixed gas flow avoids the tracheal complications that result when unhumidified gas reaches the tracheobronchial tree.

B. The ventilator jets
1. These jets are situated on the exhalation port of the ventilator. This consists of a removable block mounted on a manifold. The expiratory limb of the circuit attaches to the port.
2. The jets are supplied with the same oxygen concentration as the humidified gas supply to avoid the possibility of gas dilution in the event of tubing disconnection.
3. The pressure delivered by the jets is controlled by solenoids that are adjusted by regulators on the front panel of the ventilator. Gauges display these pressures.
4. The driving jet delivers intermittent reverse pulses of gas to the expiratory limb. This compresses the 5 LPM humidified gas into the endotracheal tube, providing the episodes of positive pressure for inspiration.
5. In a conventional ventilator, the inspiratory plateau results from occlusion of the expiratory limb of the circuit by a solenoid. The compressibility of the circuit results in an attenuation of the peak inspiratory gas flow at the endotracheal tube that can be overcome

by increasing the flow rate in the circuit. With a fixed resistance in the expiratory limb of the circuit, increases in flow result in rising inadvertent pressure during expiration.

6. The driving jet replaces the solenoid used in a conventional ventilator. The driving gas from the jet acts as a pneumatic piston, with the inspiratory pressure determined by the pressure setting on the driving jet. This has two consequences:

   a. It avoids the inadvertent positive end-expiratory pressure (PEEP) that occurs when flow rates in the circuit increase.

   b. The jet produces a higher peak inspiratory flow rate, with the inspiratory plateau being reached more rapidly. This is particularly important at the higher range of respiratory frequencies used (above 60 BPM). It results in a higher mean airway pressure, and hence improved oxygenation, at any given inspiratory time setting.

7. An electronic module determines the rate and duration of opening of the solenoid valve that controls the driving jet.

8. The PEEP jet (Figure 61) provides continuous gas flow throughout the respiratory cycle.

9. Oscillation is produced by the rotating jet drive of a motor situated at the rear of the exhaust block. This jet produces both an active inspiratory and expiratory flow of gas at the patient manifold. The rate of oscillation is variable up to 20 Hz.

10. Modes of oscillation

    a. Continuous oscillatory mode. This is used with the PEEP jet, which controls the mean airway pressure. The rotating oscillation jet regulator controls the pressure amplitude.

    b. Oscillation superimposed on the inspiratory pressure plateau, the expiratory phase, or both. This is achieved by the combined use of the driving and PEEP jets.

11. The benefits or otherwise of the combined use of oscillation and intermittent positive pressure ventilation are unknown.

C. The trigger mechanism

1. Senses the rate of change of pressure at the patient manifold

2. Detects the onset of inspiratory effort from increasing rate of reduction in pressure

3. Adjustable sensitivity within an uncalibrated range

4. Back-up breath rate adjustable in A/C mode. Each back-up breath delivered is shown on a light-emitting diode (LED) and with an optional audible beep.

D. Alarms

1. Power supply

2. Air supply

3. Oxygen supply

4. Microprocessor system failure

      5. Inspiratory gas supply failure

      6. High pressure

      7. Low pressure

      8. Cycle fail

      9. Oscillation fail (SLE 2000 HFO)

     10. Fan fail (SLE 2000 HFO)

  E. Information displayed

    1. LED displays

      a. Power on

      b. Ventilator rate

      c. Inspiratory time

      d. Inspiratory:expiratory (I:E) ratio

      e. Maximum, minimum, or mean airway pressure

      f. Inspired oxygen concentration

      g. Trigger back-up breath (and optional audible signal)

    2. Liquid crystalline display (LCD) display (SLE 2000 HFO)

      a. Pressure waveform

      b. High and low alarm settings

      c. Display time base (0.5–6 sec)

      d. Display pressure range (up to 50 cm H_2O)

      e. Variable time base for display

      f. Display can be frozen

  F. Other features

    1. The patient circuit has a restrictor fitted to the inspiratory side of the patient endotracheal manifold.

      a. The manufacturer states that this is required to ensure that it is possible to monitor the inspiratory limb of the circuit for leaks.

      b. It has also been suggested that this is required to increase the trigger sensitivity. The increased inspiratory resistance increases inspiratory effort and consequently the number of spontaneous breaths that will trigger the ventilator in small infants of <1.0 kg.

      c. However, the position of the restrictor is such that work of breathing should not be affected.

    2. A pressure waveform switch modifies the driving gas flow rate. This slows the rate of rise of pressure at the onset of inspiration.

    3. It is possible to deliver nitric oxide via the ventilator.

V. Performance of SLE 2000

  A. Trigger sensitivity

    1. In some studies, this has been defined as the proportion of infant breaths that trigger the ventilator. Caution is required in interpretation, as other factors may influence the sensitivity. These include:

inspiratory time, use of respiratory stimulants and sedation, gestational age, and the infant's neurologic state.

2. In a comparison of four neonatal ventilators, the SLE 2000 ventilator had a median sensitivity of 99% (range 90–100%) in a small number of babies with acute respiratory distress syndrome (RDS), and 96.5% (range 59–100%) in infants with chronic RDS. This was at least as sensitive as the Sechrist IV, the Infant Star, and Bear Cub ventilators (see Chapters 28, 30, and 32).

3. A study of 22 preterm infants, which monitored interactions during 67,150 spontaneous respiratory cycles in 3,592 15-second epochs, showed synchrony in only 19.5% of epochs.

4. In a study in 12 infants, the median sensitivity was 87% (range 19–100%). The sensitivity of the Infant Star ventilator using an abdominal capsule was significantly higher. In that study both ventilators had a high rate of asynchrony with the inspiratory phase of the ventilator extending into the expiratory phase of the baby's respiration.

B. Trigger delay
   1. Measurements of trigger delay should be interpreted with caution, as factors such as gestational age will also have a major influence.
   2. Median trigger delay was 80 msec (range 40–100 msec) in a patient-based study involving 13 preterm infants with RDS.
   3. Median trigger delay was 0 msec (range 0–316 msec) in 40 infants with acute or chronic respiratory distress. This was significantly shorter than with the Bear Cub II ventilator using an airflow device, particularly in babies with chronic respiratory distress. However, the infants ventilated with the Bear Cub ventilator were more immature. The delay was not significantly different from the Sechrist IV and Infant Star ventilators.
   4. In a further study of 12 infants with a gestational age of between 24 and 27 weeks, a median delay of 112 msec (range 24–270 msec) was seen. A significantly shorter delay was seen in infants ventilated with the Infant Star ventilator using an abdominal surface sensor.

C. Auto-triggering (auto-cycling)
   1. A situation where ventilator breaths occur without the infant initiating inspiratory efforts. This may occur spontaneously or, for example, because of water that has been trapped in the ventilator tubing.
   2. This is said to be common in the SLE 2000 at the highest sensitivity setting.
   3. However, a different investigator found no auto-triggering at the highest sensitivity setting in a study of 12 preterm infants with RDS. The importance of maintaining the ventilator circuit free of condensed water was emphasized.
   4. In a study of 22 preterm infants with RDS, 19.6% of 16-second epochs were associated with auto-triggering.

D. Peak inspiratory flow rate

1. We compared the SLE 2000 with the VIP BIRD and Dräger Babylog 8000 ventilators (see Chapters 25 and 26) attached to a model lung.

2. The time to plateau was significantly shorter with the SLE 2000 than for either of the other ventilators when gas flow was optimized to achieve a rapid rise to plateau.

3. With the pressure wave switch set to attenuate the rise to plateau, the time to plateau seen in the SLE 2000 was similar to the minimum obtained by the Dräger Babylog 8000 and VIP BIRD ventilators.

4. The consequences of this difference in performance are unknown.

    a. Oxygenation at any given inspiratory time setting will be improved with a short time to plateau.

    b. It is conceivable that chronic lung damage could increase with a more rapid increase in pressure.

E. Oscillation mode

A study of four neonatal ventilators delivering HFOV using a model lung showed the following:

1. The delivered volume changed little above 10 Hz, but this effect depended on lung compliance.

2. Endotracheal tube size had a major effect on delivered volume, emphasizing the importance of using the largest possible endotracheal tube.

3. The volume delivery of the SLE 2000 was comparable to that of the SensorMedics 3100A High-Frequency Oscillator (see Chapter 39) at a given setting.

4. The reduction in delivered volume with decreasing compliance was less for the SLE than for the SensorMedics oscillator.

5. The authors concluded that optimum CO_2 elimination could be achieved with relatively low frequencies and a large endotracheal tube.

F. Studies of longer-term triggered ventilation

1. A study of 68 infants ventilated for RDS with A/C ventilation demonstrated the ventilator's capability to support infants for periods of up to 28 days. No control group was available for comparison.

2. Retrospective analysis of nursing observations within 72 hours of birth, on 49 infants <28 weeks gestation with RDS, demonstrated the following:

    a. The ventilator was capable of delivering patient-triggered ventilation to infants <28 weeks gestation.

    b. With back-up rates of <40 BPM, the number of untriggered breaths was minimized.

    c. The triggered breath rate was 25% lower with an inspiratory time of 0.5 seconds compared with settings between 0.2 and 0.25 seconds.

Suggested Reading

Baumer JH, Ellis S: Patient triggered ventilation in infants under 28 weeks. Early Hum Develop 1994; 39:144.

Chan KN, Chakrabarti MK, Whitwam JG, et al: Assessment of a new valveless infant ventilator. Arch Dis Child 1988; 63:162–167.

Chan V, Greenough A: Neonatal patient triggered ventilators: performance in acute and chronic lung disease. Br J Int Care 1993; 3:216–219.

deBoer RC, Jones A, Ward PS, et al: Long term trigger ventilation in neonatal respiratory distress syndrome. Arch Dis Child 1993; 68:308–311.

Laubscher B, Greenough A, Costeloe K: Performance of four neonatal high frequency oscillators. Br J Int Care 1996; 6:148–152.

Chapter 28

Sechrist Model IV-200 SAVI® Ventilator

S. David Ferguson

I. **Modes of Ventilation**
    A. Synchronized assisted ventilation of infants (SAVI)
    B. Conventional intermittent mandatory ventilation (continuous flow, time-cycled, pressure-limited)
    C. Continuous positive airway pressure (CPAP)

II. **SAVI**
    A. Provides patient-triggered assist/control ventilation from a Sechrist Model IV-200 Ventilator (Sechrist Industries, Inc., Anaheim, CA, USA)
    B. Cannot provide synchronized intermittent mandatory ventilation (SIMV)
    C. Utilizes changes in transthoracic electrical impedance which occur during spontaneous respiration to generate a trigger signal
    D. Triggers on both active inspiration and active expiration resulting in total synchrony of breathing of baby with ventilator

III. **How SAVI Works**
    A. Changes in the ratio of gas to liquid in the thorax which occur during the respiratory cycle cause a corresponding change in transthoracic electrical impedance, which:
        1. Increases during inspiration and decreases during expiration
        2. Can be detected by conventional electrocardiogram (ECG) chest leads
        3. Can be transmitted to a neonatal cardiorespiratory monitor with a real-time analog respiratory waveform output
        4. May be affected by changes in thoracic blood volume during the cardiac cycle (cardiac artifact)
    B. Signal detection/processing

1. To obtain an optimal respiratory impedance signal
   a. Ensure chest electrodes are closely applied and changed daily.
   b. Place the positive and negative chest electrodes high up in the right anterior and left posterior axillary lines, respectively.
   c. Be prepared to alter placement if good impedance signal is not obtained on the bar graph display (see below), or if there is "false triggering" at the heart rate (cardiac artifact).
2. The neonatal cardiorespiratory monitor
   a. Processes and quantifies the inspiratory-induced impedance signal
   b. Generates a respiratory count and respiratory waveform display on the monitor screen (the impedance pneumogram)
   c. Transmits the signal via an interface cable to the impedance input socket on the Sechrist SAVI Ventilator
C. Practical points
   1. Ensure that the cardiorespiratory monitor is compatible with the Sechrist SAVI system by contacting both the manufacturer and also Sechrist Laboratories.
   2. The response time (i.e., the delay between the generation of the inspirator impedance signal and the onset of a triggered breath) will largely be determined by the monitor performance.
   3. The response time should be <80 msec.
D. Within the Sechrist SAVI Ventilator
   1. A bar graph display situated immediately above the impedance input socket on the ventilator will exhibit an ascending and descending movement to show the impedance signal is being received.
   2. An analog voltage comparator compares the voltage generated by the inspiratory impedance input signal with a trigger voltage predetermined by the setting of the ventilator sensitivity dial chosen by the operator.
   3. When the voltage of the inspiratory impedance input signal exceeds the trigger voltage, a trigger signal is generated.
   4. Through a microprocessor, the trigger signal instructs the solenoid valve of the ventilator fluidic control circuit to turn "on," unless terminated by the detection of an expiratory phase of the impedance pneumogram.
   5. At the termination of the inspiratory phase the microprocessor will not respond to any further signals for a lockout period of 200 msec to prevent breath stacking and to minimize the effects of inadvertent false triggering.
E. Initiating ventilation
   1. Set the inspiratory time at 0.3–0.4 seconds.
   2. Adjust the sensitivity dial so the bar graph display reaches but does not exceed maximum.

3. Increasing sensitivity (turning the dial clockwise) will lower the trigger voltage so a trigger signal will be generated earlier in the upward slope of the inspiratory phase.

4. If auto-cycling occurs, reduce sensitivity (turn dial counterclockwise) to increase the trigger threshold.

F. Back-up conventional mandatory ventilation

1. A trigger breath light-emitting diode (LED) will illuminate green whenever a triggered breath is delivered, and the trigger rate is displayed in real time on the ventilator.

2. If no trigger signal is generated, a control breath LED will illuminate yellow.

3. If no trigger signal is generated for a period set by the alarm "no trigger," a red LED will illuminate accompanied by an audible alarm, and conventional mandatory ventilation will be delivered at a preselected rate on the same settings of inspiratory time, peak pressure, and positive end-expiratory pressure (PEEP) as on the trigger mode.

G. Clinical points

1. Set back-up rate at 20 breaths per minute less than the infant's spontaneous respiratory rate, but never more than 60 breaths per minute.

2. If the "no trigger" alarm persists, increase sensitivity and check impedance input signal on bar graph display.

3. If still not triggering, check chest electrodes and then the clinical status of the baby for air entry, pneumothorax, and $PaCO_2$.

IV. Clinical Application of SAVI

A. Indication: respiratory failure in spontaneously breathing infants with no significant airway obstruction

B. Practical points

1. Use conventional mandatory ventilation mode for 20 minutes after administration of surfactant before commencing assist/control mode in infants with surfactant deficiency.

2. Contraindications

a. Neuromuscular disease or treatment with muscle relaxants

b. Recurrent seizures

c. Septic shock or necrotizing enterocolitis

d. Tension pneumothorax

e. Pleural effusion

f. Significant airway obstruction from pulmonary hemorrhage, meconium aspiration, or pneumonia

V. Ventilation Protocol Using SAVI

A. Position chest electrodes and connect to suitable cardiorespiratory monitor as described above.

B. Connect monitor to Sechrist SAVI Ventilator using interface cable.

C. With ventilator in conventional mechanical ventilation (CMV) mode set up as follows:

1. Flow rate: 8–12 LPM

2. Inspiratory time: 0.3–0.4 secsonds (back-up rate as described above)

3. Peak inspiratory pressure (PIP) and PEEP depending on clinical assessment of chest expansion, air entry, and arterial blood gas results

D. Switch to SAVI by turning sensitivity dial clockwise to click "on."

E. Turn SAVI toward maximum until bar graph display reaches but does not exceed maximum.

1. If cardiac artifact occurs, reduce sensitivity until it disappears.

2. If cardiac artifact persists, check, and if necessary reposition, chest electrodes.

3. Use flow rates of 10–12 LPM initially to ensure adequate tidal volume delivery.

F. Maintain target arterial blood gases by adjusting PIP and PEEP.

G. It is important to maintain $PaCO_2$ above 37.5 torr (5 kPa) to prevent trigger failure.

H. Weaning

1. Reduce PIP as tolerated depending on arterial blood gases.

2. Turn sensitivity dial counterclockwise to increase trigger threshold (but not enough to cause trigger failure).

3. Decrease bias flow from 12 LPM gradually to 8 LPM to reduce tidal volume delivered.

I. Extubate to nasal CPAP.

Suggested Reading

Visveshwara N, Freeman B, Peck M, et al: Patient-triggered synchronized assisted ventilation of newborns: report of a preliminary study of three years experience. J Perinatol 1991; 4:347–354.

Chapter 29

Newport Wave® Ventilator

Robert L. Chatburn

I. **Classification**

The Wave ventilator (Newport Medical Instruments, Newport Beach, CA, USA) is a pressure or flow controller that may be pressure-, time-, or manually triggered; pressure- or flow-limited; and pressure- or time-cycled. It has an optional compressor, an internal air-oxygen blender, and a gas outlet port that will power a nebulizer during inspiration.

II. **Input**

A. The Wave uses 100–110 volts AC at 60 Hz to power the control circuitry.

B. The pneumatic circuit operates on external compressed gas sources (i.e., air and oxygen) at 40–70 pounds per square inch gauge (psig).

C. The operator may input the mode of ventilation; pressure-triggering, pressure-limiting, and pressure-cycling thresholds; positive end-expiratory pressure/continuous positive airway pressure (PEEP/CPAP); peak inspiratory flow rate; inspiratory time; ventilatory frequency; bias flow; and FiO_2.

III. **Control Scheme**

A. Control variables

1. The Wave controls inspiratory pressure for all spontaneous breaths and for mandatory breaths whenever the peak pressure is limited using the pressure control knob.

2. At all other times, the Wave controls inspiratory flow.

B. Phase variables

1. Trigger variables

a. Inspiration is pressure-triggered when pressure in the patient circuit drops below the sensitivity setting. The threshold for triggering a mandatory breath is adjustable from 0.1–5 cm H_2O below the baseline pressure.

b. The Wave may also be manually triggered.

187

2. Limit variables
   a. Inspiration is pressure-limited during assist/control and synchronized intermittent mandatory ventilation (SIMV) modes whenever the pressure control setting (0–80 cm H_2O) is lower than the natural peak inspiratory pressure (PIP) that would result from the flow and inspiratory time settings along with the patient's lung impedance. Inspiratory pressure may also be limited by a mechanical pressure relief valve, adjustable from 0–120 cm H_2O.
   b. If the pressure control setting is high enough so that there is no pressure limit, inspiration is flow-limited. Inspiratory flow rate may be set from 1–100 L/min.
   c. The Wave can be volume-limited by setting inspiratory pause at 0%, 10%, 20%, or 30% of the ventilatory period using a switch on the back of the machine.
3. Cycle variables
   a. Inspiration may be pressure-cycled when the high inspiratory pressure alarm threshold is violated. It may be set over a range of 5–120 cm H_2O.
   b. Inspiration cannot be volume-cycled because the Wave flow control system does not measure instantaneous volume. Using the inspiratory time and flow controls, the Wave is capable of delivering tidal volumes of 5–2,000 mL.
   c. Spontaneous breaths are flow-cycled when using presure support. Actually, there is a complex mathematical control equation used for flow-cycling in this mode relating to peak flow, delivered flow, and elapsed inspiratory time. Cycling flows range from <5% to 100% of peak flow.
   d. Inspiration is normally time-cycled according to the inspiratory time setting (adjustable from 0.1–3.0 sec).
4. Baseline variables
   a. Baseline pressure may be adjusted from 0–45 cm H_2O using the PEEP/CPAP dial.
   b. Baseline continuous flow, or "bias flow," may be set from 0–30 L/min.
C. Modes
   1. Assist/control – during continuous mechanical ventilation, inspiration is pressure-triggered (depending on the presence of spontaneous breathing effort and the sensitivity setting) or time-triggered (according to the respiratory rate setting), may be pressure- or flow-limited, and is time-cycled.
   2. SIMV
      a. In SIMV, mandatory breaths are pressure-triggered (depending on the presence of spontaneous breathing effort and the sensitivity setting) or time-triggered (according to the frequency setting), may be pressure- or flow-limited, and are time-cycled. A

mandatory breath is pressure-triggered the first time a sponta-neous breathing effort is detected in each ventilatory period (the ventilatory period is equal to the reciprocal of the respiratory rate). If a breathing effort is not detected during a given venti-latory period, a mandatory breath will be delivered at the be-ginning of the next period. The ventilator will continue to deliver mandatory breaths according to the respiratory rate setting until a spontaneous breath is detected, and the sequence of events repeats itself.

   b. Spontaneous inspirations between mandatory breaths are con-trolled for baseline pressure (i.e., PEEP/CPAP) and may be assisted if the pressure support setting is above zero.

  3. Spontaneous
Inspiration is pressure-controlled in the spontaneous mode at the set PEEP/CPAP level. A pressure support level may also be set. The slope or rise time of pressure during pressure support is automat-ically controlled using "predictive learning logic" software to main-tain optimal patient synchronization.

D. Control subsystems

  1. Control circuit
The Wave uses pneumatic and electronic control components. Trig-gering and cycling signals arise from the inspiratory time and ventilatory frequency settings as well as signals from the airway pressure transducer. Output control signals from two pressure transducers (one monitors airway pressure and one monitors pres-sure in the exhalation valve) and two redundant flow transducers (monitoring the output of the master flow control valve) are used to control flow. The exhalation manifold is controlled pneumatically.

  2. Drive mechanism

   a. The Wave uses either external compressed gas (for air and oxygen) or an electric motor and compressor (for air) in conjunc-tion with a pressure regulator. Gas from supply lines is fed to an internal air-oxygen blender.

   b. Mixed gas leaves the blender at 28 psig and enters a rigid-walled vessel (the "accumulator"). The flow control system is driven by the pressure from the accumulator, reducing the instantaneous flow demand required of the blending system. This action allows a wide range of peak flow settings, reduces the flow required of the compressed gas supply, and improves response time. The accumulator also acts as a mixing chamber, which helps to stabilize the delivered oxygen concentration within a given breath.

  3. Output Control Valves

   a. All gas flow to the patient is regulated by the main flow control valve, which is a proportional solenoid valve.

   b. An electromagnetic poppet valve switches between two sources of a pneumatic signal to the exhalation valve. One source comes from the output of the master flow control valve and keeps a diaphragm-type exhalation manifold closed during assisted breaths. The other source is a pressure regulator that generates an adjustable pressure signal to control baseline pressure (i.e., PEEP/CPAP).

   c. The microprocessor coordinates the activity of both valves, such that the exhalation valve closes as the flow control valve begins to deliver flow to the patient circuit.

IV. Output

  A. Waveforms

    1. The Wave delivers a rectangular flow waveform when set for volume control, that is, if the natural PIP is below the setting of the pressure control knob or if this knob is set to "off."

    2. If PIP is limited using the pressure control knob, a variety of pressure waveforms can be achieved, ranging from rectangular to triangular depending on the respiratory system mechanics and the inspiratory flow rate.

  B. Displays

    1. In addition to the various control settings, the Wave displays include: visual alarm indicators (LEDs) and digital display of tidal volume (calculated based on flow and inspiratory time settings); minute volume; ventilatory rate; peak, mean, and baseline airway pressures; and peak flow.

    2. An electronic pressure gauge provides airway pressure measurement over the range of 0–120 cm H_2O.

    3. The Wave is usually sold with the Compass® monitor which allows monitoring of inspired tidal and expired tidal volume, inspired and expired minute volume, and peak inspiratory and expiratory flow.

V. Alarms

  A. Input power alarm: an audible alarm is activated if the electrical power is interrupted or if the air or oxygen supply falls below 32 psig.

  B. Control circuit alarms

    1. A visual "inspiratory time too long" alarm is activated if the inspiratory time and ventilatory rate settings result in an inspiratory: expiratory (I:E) ratio greater than the preset maximum. There are two selectable maximum ratios: 1:1 and 3:1.

    2. When the inspiratory time is set such that the preset maximum I:E ratio is violated, the ventilator will override the inspiratory time setting to restrict the I:E to the preset value.

    3. Audible and visual "ventilator inoperative" alarms are activated when malfunction of the integrated circuit or ventilator occurs.

    4. There are two pressure and two flow sensors in the Wave. If the

drift between the pressure or flow sensors is large, the visual display flashes automatically.

C. Output alarms: a low pressure alarm is adjustable from 0–110 cm H_2O, and a high pressure alarm is adjustable from 5–120 cm H_2O. High and low minute volume alarms are adjustable from 1–50 and 0–49 L/min, respectively.

VI. Unique Clinical feature
The Wave can ventilate any patient from the smallest newborn to the largest adult. Its pressure support and pressure triggering capabilities have been shown to be excellent.

Suggested Reading

Chatburn RL: Classification of mechanical ventilators. In Tobin MJ (Ed.): *Principles and Practice of Mechanical Ventilation, 3rd Edition.* New York, McGraw-Hill, 1994, pp. 37–64.

Goldsmith JP, Karotkin EH (Eds.): *Assisted Ventilation of the Neonate, 3rd Edition.* Philadelphia, WB Saunders, 1996.

Chatburn RL. Ventilators. In Branson RD, Hess DR, Chatburn RL (Eds.): *Respiratory Care Equipment.* Philadelphia, JB Lippincott, 1995, pp. 294–392.

Chatburn RL. Principles and practice of neonatal and pediatric mechanical ventilation. Respir Care 1991; 36:569–595.

Chapter 30

Bear Cub 750 PSV® Infant Ventilator

Cheryll K. Hagus

I. **Description**

    A. The Bear Cub 750 PSV Infant Ventilator (Bear Medical, Riverside, CA, USA) is pneumatically powered with 30–80 psig air and oxygen and electronically controlled.

    B. Designed to ventilate newborn, infant, and pediatric patients between 500 g and 30 kg in weight

    C. Provides a range of modes, controls, monitors, and alarms appropriate for the targeted patient population

    D. An optional flow sensor that may be placed at the proximal airway provides synchronized mandatory breaths and volume monitoring.

II. **Breath Types and Modes of Ventilation**

    A. Breath types

        1. The changeover from expiration to inspiration may be time-triggered based on the rate setting, or flow-triggered based on the assist sensitivity setting. Flow-triggering requires that the flow sensor be properly installed.

        2. Mandatory breaths are pressure-limited; however, the peak inspiratory pressure may be less than the inspiratory pressure setting if the volume limit function is activated.

        3. The changeover from inspiration to expiration may be time-cycled based on the inspiratory time setting or flow-cycled based on a fixed termination percentage of 5% of peak inspiratory flow. If the volume limit function is activated, mandatory breaths may be volume-cycled. When a breath is flow-cycled or volume-limited, the actual inspiratory time (T_I) may be less than the set T_I.

    B. Modes

        1. Assist/control. The patient may trigger mandatory breaths in excess of the preset rate provided the assist sensitivity threshold is met

(flow sensor must be installed). As a result, the mandatory breaths are synchronized with the patient's breathing pattern.

2. Flow-cycled assist/control. A pressure-limited breath is delivered at a preset inspiratory pressure based on the mandatory set rate or with each patient effort that meets the assist sensitivity threshold. Delivered breaths may be flow-cycled when the inspiratory flow falls to 5% of the peak flow rate, or time-cycled at the preset inspiratory time, whichever occurs first.

3. Synchronized intermittent mandatory ventilation (SIMV). In this mode, a combination of mandatory breaths and spontaneous breaths is possible. Based on "assist windows," mandatory breaths are delivered in synchrony with the patient's breathing pattern at the preset rate (flow sensor required). In between mandatory breaths, the patient may breathe spontaneously from the preset base flow.

4. Intermittent mandatory ventilation (IMV). Mandatory breaths are delivered at preset intervals based on the rate setting without regard for the patient's breathing pattern. The patient may breath spontaneously in between mandatory breaths.

5. Flow-cycled SIMV. A pressure-limited breath is delivered at a preset inspiratory pressure based on the mandatory set rate, in synchrony with the infant's spontaneous effort. These breaths may be flow-cycled when the inspiratory flow falls to 5% of the peak flow rate, or time-cycled at the preset inspiratory time limit, whichever occurs first. In between mandatory breaths, the infant may breathe spontaneously.

6. Synchronized intermittent mandatory ventilation/pressure support ventilation (SIMV/PSV). A mandatory pressure-limited breath is delivered to the patient at a preset inspiratory pressure and time-cycled at the preset inspiratory time limit, synchronized to patient effort. Any spontaneous efforts recognized by the ventilator between mandatory breaths will be supported at the preset inspiratory pressure and may be flow-cycled when the inspiratory flow falls to 5% of the peak flow rate, or time-cycled at the preset inspiratory time limit, whichever occurs first.

7. PSV. All spontaneous efforts that reach the assist sensitivity threshold will be supported by the preset inspiratory pressure and may be flow-cycled when the inspiratory flow falls to 5% of the peak flow rate, or time-cycled at the preset inspiratory time limit, whichever occurs first. There is no mandatory rate. If the patient is apneic for the duration of the apnea alarm setting, the ventilator will deliver a back-up mandatory breath at the preset pressure and inspiratory time limit. If no patient initiated breaths are taken during a time-out period based on the set ventilator rate or 10 seconds, which ever is less, another back-up breath will be delivered. This sequence will continue until a breath is recognized. An apnea alarm will be reported throughout this sequence.

8. Continuous positive airway pressure (CPAP). The patient breathes

spontaneously at a constant airway pressure determined by the positive end-expiratory pressure (PEEP) setting. When a flow sensor is installed, spontaneous breaths are monitored by the ventilator. If the patient is apneic for the duration of the apnea alarm setting, the ventilator will deliver a back-up mandatory breath at the preset pressure and inspiratory time. If no patient-initiated breaths are taken during a time-out period based on the set ventilator rate or 10 seconds, which ever is less, another back-up breath will be delivered. This sequence will continue until a breath is recognized. An apnea alarm will be reported throughout this sequence.

III. Controls

A. Ventilation

1. PEEP/CPAP 0–30 cm H_2O – sets the level of baseline pressure
2. Inspiratory pressure 0–72 cm H_2O – the primary determinant of delivered tidal volume
3. Rate 1–150 BPM – sets the number of mandatory breaths in SIMV and IMV, and the minimum number of mandatory breaths in assist/control
4. T_I 0.1–3.0 seconds – determines the maximum length of the inspiratory phase of mandatory breaths
5. Inspiratory flow 1–30 LPM – sets the flow delivered by the ventilator during the inspiratory phase of a mandatory breath
6. Base flow 1–30 LPM – sets the flow available to the patient for spontaneous breathing
7. Volume limit 5–300 mL – this patented feature is unique to the Bear Cub 750 PSV Ventilator. The preset inspiratory pressure generally determines the delivered volume. A dramatic improvement in patient compliance may result in excessive tidal volume delivery unless the inspiratory pressure is adjusted accordingly. The volume limit function allows the clinician to set a maximum tidal volume to be delivered. If the preset tidal volume should be reached prior to the achievement of the preset inspiratory pressure, the ventilator will terminate inspiration and cycle into the expiratory phase.

B. Oxygenation – FiO_2 0.21–1.0

C. Other

1. Assist sensitivity 0.2–5.0 LPM – sets the amount of flow which the patient must generate at the proximal airway flow sensor to trigger a mandatory breath in assist/control and SIMV. It also sets the threshold for monitoring the patient's total breath rate in CPAP.
2. Overpressure relief valve 15–75 cm H_2O – a mechanical valve that provides a secondary protection against excessive airway pressure. Recommended setting is 15 cm H_2O above the inspiratory pressure setting.

3. Manual breath – pushbutton control which delivers one mandatory breath according to the preset control settings

IV. Monitors
A. Timing
1. Breath rate – reflects the total breath rate in assist/control, SIMV, and CPAP (flow sensor required), and the mandatory rate in IMV
2. Patient-initiated – indicates the patient has exceeded the assist sensitivity requirement for breath delivery, either triggering a mechanical, or taking a spontaneous breath
3. Inspiratory time – displays T_I of both mandatory and spontaneous breaths
4. Expiratory time – displays T_E of mandatory breath only (i.e., time elapsed from the end of one mandatory breath to the beginning of the next)
5. I:E ratio – reflects the calculated relationship between the duration of inspiration to the duration of expiration for mandatory breaths only

B. Pressure
1. Peak inspiratory pressure – displays the maximum pressure reached during each mandatory breath
2. Mean airway pressure – reflects the average pressure applied to the proximal airway over time
3. PEEP – indicates the PEEP/CPAP measured at the proximal airway

C. Volume (requires properly installed flow sensor)
1. Minute volume – displays the measured exhaled minute volume from all breath types (i.e., mandatory and spontaneous)
2. Inspiratory tidal volume – displays the inspired tidal volume measured at the proximal airway for both mandatory and spontaneous breaths
3. Exhaled tidal volume – displays the expired tidal volume measured at the proximal airway for both mandatory and spontaneous breaths
4. Leak percent – reflects the calculated difference between delivered and exhaled tidal volume. Helpful in assessing the need for reintubation with a larger endotracheal tube

V. Alerts and Alarms
A. Alarms
1. Low PEEP/CPAP – will be activated if the measured proximal pressure falls below the set value for a minimum of 250 msec. Low PEEP/CPAP must be set within 10 cm H_2O of the PEEP setting or a prolonged inspiratory pressure alarm will sound.

2. High breath rate – will activate whenever the monitored value for breath rate exceeds the alarm setting
3. Low minute volume – will activate when the monitored minute volume falls below the set threshold (flow sensor must be attached)
4. High pressure limit – will activate when the proximal pressure exceeds the set threshold. Breath will be immediately terminated.
5. Low inspiratory pressure – this alarm is automatically set by the ventilator and indicates circuit leak or disconnect.
6. Apnea - indicates that no breath has been initiated/detected in the preset time interval (i.e., 5, 10, 20, or 30 sec)

VI. Optional Features
A. Graphics monitor – pressure, flow, and volume
B. Computer connection – RS-232
C. Analog connection – pressure, flow, and breath phase

Suggested Reading

Instruction Manual for BEAR CUB 750 PSV Infant Ventilator. Palm Springs, CA, Bear Medical Systems, Inc., 1998.

Chapter 31

Siemens Servo 300® Ventilator

Mary Dekeon

I. **The Siemens Servo 300 ventilator** (Siemens-Elema AB, Solna, Sweden) is the first ventilator with the capability to support ventilation for very low birthweight infants in the neonatal intensive care unit as well as adults.

II. **Modes**

A variety and combination of modes is available to treat severe lung injury requiring maximum support and weaning. The ventilator may be set to flow-trigger in all modes of ventilation providing options for neonatal and pediatric ventilation. All modes are synchronized with the patient's spontaneous breathing effort.

A. Control modes of ventilation: spontaneous breaths have the same characteristics (flow, inspiratory time, volume or pressure) as the set ventilator breaths.

1. Pressure control (PC)

a. This mode of ventilation employs a variable flow rate which is servo-controlled to provide a constant inspiratory pressure

(1) Tidal volume is variable

(2) Peak inspiratory pressure is constant

(3) Square pressure waveform

(4) Decelerating flow waveform (a variable flow rate differentiates this mode from time-cycled, pressure-limited ventilation, which incorporates a constant flow)

b. Indications

(1) Patients with high peak airway pressure at risk for barotrauma (e.g., respiratory distress syndrome [RDS], bronchopulmonary dysplasia [BPD], and meconium aspiration)

(2) Mode of choice for inverse inspiratory:expiratory (I:E) ratio ventilation

(3) Patients with large endotracheal tube leaks

(4) Patients with airway obstruction

c. Clinician-set parameters
   (1) Peak inspiratory pressure level (above positive end-expiratory pressure, PEEP)
   (2) Inspiratory time
   (3) Ventilator rate
   (4) PEEP
   (5) FiO_2
   (6) High and low minute ventilation alarms
   (7) High pressure alarm
   (8) Trigger sensitivity level
2. Volume control (VC)
   a. Characteristics
      (1) Tidal volume is set
      (2) Peak pressure is variable
      (3) Sinusoidal flow waveform (flow is regulated based on set tidal volume and inspiratory time)
      (4) Sinusoidal pressure waveform
   b. Indications
      (1) Postoperative patients with normal lung compliance
      (2) Other patients requiring ventilator support for nonpulmonary reasons
   c. Clinician-set parameters
      (1) Tidal volume
      (2) Inspiratory time (controls flow rate)
      (3) Pause time (added to inspiratory time, does not affect flow rate)
      (4) Ventilator rate
      (5) PEEP
      (6) FiO_2
      (7) High and low minute ventilation alarms
      (8) High pressure alarm
3. Pressure-regulated volume control (PRVC)
   a. PRVC is the hallmark of the 300 ventilator
      (1) Tidal volume is set
      (2) Peak pressure is variable
      (3) Decelerating flow waveform (the same as PC)
      (4) Square pressure waveform
   b. Indications
      (1) Patients with high peak airway pressures at risk for barotrauma (e.g., RDS, BPD, meconium aspiration)
      (2) Patients with asthma

       (3) Postoperative patients

       (4) Patients with large endotracheal tube leaks

       (5) Patients with airway obstruction

     c. Clinician-set parameters

       (1) Tidal volume

       (2) Inspiratory time

       (3) Ventilator rate

       (4) PEEP

       (5) FiO_2

       (6) High and low minute ventilation alarms

       (7) High pressure alarm

       (8) Trigger sensitivity level

B. Modes for spontaneously breathing patients (all breaths are patient-initiated)

   1. Volume support (VS)

     a. Characteristics

     Volume support is a mode for patients with an intact respiratory drive. This mode supports the patient's inspiratory effort with an assured tidal volume. Back-up ventilation is set so that if a patient becomes apneic in this mode, the ventilator alarm will activate a changeover to PRVC.

       (1) Tidal volume is set

       (2) Peak pressures are variable (based on lung compliance and respiratory effort)

       (3) Flow is decelerating

     b. Indications

       (1) Patients ready to be weaned

       (2) Patients who fail to respond to pressure support

       (3) Patients with lung disease but intact respiratory drive

     c. Clinician-set parameters

       (1) Minimum tidal volume

       (2) Inspiratory time (for back-up ventilation should apnea occur)

       (3) Ventilator rate (for back-up ventilation should apnea occur)

       (4) PEEP

       (5) FiO_2

       (6) High and low minute ventilation alarms

       (7) High pressure alarm

       (8) Trigger sensitivity level

   2. Pressure support

     a. Characteristics: pressure support is a mode for patients with an intact respiratory drive. This mode supports the patient's inspiratory effort with a set inspiratory pressure.

199

        (1) Tidal volume is variable

        (2) Peak inspiratory pressure is set

        (3) Decelerating flow

    b. Indications

        (1) Patients ready to be weaned

        (2) Patients with lung disease but intact respiratory drive

    c. Clinician-set parameters

        (1) Inspiratory pressure

        (2) FiO_2

        (3) PEEP

        (4) High and low minute ventilation alarms

        (5) High pressure alarm

        (6) Trigger sensitivity level

  3. Continuous positive airway pressure (CPAP)

    a. Characteristics

    CPAP is a mode for spontaneously breathing patients who do not require any assistance in overcoming the work of breathing imposed by lung disease or the endotracheal tube

    b. Clinician-set parameters

        (1) FiO_2

        (2) CPAP

        (3) High and low minute ventilation alarms

        (4) High pressure alarm

        (5) Trigger sensitivity level

    c. Indications

        (1) Patients ready to be weaned

        (2) Patients who need respiratory muscle strengthening

        (3) Stenting of upper airway

        (4) Postextubation support

C. Combination modes of ventilation

In addition, the above modes are offered in combination. This provides the clinician the ability to support ventilator-delivered breaths and spontaneously triggered breaths with different parameters.

  1. Synchronized intermittent mandatory ventilation (SIMV) with pressure support (volume)

  2. SIMV with pressure support (pressure)

III. Control Panel and Display

The ventilator is equipped with a state of the art control panel with digital displays; a sophisticated graphic monitoring system is an option available to provide the clinician with a wide range of flow, pressure, and volume monitoring.

A. Control panel
1. The ventilator has a "patient range selector" to set different internal parameters for adult, pediatric, and neonatal ventilation. These parameters control the following:
   a. The level of continuous flow for flow-triggering

Adult	Pediatric	Infant
32 mL/s	16 mL/s	8 mL/s

   b. Maximum inspiratory peak flow

Adult	Pediatric	Infant
200 L/min	33 L/min	13 L/min

   c. Maximum measured tidal volume

Adult	Pediatric	Infant
3,999 mL	399 mL	39 mL

   d. The apnea alarm

Adult	Pediatric	Infant
20 sec	15 sec	10 sec

2. Airway pressure panel
   A digital display of the following airway pressures is continuously displayed in the airway pressure panel:
   a. Peak
   b. Mean
   c. Pause (if applicable)
   d. End-expiratory pressure
   e. The read-out is a red digital display updated every 2 msec
   f. This panel has the following control knobs:
      (1) Upper pressure limit: 20–120 cm H_2O
      (2) Pressure control (above PEEP): 1–100 cm H_2O
      (3) Pressure support (above PEEP): 0–100 cm H_2O
      (4) PEEP: 0–50 cm H_2O
      (5) Trigger sensitivity (can be set for either flow- or pressure-triggering)
   g. Controls that are active (depending on the mode) are illuminated with an amber light.
   h. Pressures are also monitored with a bar graph with colored diodes which display the following parameters:
      (1) Upper pressure limit
      (2) Pressure control level (if applicable)
      (3) Pressure support level (if applicable)
      (4) Peak inspiratory pressure (shown with two diodes, one from the inspiratory microprocessor and one from the expiratory transducer)

(5) PEEP

(6) Trigger level below PEEP

3. Mode selection

Mode selection is made with a control knob. In addition to the modes, the ventilator may be put in standby or turned off with this control. The active mode is indicated by an amber light.

4. Respiratory pattern panel

a. This panel contains the control knobs to set the ventilator rate, inspiratory time, and inspiratory pattern.

(1) The rate knob is labeled "CMV freq. B/min"; this sets the number of breaths the ventilator will deliver in the "control modes" as well as determining the breath cycle time in the support modes. The set rate is divided into the set minute volume to obtain a tidal volume. The range is 5–150 breaths per minute.

(2) The inspiratory time control knob is set in percent of the time cycle; however, the digital read-out is in seconds. The range is from 10–80% of the total cycle time.

(3) The pause time is also in percent of the cycle time and in addition to inspiratory time percent. It is only active in VC and SIMV with PS (volume). When set, the total inspiratory time is displayed on the digital read-out.

(4) The inspiratory rise time percent may be set from 0–10%. This control ramps the inspiratory flow to "soften" it. This may be very helpful in infants with small endotracheal tubes. It is effective in all modes.

(5) The SIMV frequency knob is used to set the breath rate in the SIMV modes.

b. The respiratory control panel also contains the following digital read-outs:

(1) Measured frequency (total set breaths and spontaneous breaths)

(2) Set frequency

(3) Inspiratory period

(4) Inspiratory flow

(5) A unique feature of these digital values is the color coding: red for measured parameters and green for set values.

5. Volume panel

a. This panel contains the controls and digital readings for the following:

(1) Set tidal volume

(2) Set minute ventilation

(3) Inspiratory tidal volume

(4) Expiratory tidal volume

(5) Expiratory minute ventilation

b. A bar graph for low and high minute ventilation alarms is also contained in this panel. This bar graph continuously displays high and low alarm settings, as well as set minute ventilation and exhaled minute ventilation.

6. Oxygen panel

   a. The control to set fraction of inspired oxygen (alarms are automatically set for ±6% of set FiO_2)

   b. A knob to deliver 100% oxygen for 1 minute or 20 breaths, whichever occurs first

   c. A manual breath button for delivering manual breaths

   d. Continuous monitoring of delivered FiO_2

7. Alarm and message panel

   a. The Servo 300 has a very sophisticated alarm package containing both audible and visual readings. Visual readings are:

   (1) A digital message indicating reason for alarm

   (2) A flashing red light for an active alarm

   (3) A steady amber light indicating an alarm was violated but is no longer active

   b. Control knobs

   (1) An alarm "reset" button

   (2) A 2-minute silent button

   (3) An inspiratory pause button (maximum pause time of 5 sec)

   (4) An expiratory pause button to determine intrinsic PEEP (maximum time of 30 sec)

Suggested Reading

Keenan HT, Martin LD: Volume support ventilation in infants and children: analysis of a case series. Respir Care 1997; 42:281–287.

Piotrowski A, Sobala W, Kawczynski P: Patient-initiated, pressure-regulated, volume-controlled ventilation compared with intermittent mandatory ventilation in neonates: a prospective, randomised study. Intensive Care Med 1997; 23:975–981.

Chapter 32

Infant Star® Ventilator

Graham Bernstein

I. **Infant Star 500 and 950 Ventilators (Infrasonics, Inc., San Diego, CA, USA)**

   A. Time-cycled, pressure-limited, continuous flow ventilators. For patients <40 lbs (18 kg). Dual microprocessor controlled; demand background flow to reduce work of breathing.

      1. Upper electronics and lower pneumatics sections; rotate 270 degrees independently to facilitate patient connection and maximize visibility of displays.

      2. Electronics front panel grouped into three sections: alarm status, ventilator settings, and patient monitoring

      3. Pneumatics section has oxygen percent control (21–100%), pressure relief valve (5–120 cm H_2O), heated exhalation block housing exhalation valve diaphragm and jet venturi to minimize inadvertent positive end-expiratory pressure (PEEP), and circuit ports.

   B. Modes of ventilation

      1. Continuous positive airway pressure (CPAP) and intermittent mandatory ventilation (IMV) modes are identical between the 500 and 950 ventilators. Ventilator rate 1–150 breaths/min, peak inspiratory pressure (PIP) 5–90 cm H_2O, inspiratory time (T_I) 0.1–3 sec, PEEP 0–24 cm H_2O, flow rate 4–40 LPM, background flow 2–32 LPM.

      2. Star Sync provides patient-triggered options of synchronized intermittent mandatory ventilation (SIMV) and assist/control with both the 500 and 950 ventilators. In addition, the monitor mode and the CPAP/BACKUP mode provide self-weaning ventilation during apnea.

      3. The 950 provides two high-frequency ventilation modes (HFV ONLY and HFV + IMV). HFV rate 2–22 Hz, HFV amplitude 0–160 cm H_2O (maximum amplitude depends on ventilator circuit and settings, airway resistance, and lung compliance). Jet venturi produces "active exhalation."

II. **Star Sync Patient-Triggered Interface**

Adds modes (see above) to both the 500 and the 950. Fast response time, good reliability, and easy to use. Has mode control section, displays spontaneous and assisted breath rates, and also spontaneous inspiratory time

A. Uses a pneumatic capsule sensor, which must be taped onto the abdomen where there is visible outward movement during inspiration (below retractions). Periodically, audible "click" should be used briefly to confirm correct placement.

B. Mounted atop an Infant Star or below the ventilator base

III. Star Track Infant Graphics Monitor
Numerical and graphical (3.5 in. × 4.5 in. backlit LCD screen) windows for airway flow, tidal volume and pressure data, lung mechanics, minute volume, leak percent, and alarm settings

A. Uses a low dead space (<1 mL), heated wire anemometer placed within the endotracheal tube (ETT) adapter and circuit wye

B. Can be mounted atop the ventilator or it can be pole mounted to provide a mobile workstation

C. For infants with maximum ETT size of 5 mm and requiring a maximum of 30 LPM

Suggested Reading

Bernstein G, Mannino FL, Heldt G, et al: Randomized multicenter trial comparing synchronized and conventional intermittent mandatory ventilation in neonates. J Pediatr 1996; 128:453–463.

Bernstein G: Synchronous and patient-triggered ventilation in newborns. Neonat Intens Care 1993; 6:54–66.

Patel CA, Klein JM: Outcome of infants with birthweight <1000 gm with RDS treated with high frequency ventilation and surfactant replacement therapy. Arch Pediatr Adol Med 1995; 149:317–321.

Talbert A: Overview of high frequency ventilation and report of a multicenter clinical trial. Neonat Intens Care 1996; 9:58–66.

SECTION VII

Neonatal Apnea

Chapter 33

Apnea Syndromes

Charles A. Pohl, Alan R. Spitzer

I. **Terminology**

    A. Apnea is the absence of respiratory air flow.

    B. Pathologic apnea is the cessation of respiratory air flow for >20 seconds or a briefer pause associated with abrupt onset of pallor, cyanosis, bradycardia, or hypotonia.

    C. Apnea of infancy (AOI) is pathologic apnea that presents in an infant who is >37 weeks gestational age for which no specific cause can be identified.

    D. Periodic breathing (PB) is a respiratory pattern in which there are three or more consecutive central pauses of >3 seconds duration, separated by <20 seconds of breathing between each pause.

    E. Apnea of prematurity (AOP) is pathologic apnea or excessive periodic breathing in preterm infants.

    F. Apparent life-threatening episode (ALTE) refers to an event that is frightening to the observer and is characterized by some combination of apnea, color change, marked change in muscle tone, choking, or gagging.

    G. Sudden infant death syndrome (SIDS) is the unexpected death of an infant <1 year of age that remains unexplained after a review of the past medical records of the child, a postmortem examination, and a death scene investigation.

II. **Etiology of Apnea (Table 22)**

Apnea can be normal if it is brief, infrequent, and not associated with any underlying problems. If abnormal, apnea represents a sign rather than a specific pathologic process. Many conditions are associated with pathologic apnea.

III. **Risk Groups for Apnea**

    A. Premature infants

        1. An interplay of an immature ventilatory center, impaired central

Table 22
Medical Conditions Associated With Pathologic Apnea

Acute Conditions	Chronic Conditions
Thermal instability	Apnea of prematurity
Infection (meningitis, bacteremia, respiratory syncytial virus infection, pertussis, infantile botulism)	Gastroesophageal reflux disease
CNS pathology (seizure, intracranial hemorrhage including child abuse)	Airway obstruction (congenital anomaly, sleep apnea)
Metabolic disturbance (inborn errors of metabolism, hypernatremia, hyponatremia, hypoglycemia, hypocalcemia)	Cardiac disease (dysrhythmia, marked shunt including PDA)
Airway obstruction (neck flexion, laryngospasm)	CNS pathology (seizure, hemorrhage, malformation including Arnold-Chiari)
Necrotizing enterocolitis	Marked anemia
Postsurgical apnea	Chronic lung disease
Drug-induced	Hypoventilation syndrome (Ondine's curse)
	Idiopathic

CNS = central nervous system; PDA = patent ductus arteriosus.

nervous system chemoreceptors, and functional obstruction of the upper airway results in AOP.

   2. About 25–50% of premature infants have AOP.

   3. Apnea in premature infants is predominantly central apnea.

B. Infantile pathologic gastroesophageal reflux (GER)

   1. Peak period of onset is 1–4 months of age.

   2. Manifestations include esophagitis, failure to thrive, recurrent pneumonia, intractable wheezing, or obstructive apnea.

   3. Risk groups include premature infants, neurologically impaired children, infants with underlying lung disease (cystic fibrosis or bronchopulmonary dysplasia [BPD]), and children who require gastrostomy feedings.

C. ALTE patients

   1. Occurs in 0.5–6% of all infants

   2. Represents a clinical presentation rather than a specific disease process

   3. Causes include systemic infections, upper airway obstruction, seizures, GER, cardiac disease, or idiopathic apnea and bradycardia

   4. There is an increased incidence of SIDS, especially if vigorous resuscitation during sleep is necessary (25–30%).

D. Siblings of SIDS victims

   1. Two- to fourfold increase in SIDS rates

   2. Infanticide and hereditary disorders must be considered

E. Chronic conditions, such as BPD and tracheostomy dependency

F. Central hypoventilation syndrome (Ondine's curse)

   1. Inability to regulate ventilation during sleep secondary to inadequate output from brainstem centers

   2. Should be considered with persistent pathologic central apnea or ventilator dependency despite minimal pulmonary disease

   3. Associated with Hirschsprung's disease

IV. SIDS

A. Leading cause of postneonatal infant mortality (0.8 infant deaths per 1,000 live births)

B. Peak age is 2–4 months with the majority (95%) by age 6 months.

C. A statistically rare event, with poor predictability

D. Multiple risk factors (Table 23)

E. Etiology unknown

Table 23
Risk Factors for Sudden Infant Death Syndrome (SIDS)

Modifiable	Less Modifiable
Prone sleep position*	Prematurity
Tobacco exposure	Young mother
Inadequate health care	Less-educated mother
Lack of breast-feeding	Poverty
	Low birthweight/intrauterine retardation
	Colder climate
	Previous apparent life-threatening event

* Risk of SIDS for infants in the prone sleep position is greater if there has been a recent illness, the child sleeps on soft bedding surfaces, gas-trapping objects (e.g., pillows, stuffed animals) are present in the crib, or swaddling is used.

Suggested Reading

American Academy of Pediatrics Task Force on Prolonged Infantile Apnea: Prolonged infantile apnea. Pediatrics 1985; 76:129–131.

Fleming PJ, Blair PS, Bacon C, et al: Environment of infants during sleep and risk of the sudden infant death syndrome: results from 1993–1995 case-control study for confidential inquiry into stillbirths and deaths in infancy. Br Med J 1996; 313:191–195.

Gibson, E: Apnea. In Spitzer AR (Ed.): *Intensive Care of the Fetus and Neonate.* Philadelphia, Mosby Publishing Co., 1996, pp. 470–481.

Gibson E, Spinner S: A critical assessment of the relationship of infant sleep position and SIDS. Foc Opin Pediatr 1996; 2:94–107.

Kraus JF, Grenland S, Bulterys M: Risk factors for sudden infant death syndrome in the United States collaborative perinatal project. Int J Epidemiol 1989; 18:113–120.

National Institutes of Health Consensus Development Conference on Infantile Apnea and Home Monitoring. Sept. 29 to Oct. 1, 1980. Pediatrics 1987; 79:292–299.

Oyen N, Markestad T, Skjaerven R, et al: Combined effects of sleeping position and prenatal risk factors in sudden infant death syndrome: the Nordic epidemiological SIDS study. Pediatrics 1997; 100:613–621.

Ponsonby AL, Dwyer T, Gibbons LE, et al: Factors potentiating the risk of SIDS associated with prone sleeping position. N Engl J Med 1993; 329:377–382.

Willinger M, Hoffman HJ, Hartford RB: Infant sleep position and risk for sudden infant death syndrome: report of meeting held January 13 and 14, 1994. National Institutes of Health, Bethesda, Maryland. Pediatrics 1994; 93:814–819.

Chapter 34

Diagnosis of Apnea

Charles A. Pohl, Alan R. Spitzer

I. **Approach to the Apneic Infant (Table 24)**
Apnea is a sign rather than a specific pathologic process.

   A. Cardiopulmonary stabilization

   B. Detailed history and physical exam

   C. The diagnostic evaluation is directed by the infant's associated findings.

II. **Indications for Hospitalization of Apneic Infants (Table 25)**

III. **Diagnostic Considerations**

   A. Complete blood count and cultures of blood, urine, and spinal fluid are necessary if a serious bacterial infection is suspected.

   B. Continuous multichannel recording (Figures 62 and 63)

   1. Measures chest wall movement, nasal/oral airflow (or change in air temperature), oxygen saturation, and heart rate trend

   2. Categorizes apnea

   a. Central apnea: absence of nasal airflow and chest wall movement

   b. Obstructive apnea: lack of airflow in the presence of chest wall movement

   c. Mixed apnea: combinations of central and obstructive apnea

   3. Sensitivity is improved if the child is continuously recorded for at least 18–24 hours.

   4. A two-channel pneumogram (which measures only chest wall excursion and heart rate trend) provides insufficient information.

   C. Intraesophageal pH recording with a multichannel recording if gastroesophageal reflux is suspected (Figure 64)

   D. A barium swallow study is useful if the infant has signs of swallowing dysfunction or anatomic anomalies such as esophageal web or tracheoesophageal fistula.

   E. A gastric emptying study and an abdominal sonogram are useful if there is a clinical picture of a generalized gastrointestinal motility disorder or pyloric stenosis.

Table 24
Diagnostic Clues for Infants with Apnea or Apparent
Life-Threatening Episodes

Clinical Features	Underlying Pathology
Choking during a feed	Pharyngeal dyscoordination, laryngospasm, GERD
Postfeed spitting, color change, posturing (back arching)	GERD
Abnormal eye movement, muscle tone change and post-ictal activity; abnormal neurologic findings, developmental delay	Seizures
Fever, activity change, or recalcitrant apnea	Serious bacterial infection
Family history of SIDS or ALTE; presence of bruising	Familial disorder (inborn error of metabolism) or child abuse

ALTE = apparent life-threatening event; GERD = gastroesophageal reflux disease; SIDS = sudden infant death syndrome.

F. A chest radiograph and/or radionuclide milk scan are helpful if the child has persistent, yet unexplained, lower airway signs.

G. Upper airway evaluation (including a lateral neck radiograph and otolaryngology evaluation) is useful if there is fixed or recurrent stridor, as well as unexplained pathologic obstructive apnea.

H. An electroencephalogram (EEG) should be considered in infants suspected of apneic seizures or having persistent pathologic central apnea without an identifiable cause.

I. Imaging studies of the brain are necessary in the presence of develop-

Table 25
When to Hospitalize an Apneic Infant

Ill appearance
Frequent clinical episodes or monitor alarms
Initiation of resuscitation
Color change (i.e., cyanosis or duskiness)
Change in muscle tone
Discrepancy in medical history
Parental anxiety

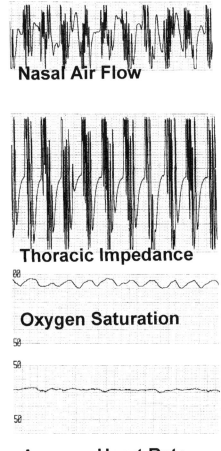

Nasal Air Flow

Thoracic Impedance

Oxygen Saturation

Average Heart Rate

Figure 62. Multichannel recording of an asymptomatic 3-week-old, formerly 34 weeks gestation, preterm infant. The event shows periodic breathing associated with fluctuation in oxygenation, with saturation decreasing to as low as 90%. The heart rate is stable.

     mental delay, suspicion of an intracranial hemorrhage (including child abuse), dysmorphic features, an abnormal neurologic examination, or mental status changes.

J. Serum ammonia, as well as urine and serum amino acids and organic acids, are useful if a metabolic disorder is suspected.

K. Serum electrolytes and glucose can help diagnose a recent stressful condition, a metabolic process, or chronic hypoventilation.

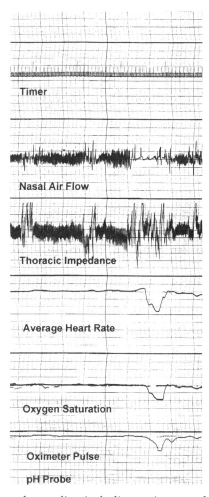

Figure 63. Multichannel recording including an intraesophageal pH tracing in a child with a 26-second obstructive apnea episode associated with a 40% decrease in heart rate and a desaturation to 75%. No decrease in pH is noted. There is also a channel for pulse detection from the pulse oximeter, which measures averaged heart rate.

  L. An echocardiogram and a cardiology referral are necessary if the history or physical examination suggests cardiac disease (e.g., feeding difficulties, heart murmur, and cyanosis).
  M. An electrocardiogram (ECG) is useful when severe unexplained tachycardia or bradycardia exists. Cardiac conduction abnormalities (e.g., prolonged QT syndrome) are rare, but important, causes of infant apnea.

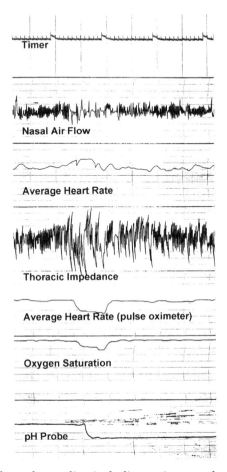

Figure 64. Multichannel recording including an intraesophageal pH tracing in a 6-week-old, formerly 28 weeks gestation, preterm infant with episodes of bradycardia and choking during feeding. The decrease in pH is associated with brief periods of obstructive apnea and desaturation to 80%, and indicates a significant gastroesophageal reflux event. Tachycardia is observed during the episode.

N. A stool specimen for botulism is helpful if the apneic infant has associated constipation and hypotonia.

O. The polysomnogram is useful in older children with sleep apnea associated with features such as bizarre behaviors, abnormal body movements, or nocturnal enuresis. This multichannel recording includes an EEG, a chin muscle electromyogram, and an electrooculogram

Suggested Reading

American Academy of Pediatrics Task Force on Prolonged Infantile Apnea: Prolonged infantile apnea. Pediatrics 1985; 76:129–131.

Dransfield DA, Spitzer AR, Fox WW: Episodic airway obstruction in premature infants. Am J Dis Child 1983; 137:441–443.

Gibson E: Apnea. In Spitzer AR (Ed): *Intensive Care of the Fetus and Neonate.* Philadelphia, Mosby Publishing Co., 1996, pp. 470–481.

National Institutes of Health Consensus Development Conference on Infantile Apnea and Home Monitoring. Sept. 29 to Oct. 1, 1980. Pediatrics 1987; 79:292–299.

Spitzer AR, Boyle JT, Tuchman D, et al: Awake apnea associated with gastroesophageal reflux: a specific clinical syndrome. J Pediatr 1984; 104:200–205.

Chapter 35

Treatment of Apnea

Charles A. Pohl, Alan R. Spitzer

The therapy of an apneic infant, as with the evaluation, must be directed at identifying and subsequently managing the underlying cause.

I. **Apnea of Prematurity**
   A. Xanthine derivatives (i.e., caffeine or theophylline)
      1. Proposed mechanisms include stimulation of skeletal and diaphragmatic muscle contraction, increase of the ventilatory center's sensitivity to carbon dioxide, and stimulation of the central respiratory drive.
      2. Dosage
         a. Active caffeine alkaloid: 2.5 mg/kg daily (5 mg/kg/day of caffeine citrate), 24 hours after a loading dose of 10 mg/kg of active caffeine
         b. Theophylline: 1–2 mg/kg every 8 hours after a loading dose of 5–6 mg/kg
      3. Therapeutic serum concentrations
         a. Caffeine: 5–25 mg/L
         b. Theophylline: 5–10 mg/L. Higher concentrations may be necessary.
      4. Side effects include nausea, vomiting, central nervous system excitability, seizures, tachycardia, and cardiac arrhythmia. Serious toxic effects are rare at serum levels below 20 mg/L.
      5. Caution is necessary if intercurrent viral illness and certain drugs (primarily metabolized by the liver), coexisting seizures (lowers the seizure threshold), or coexisting gastroesophageal reflux (GER; lowers the esophageal sphincter tone) are present.
      6. The wider therapeutic range and longer half-life of caffeine over theophylline results in less frequent monitoring of drug concentrations and in less serious toxicity.
   B. Continuous positive airway pressure (CPAP)
      1. Proposed mechanism

    a. Improvement in oxygenation

    b. Stabilization of upper airway patency

    c. Reduction in intercostal-phrenic inhibitory reflex

    d. Alteration of Hering-Breuer deflation reflex

  2. Indications

    a. Poor response to xanthine derivatives

    b. Inability to maintain airway patency and obstructive apnea

  3. Low positive pressure (2–5 cm H_2O) by nasal prongs is suggested as a starting point.

II. Pathologic GER

A. Nonpharmacologic therapy

  1. Small, frequent thickened feeds (e.g., rice cereal in formula)

  2. Postprandial prone-elevated position

  3. Avoid the use of an infant car seat immediately following a feeding.

B. Pharmacologic therapy

  1. Consider in any child who does not respond to traditional therapy or who has documented gastroesophageal reflux disease (GERD).

  2. Metoclopramide

    a. Stimulates gastroesophageal motility and increases lower esophageal sphincter tone

    b. Side effects include restlessness, drowsiness, and extrapyramidal symptoms.

    c. Avoid in the presence of bowel obstruction

    d. Dosage: 0.1 mg/kg/dose up to 4 times daily (30 minutes prior to meals and at bedtime)

  3. Cisapride

    a. Increases peristalsis and lowers esophageal tone by stimulating smooth muscle contraction of entire intestinal tract

    b. Side effects include gastroesophageal discomfort, diarrhea, severe photosensitivity reaction, and potentially life-threatening cardiac arrhythmias.

    c. Avoid in the following situations:

      (1) Concomitant use of cytochrome P450 medication (e.g., erythromycin, clarithromycin)

      (2) Predisposition to arrhythmias (e.g., history of prolonged QT interval, uncorrected electrolyte imbalance, underlying renal failure, ischemic heart disease, respiratory failure)

      (3) Bowel obstruction

    d. Dosage: 0.1–0.3 mg/kg/dose 3 or 4 times daily. *Do not exceed the recommended daily dose.*

   e. Consider an electrocardiogram (ECG), serum electrolytes, and serum magnesium level prior to starting Cisapride.

4. Histamine H_2 receptor antagonists are useful with symptomatic esophagitis (e.g., back arching, irritability) or if the patient has had a protracted medical course).

5. Omeprazole
   a. Proton pump inhibitor
   b. Useful if there has been a poor response to traditional pharmacologic agents
   c. Long-term safety is unknown

III. **Protective Strategies for Sudden Infant Death Syndrome (SIDS) (Table 26)**

A. Good health care

B. Supine sleep position for healthy infants
   1. Reduces SIDS rates by 40–50%
   2. Proposed harmful mechanisms that may enhance SIDS risk in the prone position
      a. Airway obstruction
      b. Inadequate oxygenation from rebreathing
      c. Thermal stress
      d. Decreased cerebral blood flow
      e. Efficient or deeper sleep
      f. Poor oxygenation with respiratory distress
   3. No proven increased risk of aspiration, GER, apparent life-threatening event (ALTE)
   4. Consider prone position if any of the following are present
      a. Severe GER
      b. Certain upper airway anomalies (e.g., Pierre-Robin syndrome)
      c. Premature infants with serious respiratory disease

Table 26
Protective Strategies for Sudden Infant Death Syndrome

Good health care
Supine sleep position for healthy infants
Avoid soft bedding (e.g., sheep skin)
Avoid gas-trapping objects (e.g., pillows, stuffed animals)
Smoke-free environment
Documented home monitors
Avoid alcohol and drug use if co-sleeping

---

5. Factors that exacerbate SIDS in the prone position
   a. Recent illness
   b. Soft bedding (e.g., sheep skin)
   c. Thermal insulation (i.e., swaddling, no central heating)
C. Avoid soft bedding (e.g., sheep skin)
D. Avoid gas-trapping objects near the baby's head (e.g., pillows, stuffed animals)
E. A smoke-free environment is very beneficial.
F. Documented home monitors (Figure 65)
   1. Measure
      a. Chest wall movement (central apnea) and heart rate trends
      b. Monitor compliance

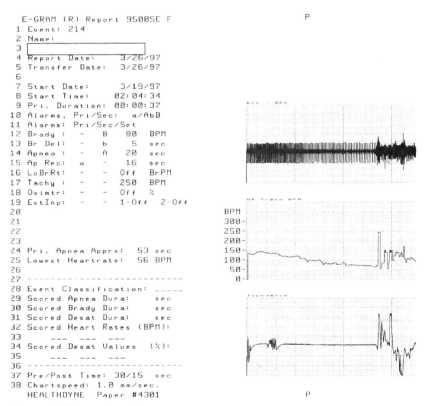

Figure 65. Documented home monitor recording of a 3-month-old, formerly 32 weeks' gestation, preterm infant. The event shows a 53-second central apnea associated with decrease in the heart rate to 62 BPM. The pathologic apnea resolved after the initiation of caffeine therapy.

2. Benefits/uses
   a. Alert caregivers to potentially serious central apnea or bradycardia
   b. Transition of a technology-dependent child
   c. Shortening the hospital stay for a symptomatic premature apneic infant
   d. Guidance of pharmacologic therapy
   e. Alleviation of family anxiety
   f. Reduction of SIDS (controversial)
3. Indications
   a. Premature infants with pathologic apnea or very young gestational age
   b. Infant with GERD and associated apnea or bradycardia
   c. Infant with ALTE
   d. Sibling of infant who died of SIDS
   e. Infant with certain underlying neurologic, cardiac, or pulmonary conditions (e.g., tracheostomy, central alveolar hypoventilation syndrome)
4. Indications: special consideration cases
   a. Infant with oxygen dependency
   b. Infant with apneic seizures
   c. Technology-dependent children
   d. Infants with a critically ill medical course
5. Limitations
   a. False alarms (especially with advancing age)
   b. Misguided faith and overdependence on monitor technology
   c. Additional family stress in some cases
   d. Poor compliance
   e. Limitation as a diagnostic tool (e.g., obstructive apnea)
   f. Dermatologic problems (skin irritation) from the monitor leads
   g. Vulnerable child syndrome
   h. Sibling jealousy
4. Criteria for discontinuation of monitoring
   a. Six to eight weeks after last significant clinical or documented event, once methylxanthines have been discontinued
   b. Four weeks free of events if the infant has a self-limited or treated condition (e.g., GER, respiratory syncytial virus)
   c. Age 6 months or until 1 month after the age of previous sibling's death if the child is an asymptomatic sibling of a SIDS victim
5. Key to safe, yet less stressful, use of a home monitor: a comprehensive program of evaluation, treatment, and follow-up

 a. Cardiopulmonary resuscitation (CPR) and monitor training for primary caregivers
 b. Twenty-four hour availability of vendor repair team and qualified support staff
 c. Regular review of recordings by an experienced professional
 d. Frequent communication among the experienced monitor professional, the family, and the primary medical provider
 G. Avoid parental alcohol and drug use if co-sleeping.

Suggested Reading

American Academy of Pediatrics Task Force on Infant Positioning and SIDS: positioning and SIDS. Pediatrics 1992; 89:1120–1126.

American Academy of Pediatrics Task Force on Infant Positioning & SIDS Update. Pediatrics 1996; 98:1216–1218.

Gibson E, Spinner S, Cullen JA, et al: Documented home apnea monitoring: effect on compliance, duration of monitoring, and validation of alarm reporting. Clin Pediatr 1996; 35:505–513.

Guilleminault C, Pelayo R, Clerk A, et al: Home nasal continuous positive airway pressure in infants with sleep disorders breathing. J Pediatr 1995; 127:905–912.

Gunasekaran TS, Hassall EG: Efficacy and safety of omeprazole for severe gastroesophageal reflux in children. J Pediatr 1993; 123:148–154.

Light MJ, Sheridan MS: Home monitoring in Hawaii: the first 1,000 patients. Hawaii Med J 1989; 48:304–310.

National Institutes of Health Consensus Development Conference on Infantile Apnea and Home Monitoring. Sept. 29 to Oct. 1, 1980. Pediatrics 1987; 79:292–299.

Spitzer AR, Gibson E: Home monitoring. Clin Perinatol 1992; 19:907–926.

SECTION VIII

High-Frequency Ventilation

Chapter 36

General Concepts of High-Frequency Ventilation

J. Bert Bunnell

I. **High-Frequency Ventilation (HFV) is Different from all other Forms of Mechanical Ventilation.**

A. HFV can ventilate patients who are virtually impossible to ventilate almost any other way.

B. HFV does not try to mimic normal breathing.

   1. HFV allows one to use small tidal volumes, even smaller than anatomic dead space.

   2. HFV provides a different distribution of gas within lungs.

      a. Airway resistance is the primary determinant of distribution.

      b. Unlike in conventional ventilation (CV), lung compliance is not an important factor.

C. HFV enables safe use of positive end-expiratory pressure (PEEP) that is higher than that used during CV.

   1. Higher PEEP better stabilizes surfactant-deficient alveoli.

   2. If PEEP is too high, it interferes with cardiac output, but risk of lung injury is associated more with the tidal volume (V_T) provided on top of PEEP, rather than PEEP itself.

D. Clinical comparisons of airway pressures monitored during HFV versus CV only approach relevancy at the distal end of the endotracheal tube (ETT).

   1. Distal airway pressure more closely approximates alveolar pressure.

   2. Distal pressure monitoring enables feedback control of gas delivery.

E. Proximal airway pressure monitoring can be very misleading during HFV.

   1. High-velocity gas flows create large pressure drops across the ETT.

   2. Thus, proximal pressure amplitude (i.e., $\Delta P = PIP - PEEP$) is misleadingly large compared to CV.

3. Meaningful proximal pressure monitoring during HFV is limited to mean airway pressure (Pāw).
4. However, if airways collapse, mean alveolar pressure can be greater than mean Paw.

II. **How HFV Works**

A. Resonant frequency phenomena
  1. Forced oscillations pulmonary function experiments revealed that the lungs have a natural or "resonant" frequency (e.g., 4–8 Hz [cycles per second] in adult humans). At resonance:
    a. Gas momentum supplies the energy to overcome lung compliance, and lung recoil supplies the energy to send gas back out of the lungs.
    b. Timing and energies are perfectly matched to conserve energy.
    c. Outside force is required *only* to overcome airway resistance.
  2. Therefore, less pressure is required to move gas in and out of the lungs at resonant frequency.
B. Asymmetric gas flow streaming, dead space reduction, and direct alveolar ventilation
  1. High-velocity inspiratory gas flows into the lungs down the central core of airways, or along one wall of some airways, as it passes bifurcations in short, abrupt bursts.
    a. The higher the velocity, the sharper the point on the bullet-shaped velocity profile of the in-rushing gas.
    b. *Effective* dead space volume (V_D) is reduced since only portions of the anatomic dead space are used.
    c. Fresh gas penetrates some alveoli directly even when $V_T <$ anatomic V_D.
  2. In high-frequency oscillatory ventilation (HFOV), gas is sucked from many airways into one (the trachea), causing a turbulent, *flat* expiratory wave front.
  3. In high-frequency jet ventilation (HFJV), gas flows out passively, seeking its path of least resistance in the annular or "unused" spaces around the highly accelerated inspired gas
  4. The net effect of several oscillations or HFJV cycles: fresh gas advances down the core of airways while exhaled gas moves out along airway walls.
C. Increased bulk flow (convection) and enhanced diffusion
  1. When one reduces HFV V_T but maintains constant $PaCO_2$, *minute* volume rises dramatically.
  2. The abundant fresh gas effectively washes out expired gas from the airways.
  3. Increased washout of expired gases increases O_2 and decreases

227

CO_2 partial pressures at the intra-airway gas exchange boundary, thereby increasing diffusion.

4. Examples of enhanced intrapulmonary gas exchange in nature occur in running and panting animals, and birds during vigorous flight.

III. Using HFV in the Neonatal Intensive Care Unit

A. Safe and reliable devices are available.

1. HFV devices were the first and are still the only type of mechanical ventilator required to be proven safe and effective before they can be marketed in the USA.

   a. The Food and Drug Administration (FDA) administers this *Premarket Approval (PMA)* process.

   b. All other ventilators are approved via the *510(k)* process whereby new equipment must be shown to be "substantially equivalent" to devices that are currently being legally sold in the USA. (Bases for comparison are products legally marketed in the USA before May 28, 1976.)

2. Three HFV devices have been FDA approved via this PMA process for use on newborns in the USA.

3. Several other devices are in use outside the USA.

B. What clinical disorders are theoretically amenable to HFV treatment?

1. Restrictive lung diseases (conditions accompanied by low lung compliance) such as pneumonia, tension pulmonary interstitial emphysema, diaphragmatic hernia, pulmonary hypoplasia, etc.

2. Atelectatic lung diseases such as respiratory distress syndrome (RDS), where alveoli can be safely opened through the use of high mean Paw HFV or HFV in conjunction with conservative intermittent mandatory ventilation (IMV) and optimal PEEP.

3. Some obstructive lung disorders, such as aspiration pneumonia, where the HFV modality applied is effective in facilitating removal of aspirated material and mucus (e.g., HFJV for meconium aspiration) and some airway stenoses where HFV improves ventilation/perfusion matching.

4. Pulmonary airleak syndromes and cardiac surgery patients benefit from low mean Paw HFV with its smaller tidal volumes and lower intrapulmonary pressure amplitudes.

5. Abrupt, high-velocity HFJV insufflations "shoot" inspired gas right past large, upper airway leaks and fistulas, allowing them to heal.

C. In what clinical conditions might HFV treatment be contraindicated?

1. Disorders such as asthma, wherein airway resistance is uniformly increased. (Very low rates and long expiratory times should be more effective here.)

2. Some nonhomogeneous lung disorders may not respond well to HFOV because of its active exhalation, which can further aggravate an already unfortunate distribution of ventilation.

IV. **Three Major Types of HFV Are Used Routinely**
   A. HFJV
      1. Inspired gas is injected into the ETT through a jet nozzle (typical frequency range: 150–660 bpm, or 2.5–11 Hz).
      2. Present-day devices use either a special ETT (e.g., Mallinckrodt Hi-Lo Jet® ETT, Mallinckrodt, Inc., St. Louis, MO, USA) or a special 15-mm ETT adapter (e.g., Bunnell LifePort,® Bunnell, Inc., Salt Lake City, UT, USA) with two side ports for gas injection and distal airway pressure monitoring, and the main lumen for spontaneous breathing, concomitant IMV, and HFV exhalation.
   B. HFOV
      1. HFOV provides sinusoidal, push-pull, piston-type ventilation from 180–900 bpm (3–15 Hz).
      2. Some devices allow inspiratory:expiratory (I:E) ratio (or percent inspiratory time [T_I]) to be adjusted from 1:1 to approximately 1:2.33.
   C. Hybrids (high-frequency positive pressure ventilators, "flow-interrupters," and combined HFV/IMV devices) may provide jet, oscillatory, or conventional ventilation over similar frequency ranges.

V. **How HFV Devices Differ from Conventional Ventilators and Each Other**
   A. Active versus passive exhalation
      1. HFOVs actively "suck" gas back out of the patient's lungs during exhalation.
         a. In cases where high mean Paw is useful, active exhalation allows higher frequencies to be used with fewer gas-trapping problems.
         b. When lower mean Paw(s) are used, the sucking action may promote airway collapse ("choke points") and more gas trapping, and mean *alveolar* pressure > mean *airway* pressure.
      2. All other types of HFV rely on the patient's passive exhalation.
         a. Must minimize I:E and limit rate to allow sufficient time for exhalation and avoid gas trapping.
         b. Works well when lower Paw is desired (e.g., airleaks, postcardiac surgery)

B. Interdependency of controls, fixed I:E, and their effects

 1. Many devices, particularly HFOV, exhibit direct interdependency between rate and delivered V_T when I:E ratios are held constant.

  a. As rate is increased, T_I decreases, so less V_T is delivered, and conversely.

  b. Since V_T is much more important for ventilation compared to rate (see below), $PaCO_2$ rises when rate is increased, which is counterintuitive.

 2. Other HFV devices maintain constant V_T when rate is changed.

  a. T_I is held constant.

  b. $PaCO_2$ rises and falls intuitively as rate is lowered and raised, respectively.

C. Proximal versus distal airway pressure monitoring (see above).

VI. How all HFV Devices are Similar

A. Effective frequencies

 1. Primary determinant of appropriate frequency is patient's weight.

 2. Optimal frequency produces best ventilation with lowest ΔP and V_T and no gas trapping.

 3. Venegas and Fredberg recommend finding and using the "corner frequency" (Figure 66).

  a. Plot peak pressure or pressure amplitude measured at the carina versus frequency.

  b. The "corner" occurs where pressure changes from falling rapidly to flattening out or rising.

  c. At this frequency, the lowest pressure for ventilation is required while avoiding gas trapping.

  d. Their analysis indicates that the smallest premature infant, with the stiffest lungs and highest airway resistance, has an optimal frequency of 10–12 Hz or 600–720 bpm.

  e. As compliance goes up, optimal frequency goes down. (Thus, any infant larger than the smallest would require a frequency <600–720 bpm.)

  f. As airway resistance improves (decreases), optimal frequency increases, because it is easier for the insufflated gas to get back out quickly.

B. Determinants of ventilation

 1. Several HFV investigators have found CO_2 elimination to be proportional to frequency times $(V_T)^2$.

 2. Thus, a frequency that is consistent with patient's size and condition (i.e., lung impedance) should be chosen, and ΔP or V_T should be adjusted to produce the desired $PaCO_2$.

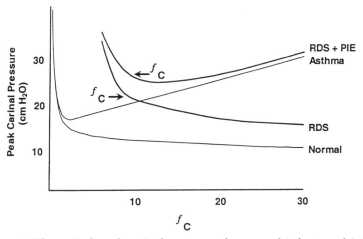

Figure 66. Theoretical peak carinal pressures for normal infants and infants with decreased compliance (RDS), increased airway resistance (asthma), and both low compliance and high airway resistance (RDS and PIE) with PEEP = 10 cm H_2O. Note how increased resistance reduces optimal frequency; however, most infants with RDS are well served using the corner frequency (f_C) of about 10 Hz in these examples. Using higher frequencies increases the risk of gas trapping. RDS = respiratory distress syndrome; PIE = pulmonary interstitial emphysema; PEEP = positive end-expiratory pressure. (Modified with permission from Venegas JG, Fredberg JJ: Understanding the pressure cost of high-frequency ventilation: why does high-frequency ventilation work? Crit Care Med 1994; 22:S49–S57, ©Williams & Wilkins.)

C. Determinants of oxygenation

    1. As in every form of mechanical ventilation, mean Paw and appropriate management of lung volume are the primary determinants of oxygenation.

    2. Since HFV offers the opportunity to use higher PEEP, it is very useful to separate alveolar recruitment from alveolar stabilization maneuvers *especially after successful recruitment.*

        a. Raise mean Paw (via increased baseline pressure or PEEP) or by adding concomitant IMV at rates up to 10 bpm to recruit collapsed alveoli.

        b. Once alveolar recruitment is evident by improved oxygenation (SaO_2), *discontinue the recruitment maneuver* (i.e., lower mean Paw) and rely on PEEP for maintenance of adequate alveolar volume.

        c. If SaO_2 subsequently falls, PEEP or mean Paw is evidently too low, so raise it immediately. (You may also have to re-recruit collapsed alveoli if you wait too long.)

3. To recruit lung volume in the absence of atelectasis, just raise mean Paw via baseline pressure or PEEP.

    a. Many neonatologists are very reluctant to use PEEP > 6 cm H_2O.

    b. Most preterm infants, however, need PEEP $\cong$ 7–8 cm H_2O, and it is usually safe and effective during HFV!

4. With nonhomogeneous lung disease where spotty atelectasis may be present, concomitant IMV at low rates (2–5 bpm) may be helpful to improve ventilation/perfusion matching.

VII. HFV Device Limitations

  A. HFJV

    1. Passive exhalation

      a. Must keep frequency tuned to patient size: larger patients require lower rates.

      b. Must pay attention to lung time constants: more compliant lungs require lower rates.

    2. Must be ready to suction right after initiation of HFJV.

      a. HFJV very effectively facilitates mucociliary clearance; be ready to take advantage of it!

      b. Do not suction as often after initial airway clearance; it just collapses alveoli.

  B. HFOV

    1. Active exhalation

      a. Watch out for choke points (gas trapping):

        (1) airway collapse caused by sucking action

        (2) evident when high $PaCO_2$ cannot be reduced

      b. Keep mean Paw up (select HFOV patients who will benefit from higher mean Paw).

    2. May not work well with nonhomogeneous lung disorders

    3. Watch out for mucus impaction.

      a. HFOV with I:E = 1:1 or 1:2 may hamper mucociliary clearance.

      b. Do not suction unless necessary; it just collapses alveoli.

  C. Hybrids and combined HFV and CV

    1. Compressible volume of conventional-style circuits limits ventilator power and effectiveness.

    2. Concomitant IMV must be managed appropriately.

      a. Increase IMV rate to actively recruit collapsed alveoli (5–10 bpm).

      b. Decrease IMV rate (0–3 bpm) when atelectasis resolves.

      c. Cease IMV (i.e., use only continuous positive airway pressure [CPAP]) when airleaks are present.

VIII. Weighing the Risks and Benefits of HFV

A. Use of appropriate ventilator strategies for specific lung disorders is more important than which ventilator is used.

B. Proper alveolar volume recruitment is critical for good oxygenation.

C. Finding and using optimal PEEP or mean Paw is also crucial.

D. It is still not certain what causes adverse side effects (intraventricular hemorrhage, periventricular leukomalacia, airleaks, mucus plugs) and how they can be mitigated.

IX. How to Optimize HFV

A. Learn when to start HFV without hesitation (when indicated by pathophysiology; weighing risks vs. benefits; associating ventilator patterns with potential injuries; etc.).

B. Match ventilator strategy to patient's pathophysiology and the availability of an appropriate device.

C. Choose HFV rate based on patient size and lung time constant.

D. Use minimum T_I or I:E ratio to maximize inspired gas penetration and minimize gas trapping.

    1. Shorter T_I allows more time for passive exhalation with HFJV.

    2. Greater percent expiration with HFOV means less force is required to suck gas back out (which means less chance of creating choke points).

E. Find and use optimal PEEP or mean Paw, paying particular attention to whether you need to recruit more lung volume or just stabilize the volume you have.

    1. Recruit collapsed alveoli by *temporarily* increasing concomitant IMV rate (if available).

    2. Once recruitment is successful, IMV rate should be reduced and PEEP must be optimized to support the open alveoli without compromising cardiac output.

F. Keep $PaCO_2$ in proper range using ΔP or V_T.

G. Adjust settings as patient's condition changes.

H. Do not stop prematurely.

    1. If an unacceptable blood gas results, reassess and adjust strategy.

    2. If an acceptable good blood gas is achieved, wean appropriately.

        a. Do not change back to conventional ventilation too soon. (Injured lungs take time to heal!)

        b. Do not drop PEEP or mean Paw when FiO_2 is still high.

X. Conclusions

A. HFV is not for every patient, but it may provide incredible benefits if the appropriate device is used on the appropriate patient in the appropriate way at the appropriate time.

B. Let comprehensive knowledge of pulmonary pathophysiology and respiratory therapy, and common sense, be the guides.

Suggested Reading

Bandy KP, Donn SM, Nicks JJ, Naglie RA: A comparison of proximal and distal high-frequency jet ventilation in an experimental animal model. Pediatr Pulmonol 1986; 2:225–229.

Boynton BR, Villanueva D, Hammond MD, et al: Effect of mean airway pressure on gas exchange during high-frequency oscillatory ventilation. J Appl Physiol 1991; 70:701–707.

Clark RH: High-frequency ventilation. J Pediatr 1994; 124:661–670.

Harris TR, Bunnell JB: High-frequency jet ventilation in clinical neonatology. In Pomerance JJ, Richardson CJ (Eds.): Neonatology for the Clinician. Norwalk, CT, Appleton & Lange, 1993, pp. 311–324.

Haselton FR, Scherer PW: Bronchial bifurcations and respiratory mass transport. Science 1980; 208:69–71.

Henderson Y, Chillingworth FP, Whitney JL: The respiratory dead space. Am J Physiol 1915; 38:1–19.

Perez Fontan JJ, Heldt GP, Gregory GA: Mean airway pressure and mean alveolar pressure during high frequency jet ventilation in rabbits. J Appl Physiol 1986; 61:456–463.

Venegas JG, Fredberg JJ: Understanding the pressure cost of high frequency ventilation: why does high frequency ventilation work? Crit Care Med 1994; 22:S49–S57.

Chapter 37

High-Frequency Jet Ventilation and the Bunnell Life Pulse® High-Frequency Jet Ventilator

Martin Keszler

I. **Indications**

   A. Late rescue: high-frequency jet ventilation (HFJV) has been extensively used for the treatment of refractory respiratory failure unresponsive to conventional ventilation (CV). Airleak syndrome has been the most commonly treated underlying disorder, but infants with severe diaphragmatic hernia, respiratory distress syndrome (RDS), meconium aspiration, and pneumonia have also been successfully rescued.

   B. Early rescue: HFJV has documented efficacy in the treatment of moderate to severe RDS, pulmonary interstitial emphysema (PIE), large leak through a bronchopleural fistula (intractable pneumothorax) or tracheoesophageal fistula, abdominal distention with poor chest wall compliance, congenital diaphragmatic hernia, and selected patients with meconium aspiration syndrome (MAS) with or without pulmonary hypertension.

   C. Prophylactic use: despite evidence of effectiveness of HFJV in lowering incidence of chronic lung disease (CLD), first-line treatment of infants with RDS at high risk for developing CLD is not yet widely practiced.

II. **Mechanism of Gas Exchange**

   A. Pulses of high-velocity jet stream of gas move down the center of the airway penetrating through the dead space gas which simultaneously moves outward along the periphery of the airway.

   B. Enhanced molecular diffusion probably plays an important role in the distal airways.

   C. Gas exchange is achieved with smaller tidal volumes and pressure amplitude than with CV.

III. **Benefits of HFJV**

   A. Lower pressure amplitude (ΔP = PIP - PEEP), where P is pressure, PIP is peak inspiratory pressure, PEEP is positive end-expiratory pressure.

B. Improved CO_2 elimination

C. Ability to use low mean airway pressure (Pāw) when indicated

D. Resolution of airleaks

E. Decrease in airflow through points of airway disruption

F. Ability to use high PEEP safely when indicated

G. Improved recruitment and maintenance of lung volume

H. Improved hemodynamics because of less interference with venous return

I. Mobilization of secretions and aspirated material

J. Decreased risk of chronic lung disease

IV. Possible Complications of HFJV

A. Mucosal damage was reported in some early studies when inadequate humidification was used. This is no longer a problem.

B. Increased incidence of periventricular leukomalacia and intraventricular hemorrhage (IVH) reported in one study – likely related to inadvertent hyperventilation. Similar findings were seen in some oscillatory ventilation studies and with conventional hyperventilation.

C. Air trapping is possible if inappropriately high ventilator rate is used.

V. Available Devices

A. The Bunnell Life Pulse (Bunnell Inc., Salt Lake City, UT, USA) is the only Food and Drug Administration (FDA) approved neonatal HFJV device currently available in the USA. Other HFJV devices manufactured in the USA are used in Europe and elsewhere.

B. The Life Pulse is a microprocessor-based ventilator that continuously monitors Paw and automatically adjusts the pressure that drives pulses of gas across the injector cannula to achieve the set PIP (range, 8–50 cm H_2O).

C. Ventilator rate (240–660 breaths/min = 4–11 Hz) and inspiratory time (T_I) (range, 0.02–0.034 sec) are set independently.

D. PEEP and superimposed low-rate intermittent mandatory ventilation (IMV) are generated by a conventional ventilator used in tandem with the Life Pulse.

E. The FiO_2 of the two ventilators can be adjusted separately (but should be maintained at the same level), or both ventilators can be supplied from a common source using a single blender.

F. PIP, mean Paw, pressure amplitude, and servo pressure are displayed on the face of the ventilator.

G. Alarms are automatically set 15% above and below current levels for PIP, mean Paw, and servo pressure once the values stabilize and the ventilator reaches the "ready" state. Subsequently, the alarm limits can be adjusted manually.

H. An efficient low volume humidifier is built into the device assuring optimal heating and humidification of inspired gases.

I. The delivery of gas is controlled by a pinch valve located in a "patient box" placed near the patient's head. The box also houses the pressure sensor. This arrangement ensures accurate pressure monitoring and efficient ventilation.

J. Reintubation is no longer required, because a special endotracheal tube adapter (LifePort®) containing a pressure-sensing lumen and the injector port has replaced the original triple lumen endotracheal tube formerly required for HFJV.

K. Suctioning can be done in one of two ways. The jet ventilator can be placed in standby mode and suctioning done in the usual fashion. Alternately, suctioning is done with the ventilator continuing to operate and constant suction is applied while the suction catheter is advanced and then withdrawn. This is necessary because the jet ventilator will force gas past the suction catheter and cause overpressure, unless continuous suction is applied.

VI. Clinical Use

A. Patient selection
1. Risks and benefits should be carefully considered before initiating HFJV (see above).
2. Early, rather than late, initiation is preferable in most situations.
3. Patient selection should be based on experience and published evidence of efficacy (see "Indications").
4. However, clinicians in the USA should be aware that, as of this writing, the FDA has only officially approved the Life Pulse for the treatment of PIE and for rescue of infants with refractory respiratory failure complicated by airleak.

B. Basic control of blood gases
1. Oxygenation is determined by FiO_2 and mean Paw (increased mean Paw = improved oxygenation).
2. Mean Paw is determined by PIP, PEEP, and T_I.
3. Ventilation (CO_2 elimination) is primarily determined by pressure amplitude ($\Delta P = PIP - PEEP$).
4. Rate has a relatively minor effect on ventilation. The usual range is 360–500 breaths/min, depending on the size of the baby and time constants. A rate that is too fast may increase $PaCO_2$ because of air trapping.
5. Background IMV rate of 2–5 breaths/minute is superimposed on the HFJV pulses to maintain lung volume (periodic sigh). The PIP should be the same as the HFJV PIP or slightly lower so as not to interrupt the jet. The T_I of the sigh breaths should be 0.3–0.5 seconds.

6. Note that sighs recruit lung volume but adequate mean Paw (PEEP) is needed to maintain it.

7. Weaning from HFJV is accomplished primarily by weaning PIP, leaving rate unchanged, except as dictated by changes in time constants (see below).

8. Note that decreasing amplitude by lowering PIP also lowers mean Paw and thus affects oxygenation. This problem can be avoided by increasing PEEP to compensate.

C. Matching ventilator strategy to disease pathophysiology

1. Choosing the appropriate ventilator strategy is critical – the wrong strategy may lead to lack of improvement and/or complications.

2. Ventilator settings must be selected according to the patient's specific needs.

3. The underlying disease, postnatal age, and patient size all must be considered in choosing an appropriate strategy and settings.

D. Low pressure strategy

1. This approach is appropriate when airleak is a major problem (i.e., PIE, pneumothorax) and the imperative is to reduce Paw(s) in an effort to resolve the airleak.

2. PIP should be set 10–15% below current levels on CV.

3. PEEP should be 3–5 cm H_2O, depending on severity of airleak and coexisting lung disease (may need to be higher if severe atelectasis coexists with PIE).

4. Remember that oxygenation is related to mean Paw and that it may deteriorate with the drop in pressure. Marginal PaO_2 may have to be accepted and generous FiO_2 is often needed.

5. T_I should be kept at the minimum value of 0.02 seconds.

6. Background IMV should be omitted if the lungs are overexpanded and severe PIE is present.

7. Optimal HFJV rate depends on an estimation of the patient's time constants (usual range, 360–420 breaths/min to allow adequate expiratory time).

8. If marginal oxygenation prevents further decrease in PIP but $PaCO_2$ is low, narrow the pressure amplitude by increasing PEEP to avoid hypocarbia and maintain oxygenation.

9. If diffuse atelectasis develops and oxygenation is inadequate, an increase in mean Paw, usually by increasing PEEP, is indicated, provided ventilation is adequate. The background IMV may be (re)started at this time.

10. If ventilation is also inadequate, PIP should be increased as well.

11. When airleak resolves and atelectasis becomes the dominant problem, switch to the optimal volume strategy (see below).

E. Optimal volume strategy

1. This strategy is appropriate in most situations, especially in RDS.

2. The goal is to optimize lung volume, thereby improving ventilation/perfusion matching and to avoid the recruitment/de-recruitment cycle typical of conventional large tidal volume (V_T) ventilation.

3. When switching from CV, mean Paw should be increased 10–15% by increasing PEEP.

4. The following rules of thumb can be used for initial PEEP settings:
set PEEP at 5 cm H_2O if FiO_2 is <0.30
set PEEP at 6–7 cm H_2O if FiO_2 is 0.30–0.50
set PEEP at 8 cm H_2O if FiO_2 is >0.50

5. PIP should initially remain the same as on CV. If starting HFJV without prior CV, choose a pressure that results in adequate chest wall movement.

6. Background sigh rate is set at 2–5/min with T_I of 0.3–0.5 seconds and PIP is set as high as possible without interrupting the jet ventilator.

7. Ventilator rate of 420–500 breaths/min with T_I of 0.02 seconds is appropriate early in the course of RDS, because time constants are short. Later, as compliance improves, rate should be lowered to avoid air trapping.

8. Optimization of lung volume is reflected by marked improvement in oxygenation. If the initial settings do not allow weaning of FiO_2 to <0.35, PEEP should be increased further.

9. *Rarely,* when severe atelectasis is present and not resolving with the above approach, conventional PIP may need to be increased above the jet PIP for a *brief* period and be allowed to interrupt the jet in order to re-expand the lungs. Remember that without sufficient PEEP to maintain lung volume, this will be ineffective and potentially damaging.

10. The background sigh rate or PIP should *not* be increased as a primary means of increasing mean Paw. This is more safely accomplished by raising PEEP. Remember that the large V_T of CV is the very thing you are trying to avoid!

11. Once lung volume is optimized, compliance will improve rapidly. This will be reflected in improved chest wall movement and CO_2 elimination. *PIP must be lowered promptly to avoid hypocarbia.*

12. Mean Paw should not be weaned until the FiO_2 is ≤0.30. Remember to compensate for decreasing PIP by raising PEEP.

13. Periodic chest radiographs are helpful in verifying adequate lung expansion/detecting overexpansion.

F. Treatment of meconium aspiration syndrome (MAS) and persistent pulmonary hypertension of the newborn (PPHN)

1. MAS is a heterogeneous disorder and evolves rapidly over time. The effectiveness of HFJV in this syndrome is variable, ranging from poor to dramatic.

2. In the acute phase, when large airways are obstructed with par-

ticulate meconium, HFJV may be ineffective as the jet stream is broken up by the obstructing debris.

3. When the surfactant inactivation or inflammatory effect predominates, HFJV is usually quite effective and the high volume strategy is appropriate. However, beware of overexpansion and air trapping. Remember: larger infants need slower rates; higher airway resistance requires slower rates. Typical range is 340–380 breaths/min.

4. HFJV provides a sort of internal vibration that helps to mobilize secretions/aspirated material. The expiratory flow along the periphery of the large airways brings the secretions proximally. Be ready to suction when initiating HFJV!

5. HFJV is an effective and relatively gentle means of hyperventilation, if this is desired to treat PPHN. Avoid extremes of $PaCO_2$ and pH which are easily achieved with HFJV, but may be dangerous.

G. Miscellaneous conditions responsive to HFJV

1. When diaphragmatic excursion is impaired by increased intraabdominal pressure, the small V_T of HFJV with sufficiently high PEEP to apply counterpressure on the diaphragm and maintain lung volume is advantageous. Babies with acute abdominal distention from necrotizing enterocolitis or similar conditions and those post-repair of gastroschisis, diaphragmatic hernia, or omphalocele often respond dramatically with improved gas exchange and hemodynamics.

2. Infants with airway disruption such as intractable pneumothorax with constant large flow through chest tubes, tracheoesophageal fistula, or tracheal tear respond with improved gas exchange and decreased flow through the point of airway disruption. This is because the jet stream moves down the center of the airway with virtually no lateral pressure on the airway wall. The gas that does escape is probably expiratory gas. The low pressure strategy is indicated.

3. Infants with lung hypoplasia benefit from the more gentle, small V_T ventilation possible with HFJV. Gentle hyperventilation is easily achieved in most cases where PPHN is present. An intermediate approach between the optimal volume and low pressure strategy works best.

H. Weaning from HFJV

1. Weaning is accomplished by lowering FiO_2 first and PEEP second, once the FiO_2 is ≤0.30.

2. PIP is lowered in response to low normal $PaCO_2$ or excessive chest wall movement. Remember to compensate for decreasing PIP by increasing the PEEP, if necessary, to maintain mean Paw.

3. Ventilator rate is not decreased as a means of weaning. However, if initially >420 breaths/min, it may need to be lowered to accommodate lengthening time constants because of increasing compliance and/or increasing resistance as RDS evolves.

4. It is possible to wean directly to continuous positive airway pressure (CPAP). This is often possible, once PIP is ≤10–12 cm H_2O and PEEP ≤6 cm H_2O.

5. Alternately, once the pressure is ≤14–18 cm H_2O and PEEP ≤6 cm H_2O, you can switch to CV. Usually a 10–15% higher PIP is needed after switching.

Suggested Reading

Gonzalez F, Harris T, Black P, et al: Decreased gas flow through pneumothoraces in neonates receiving high-frequency jet versus conventional ventilation. J Pediatr 1987; 110:464–466.

Harris TR, Bunnell JB: High-frequency jet ventilation in clinical neonatology. In Pomerance JJ, Richardson CJ (Eds.): *Neonatology for the Clinician.* Norwalk, CT, Appleton & Lange, 1993, pp. 311–324.

Keszler M, Donn S, Bucciarelli R, et al: Multi-center controlled trial of high-frequency jet ventilation and conventional ventilation in newborn infants with pulmonary interstitial emphysema. J Pediatr 1991; 119:85–93.

Keszler M, Modanlou HD, Brudno DS, et al: Multi-center controlled clinical trial of high frequency jet ventilation in preterm infants with uncomplicated respiratory distress syndrome. Pediatrics 1997; 100:593–599.

Sugiura M, Nakabayashi H, Vaclavik S, Froese AB: Lung volume maintenance during high frequency jet ventilation improves physiological and biochemical outcome of lavaged rabbit lung. Physiologist 1990; 33:A123.

Wiswell TE, Graziani LJ, Kornhauser MS, et al: High-frequency jet ventilation in the early management of respiratory distress syndrome is associated with a greater risk for adverse outcomes. Pediatrics 1996; 98:1035–1043.

Wiswell TE, Graziani LJ, Kornhauser MS, et al: Effects of hypocarbia on the development of cystic periventricular leukomalacia in premature infants treated with high-frequency jet ventilation. Pediatrics 1996; 98:918–924.

Chapter 38

High-Frequency Oscillatory Ventilation

Reese H. Clark, Dale R. Gerstmann

I. **Background**

  A. Definition – high-frequency oscillatory ventilation (HFOV) is rapid rate, low tidal volume form of mechanical ventilation

  B. Reasons for development of HFOV:

    1. To improve gas exchange in patients with severe respiratory failure

    2. To reduce ventilator-associated lung injury

      a. Prevention of volutrauma. HFOV dramatically reduces the tidal volume needed to maintain ventilation (normocarbia). During HFOV, the lung is held close to mean lung volume. There is minimal change in lung volume with each delivered breath. Visually, this translates to chest wall vibration that is barely perceptible. In contrast, during conventional ventilation (CV) the lung is cycled from low to high volume with each breath and chest rise and fall easily visible.

      b. Reduced exposure to inspired oxygen. HFOV improves the uniformity of lung inflation, reduces intrapulmonary shunt, and improves oxygenation. The need for supplemental oxygen is reduced and exposure to oxygen free radicals is decreased.

    3. To decrease pulmonary morbidity in patients who require assisted ventilation

    4. To provide a method of assisted ventilation that allows severe pulmonary airleaks to heal.

II. **Difference Between HFOV and CV**

A. Parameter	CV	HFOV
1. Rate (BPM)	0–60	180–1,200
2. Tidal volume (mL/kg)	4–20	0.1–5
3. Alveolar pressure (cm H_2O)	5–50	0.1–20
4. End-expiratory lung volume	low	high

B. Advantages of HFOV

   1. Improves ventilation at lower pressure and volume swings in the lung

   2. Safer way of using "super" positive end-expiratory pressure (PEEP). The lung can be inflated to higher mean volumes without having to use high peak airway pressures (Paw) to maintain ventilation (CO_2 removal).

   3. Produces more uniform lung inflation

   4. Reduces airleak

C. Disadvantages of HFOV

   1. Compared to CV there is a greater potential for gas trapping and the development of inadvertent PEEP. The time for exhalation during HFOV is *very short.* Gas delivered to the lung during the inspiratory cycle may become trapped in the lung. This "trapped" gas can cause overinflation of the lung and lung injury (stretch injury, e.g., pulmonary interstitial emphysema [PIE], pneumothorax). The propensity for gas trapping is dependent on the device being used. Devices that facilitate exhalation are less likely to cause gas trapping than devices that depend on the passive recoil of the chest and lung.

   2. Defining optimal mean lung volume is difficult yet crucial to the safe use of HFOV.

   a. Lung overinflation is associated with decreased venous return and compromised cardiac output. It can also cause acute lung injury especially if cardiac output is compromised.

   b. Underinflation of the lung is equally dangerous. Collapsed lungs are difficult to recruit and recruitment of collapsed lungs can be associated with significant lung injury. Atelectasis is also associated with increased pulmonary vascular resistance, increased intra- and extrapulmonary shunts, and life-threatening hypoxemia.

III. Types of HFOV

   A. Diaphragm HFOV with a variable fractional inspiratory time. The SensorMedics 3100A® (SensorMedics Inc., Yorba Linda, CA, USA) oscillatory ventilator is the only HFOV device approved for use in newborns in the USA. It is an electronically controlled diaphragm that produces pressure oscillation in the patient circuit. The mean Paw is set independently from the pressure oscillations. Adjusting the bias flow or the outlet resistance in the patient circuit controls mean Paw.

   B. Piston HFOV with a fixed fractional inspiratory time. These types of HFOV have used a 1:1 inspiratory:expiratory (I:E) ratio. In healthy adult rabbits, the use of a 1:1 I:E ratio has been shown to be associated with gas trapping and inadvertent PEEP. Newer devices allow for 1:2 and 1:1 I:E ratios. The Hummingbird (Medtran, Tokyo, Japan) is the best example of this type of HFOV. This ventilator is used widely in Japan.

C. Hybrid devices employ a Venturi device to generate negative pressure during the expiratory cycle of ventilation.

IV. **Calculations of Minute Ventilation (i.e., quantity of CO_2 removed from the lung)**

A. For CV: rate $\times$ tidal volume

B. For HFOV: rate$^{(0.5-1)} \times V_T^{(1.5-2)}$

　　1. This equation predicts that factors effecting tidal volume (V_T) delivery have a larger impact on ventilation during HFOV than they do for CV. Changes in endotracheal tube size, lung compliance, airway resistance, and chest wall rigidity all impact delivery of "tidal volume."

　　2. It is also important to remember that the impedance of the respiratory system increases with frequency. During HFOV, as frequency is increased, tidal volume delivery and minute ventilation may decrease.

　　3. Some devices, such as the SensorMedics 3100A, decrease V_T output at higher frequencies, which can be compensated for by increasing the power setting.

C. Theory for improved ventilation during HFOV

　　1. Enhanced molecular diffusion

　　2. Enhanced convection (Pendelluft effect)

　　3. Taylor dispersion

　　4. Reduced dependence on bulk convection

D. Oxygenation

　　1. Directly related to the degree of lung inflation

　　2. Dependent on FiO_2

E. Physiologically targeted strategies of HFOV

　　1. Poor lung inflation. HFOV has its most dramatic effects in infants and children whose primary pathophysiology is decreased lung inflation. When used with continuous distending pressure (CDP) directed at recruiting lung volume, and followed by careful weaning of the CDP once lung inflation is improved and FiO_2 is decreased, HFOV reduces lung injury and promotes healthy survival. This approach exploits the concept of pressure-volume hysteresis, assuming the lung still has some recruitable volume. By using a CDP that is higher than the lung opening pressure, and usually greater than that which could be safely applied during CV, HFOV recruits collapsed lung units. Once open, these lung units can usually be maintained open at a lower mean Paw.

　　2. Pulmonary hypertension. HFOV can be effective in patients with pulmonary hypertension if the process leading to pulmonary hy-

pertension is poor lung inflation and regional hypoxia and hypercarbia. Improving lung inflation improves ventilation/perfusion matching and gas exchange, thereby relaxing the pulmonary vascular bed and decreasing pulmonary arterial pressure. HFOV is not as effective in patients with airway obstruction or in patients with poor cardiac output. Airway obstruction attenuates the pressure signal as it is propagated across the airways to the alveolus. This attenuation decreases the alvelolar ventilation and reduces ventilator efficiency. In patients with poor cardiac output, the constant high end-expiratory pressure can decrease venous return and impair cardiac output.

3. Reported indications for HFOV. Numerous clinical reports of uncontrolled trials of the use of HFOV as a rescue technique have been published. The absolute indications and contraindications remain to be established by carefully controlled clinical trials. The following list represents reported indications for HFOV:

    a. Persistent airleak (e.g., bronchopleural fistula, pulmonary interstitial emphysema [PIE])

    b. Persistent neonatal respiratory failure associated with:

        (1) Respiratory distress syndrome (RDS)

        (2) Pneumonia

        (3) Adult respiratory distress syndrome (ARDS)

        (4) Meconium aspiration syndrome (MAS)

        (5) Lung hypoplasia syndromes

        (6) Congenital diaphragmatic hernia (CDH)

        (7) Hydrops fetalis

        (8) Potter's variant

    c. Tracheoesophageal fistula in patients who are not surgical candidates (e.g., premature infants)

    d. Primary pulmonary hypertension which is responsive to reversal of atelectasis and controlled alkalosis. HFOV may be able to produce alkalosis with less barotrauma than CV.

4. Reported contraindications

    a. Airway disease associated with gas trapping. Most authors agree that HFOV is not effective in patients with airway obstruction. The use of HFOV in patients with airway disease can accentuate problems with gas trapping.

    b. Shock. Appropriate use of HFOV increases mean lung volume. As lung volume increases, right atrial volume will decrease. These changes impede venous return. Reduced venous return may amplify problems with hypotension unless preload is increased. These problems are similar to the problems seen with increasing levels of PEEP.

F. Specific reports and summary of results of clinical trials

    1. RDS

The largest prospective study involving HFOV was reported by the HIFI Study Group. Of 673 preterm infants weighing between 750 g and 2,000 g, 346 were assigned to receive CV and 327 to receive HFOV. No infant received surfactant. The incidence of bronchopulmonary dysplasia (BPD) was nearly identical in the two groups. HFOV did not reduce mortality or the level of ventilatory support during the first 28 days. HFOV was associated with an increased incidence of pneumoperitoneum of pulmonary origin, grades 3 and 4 intracranial hemorrhage, and periventricular leukomalacia. These results suggested that HFOV, as used in this trial, did not offer any advantage over CV, and it might be associated with undesirable side effects.

2. In a much smaller study (n = 98), also in non-surfactant-treated infants, Clark et al. showed that HFOV could be used to reduce the incidence of chronic lung disease in premature infants with hyaline membrane disease (HMD) without increasing the incidence of intraventricular hemorrhage (IVH), when used with strategies designed to recruit lung volume. The average CDP used during HFOV was 2–3 cm H_2O higher than the mean Paw used during CV.

3. In a multicenter trial (n = 176), the HIFO study group showed that rescue HFOV could be used to reduce the incidence of airleak syndromes in infants with established severe lung disease. There was a slight increase in incidence of grades 3 and 4 IVH in those treated with HFOV.

4. In the most recent clinical trial, all infants received surfactant. The purpose of this study was to compare the hospital course and clinical outcome of preterm infants with RDS treated with surfactant and managed with HFOV or CV as the primary mode of ventilator support. One-hundred twenty-five infants of ≤35 weeks estimated gestation with arterial to alveolar oxygen ratio <0.5 were studied. HFOV was used in a strategy to promote lung recruitment and maintain lung volume. Patients randomized to HFOV demonstrated the following significant findings compared with CV-treated patients: vasopressor support was less intensive; surfactant redosing was not as frequent; oxygenation improved more rapidly and remained higher during the first 7 days; fewer infants required prolonged supplemental oxygen or ventilator support; treatment failure was reduced; more patients survived without chronic lung disease at 30 days; need for continuous supplemental oxygen at discharge was less; frequency of necrotizing enterocolitis was lower; there were fewer abnormal hearing tests; and hospital costs were decreased. When used early with a lung recruitment strategy, HFOV after surfactant replacement resulted in clinical outcomes consistent with a reduction in both acute and chronic lung injury.

5. Using the Infant Star® HFOV (Infrasonics, Inc., San Diego, CA, USA) and a volume recruitment strategy, Thome et al. were unable to reproduce the results reported by Gerstmann et al. (HFOV) or Keszler et al. (high-frequency jet ventilation [HFJV]).

G. Current status

1. Animal studies show that HFOV reduces lung injury, promotes more uniform lung inflation, improves gas exchange, and prolongs the effectiveness of exogenous surfactant in experimental models of acute lung injury.

2. Clinical studies show that the results are strategy specific. When used with a strategy designed to optimize lung inflation, HFOV can be used safely to reduce the occurrence of chronic lung disease. However, technology is everchanging and the debate over the best surfactant and the most gentle mode of conventional ventilation rages on.

H. Airleak syndromes

1. PIE. Two large series of patients have been reported.

   a. Keszler et al. (n = 144). Patients were randomly assigned to rapid-rate CV or HFJV. Using defined crossover criteria, HFJV was more successful than CV (61% vs. 37%, p <0.01). PIE resolved more quickly; oxygenation and ventilation were improved, and patients managed with HFJV could be weaned to lower ventilator settings more rapidly.

   b. Clark et al. showed that HFOV improved gas exchange in premature infants with severe respiratory failure and PIE. Compared with previously reported data involving CV, HFOV also appeared to improve survival.

   c. In both studies, infants with severe disease and infants <1.0 kg were less responsive than those treated more proactively and who were more mature.

   d. Current status: PIE remains a serious complication of assisted ventilation. The introduction of surfactant has reduced the incidence of PIE but has not eliminated the disease process. HFOV improves gas exchange and appears to improve the outcome of patients with PIE. However, affected infants are at high risk for long-term pulmonary and neurological morbidity.

2. Pneumothoraces

   a. Blum-Hoffman showed that HFOV was effective in improving oxygenation and ventilation in patients with airleak syndromes. Carter et al. reported similar results.

   b. Current status: both HFJV and HFOV appear to improve gas exchange and allow for more rapid resolution of pneumothoraces.

3. Extracorporeal membrane oxygenation (ECMO) candidates

   a. Paranka et al. demonstrated that 50% of the ECMO-eligible patients could be rescued with HFOV alone. The outcome of patients rescued with HFOV was as good as for those who went on to require ECMO. Patients with CDH (30%) and MAS (50%) were not as likely to respond to HFOV as were patients with pneumonia (85%) and/or RDS (90%).

   b. Vaucher et al., using a different type of HFOV and a different clinical strategy, did not demonstrate results as encouraging as the Paranka et al. study. This study suggested that patients who met criteria for treatment with ECMO and were treated with ECMO had less chronic lung disease than infants who were "rescued" with alternate therapies. Walsh-Sukys presented similar findings. Both of these studies show that prolonged use of HFOV or CV to avoid ECMO may increase the risk for development of chronic lung disease.

c. Kinsella et al. reported that treatment with HFOV and nitric oxide was more effective than either therapy alone in the management of babies with lung disease and pulmonary hypertension. This finding was particularly true for infants with RDS or MAS.

d. Current status: as in RDS, the results achieved with HFOV are likely to be device and strategy specific. The relative role that surfactant, nitric oxide, liquid ventilation, HFOV and ECMO play in the management of full-term infants with severe respiratory failure has not yet been determined. It is clear that HFOV improves gas exchange and may reduce the need for ECMO in patients who are considered to be ECMO candidates. There are also data to suggest that HFOV can be used to improve the effectiveness of inhaled nitric oxide.

I. Reported complications of HFOV

1. Adverse cardiopulmonary interactions – increasing mean Paw during any form of ventilation increases lung volume. As lung volume increases, intrathoracic pressure increases and right atrial size decreases. As a result, venous return and thus cardiac output can be reduced. This problem is analogous to the reduction of cardiac output that is seen when a high level of PEEP is used. The interaction of mean Paw with cardiac output and organ blood flow is intimately related to lung compliance and lung volume. As lung compliance improves, lung volume increases even if mean Paw is not changed. It is essential to maintain the balance between adequate lung volume and cardiac preload. During HFOV, lung volume is nearly constant. Failure to maintain adequate preload and/or optimal lung volume can result in progressive hypotension.

2. Necrotizing tracheobronchitis has not been a reported complication of HFOV, but was seen earlier in other forms of HFV.

3. Mucostasis

a. The HFOV I:E setting effects mucus clearance from the lung. Mucus can build up in the airways during HFOV. When weaned from HFOV and returned to CV, some patients will rapidly mobilize these secretions. Airways can become occluded and frequent suctioning may be required during the 24–48 hour period following HFOV. Airway trauma associated with suctioning should be avoided by passing the suction catheter only 1 centimeter below the endotracheal tube. While mucostasis is an uncommon complication of HFOV, it can be life threatening.

    b. Gerstmann et al. found that premature patients with RDS who were treated with HFOV actually required less suctioning.

    c. Management of airway secretions must be individualized. Try to avoid suctioning unless clinically indicated (increasing $PaCO_2$, visible airway secretions, or decreasing oxygen saturation).

  4. Gas trapping – see above

  5. Intraventricular hemorrhage and periventricular leukomalacia. Recent meta-analysis suggests that the association between HFOV and poor neurologic outcome is more related to how HFOV is used rather than whether it is used. HFOV can cause rapid reduction in $PaCO_2$, which can cause sudden changes in cerebral blood flow. To use HFOV safely, acute changes in ventilation, especially overventilation (i.e., hypocarbia and alkalosis), must be avoided.

J. General and disease-specific recommendations

  1. Atelectasis with diffuse radiopacification of the lung (RDS or pneumonia)

    a. The CDP required to optimize lung inflation is higher than that which can be achieved on CV. Mean Paw can be increased in 1–2 cm H_2O increments until PaO_2 improves or the chest radiograph shows normal inflation. Evidence of overinflation or signs of cardiac compromise should be avoided. Radiographic signs of overinflation include extra clear lung fields, a small heart, flattened diaphragms, and more than nine posterior ribs of lung inflation. Signs of cardiac compromise include increased heart rate, decreased blood pressure, poor peripheral perfusion, and metabolic acidosis.

    b. Mean Paw used in the management of uncomplicated RDS in premature infants is generally lower than that used to treat term newborns. The severity of the lung disease, the age at start of HFOV, the use of surfactant, and the presence of infection will all influence the amount of pressure that is required. CDPs commonly reported are:

      (1) For infants <1 kg, 5–18 cm H_2O

      (2) For infants 1–2 kg, 6–20 cm H_2O

      (3) For infants >2 kg, 10–25 cm H_2O

    c. Frequency is generally held constant at 10–15 Hz. Most clinical data report the use of 10 Hz. In infants who are <1 kg, extreme caution must be taken to avoid hyperventilation and alkalosis. If $PaCO_2$ is low and the pressure amplitude is <20 cm H_2O, the frequency may need to be increased in order to decrease minute ventilation and allow the $PaCO_2$ to rise to a normal range. Also, if small changes in power settings result in larger changes in $PaCO_2$, ventilation control will be improved by increasing the frequency from 10 to 15 Hz.

  2. MAS

    a. Some MAS patients present with diffuse lung injury with limited pulmonary hypertension and minimal airway obstruction. These patients respond as described above.

    b. In contrast, some newborns with MAS have severe airway obstruction and pulmonary hypertension. These infants are not as responsive to HFOV.

    c. During the initiation of HFOV in patients with MAS, a chest radiograph should be taken to assess lung inflation and to rule out evidence of gas trapping. Lowering the frequency and increasing CDP may reduce gas trapping from narrowed airways.

    d. Patients who have poor lung inflation, minimal improvement in gas exchange during HFOV, and clinical evidence of pulmonary hypertension are more likely to respond to a combination of HFOV and inhaled nitric oxide than to either therapy alone.

3. Lung hypoplasia syndromes

    a. Similar to patients with MAS, the patients most likely to respond to HFOV are those in whom the primary pathophysiologic process is poor lung inflation.

    b. Patients whose lung volumes have been optimized on HFOV as evidenced by clear lung fields, but who still have severe pulmonary hypertension, are less likely to respond to HFOV alone.

    c. Patients with both poor lung inflation and pulmonary hypertension may be best treated with a combination of HFOV and inhaled nitric oxide.

4. Airleak syndrome

    a. Patients who have severe persistent airleak (like PIE or recurrent pneumothoraces) require a different approach. The goal of assisted ventilatory support must be to allow the airleak to resolve. If the airleak is unilateral, placing the involved lung in the dependent position will increase the resistance to gas flow to this lung and promote atelectasis. Both lung collapse and decreased ventilation of the dependent lung will promote airleak resolution.

    b. In addition to dependent positioning, using a strategy of HFOV that emphasizes decreasing mean Paw over decreasing FiO_2 will facilitate airleak resolution.

5. Idiopathic pulmonary hypertension with normal lung inflation
These patients are easy to ventilate on low levels of conventional support. HFOV is not as effective in these patients and can be associated with the development of life-threatening hypoxemia if the balance between preload and lung volume is not carefully addressed.

Suggested Reading

Anonymous: Randomized study of high-frequency oscillatory ventilation in infants with severe respiratory distress syndrome. HIFO Study Group. J Pediatr 1993; 122:609–619.

Anonymous: High-frequency oscillatory ventilation compared with conventional mechanical ventilation in the treatment of respiratory failure in preterm infants. The HIFI Study Group. N Engl J Med 1989; 320:88–93.

Blum-Hoffman E, Kopotic RJ, Mannino FL: High-frequency oscillatory ventilation combined with intermittent mandatory ventilation in critically ill neonates: 3 years of experience. Eur J Pediatr 1988; 147:392–398.

Carter JM, Gerstmann DR, Clark RH, et al: High-frequency oscillatory ventilation and extracorporeal membrane oxygenation for the treatment of acute neonatal respiratory failure. Pediatrics 1990; 85:159–164.

Clark RH, Dykes FD, Bachman TE, et al: Intraventricular hemorrhage and high-frequency ventilation: a meta-analysis of prospective clinical trials. Pediatrics 1996; 98:1058–1061.

Clark RH, Gerstmann DR, Null DM, et al: Prospective randomized comparison of high-frequency oscillatory and conventional ventilation in respiratory distress syndrome. Pediatrics 1992; 89:5–12.

Clark RH, Gerstmann DR, Null DM, et al: Pulmonary interstitial emphysema treated by high-frequency oscillatory ventilation. Crit Care Med 1986; 14:926–930.

Clark RH, Yoder BA, Sell MS: Prospective, randomized comparison of high-frequency oscillation and conventional ventilation in candidates for extracorporeal membrane oxygenation. J Pediatr 1994; 124:447–454.

Clark RH: High-frequency ventilation. J Pediatr 1994; 124:661–670.

Fredberg JJ, Allen J, Tsuda A, et al: Mechanics of the respiratory system during high frequency ventilation. Acta Anaesthesiol Scand 1989; 90:39–45.

Gerstmann DR, Minton SD, Stoddard RA, et al: The Provo multicenter early high-frequency oscillatory ventilation trial: improved pulmonary and clinical outcome in respiratory distress syndrome. Pediatrics 1996; 98: 1044–1057.

Gerstmann DR, deLemos RA, Clark RH: High-frequency ventilation: issues of strategy. Clin Perinatol 1991; 18:563–580.

Keszler M, Modanlou HD, Brudno DS, et al: Multicenter controlled clinical trial of high-frequency jet ventilation in preterm infants with uncomplicated respiratory distress syndrome. Pediatrics 1997; 100:593–599.

Keszler M, Donn SM, Bucciarell RL, et al: Multicenter controlled trial comparing high-frequency jet ventilation and conventional mechanical ventilation in newborn infants with pulmonary interstitial emphysema. J Pediatr 1991; 119:85–93.

Kinsella JP, Truog WE, Walsh WF, et al: Randomized, multicenter trial of inhaled nitric oxide and high-frequency oscillatory ventilation in severe, persistent pulmonary hypertension of the newborn. J Pediatr 1997; 131: 55–62.

Paranka MS, Clark RH, Yoder BA, et al: Predictors of failure of high-frequency oscillatory ventilation in term infants with severe respiratory failure. Pediatrics 1995; 95:400–404.

Thome U, Kossel H, Lipowsky G, et al: Randomized comparison of high-frequency ventilation with high-rate intermittent positive pressure ventilation in preterm infants with respiratory failure. J Pediatr 1999; 135:39–46.

Vaucher YE, Dudell GG, Bejar R, et al: Predictors of early childhood outcome in candidates for extracorporeal membrane oxygenation. J Pediatr 1996; 128:109–117.

Wiswell TE, Clark RH, Null DM, et al: Tracheal and bronchial injury in high-frequency oscillatory ventilation and high-frequency flow interruption compared with conventional positive-pressure ventilation. J Pediatr 1988; 112:249–256.

Chapter 39

SensorMedics 3100A® High-Frequency Oscillatory Ventilator

David J. Durand, Jeanette M. Asselin

I. **Physiology of High-Frequency Oscillatory Ventilation (HFOV)**
   A. Conceptual difference between conventional and high-frequency ventilation
      1. With conventional ventilation (CV), gas is moved from the upper airway to the alveoli primarily by *bulk flow* ("pouring gas into and out of the alveoli").
      2. With HFOV, gas movement is accomplished primarily by the *mixing* of gas in the upper airway with gas in the alveoli ("shaking gas into and out of the alveoli").
      3. This *mixing* phenomena occurs as the result of some very complex mechanisms.
   B. Characterizing HFOV breaths
      1. The SensorMedics 3100A (SensorMedics, Inc., Yorba Linda, CA, USA) generates a pressure wave which, when measured at the hub of the endotracheal tube, is approximately a sine wave.
      2. This pressure pattern is characterized primarily by three factors, each of which can be independently adjusted:
         a. Mean airway pressure (Pāw) – the average pressure throughout the respiratory cycle
         b. Amplitude – the size of the pressure wave, or tidal volume
         c. Frequency – the number of breaths per minute
   C. Oxygenation and ventilation
      1. Oxygenation is proportional to mean Paw.
         a. The higher the mean Paw, the greater the number of alveoli that are open throughout the respiratory cycle. This decreases atelectasis and improves ventilation/perfusion matching.
         b. Increasing mean Paw increases average lung volume, and is reflected by increased lung volume on chest radiography.
      2. Ventilation (or CO_2 removal) is approximately proportional to (frequency) $\times$ (amplitude)^2.

    a. The primary implication of this is that changes in amplitude have a greater impact on CO_2 exchange than do changes in frequency.

    b. For most patients a frequency is chosen and left constant, while CO_2 exchange is affected by changing the amplitude.

  3. Effect of frequency on amplitude

    a. The endotracheal tube and upper airway act as a *low pass filter*. This means that low-frequency pressure waves are passed from the ventilator to the alveoli without being attenuated, while high-frequency pressure waves are attenuated. The higher the frequency, the greater the attenuation.

    b. A simplified example of the attenuation of pressure amplitude at high frequencies is outlined below. Imagine a ventilator that is set to deliver an amplitude of 20 cm H_2O (e.g., peak inspiratory pressure [PIP], 25 cm H_2O; positive end-expiratory pressure [PEEP], 5 cm H_2O).

      (1) At a low frequency (e.g., 30 breaths/min), this pressure amplitude of 20 cm H_2O is completely transmitted to the alveoli. The alveolar pressure changes from 5 to 25 cm H_2O as the ventilator cycles.

      (2) At an intermediate frequency (e.g., 120 breaths/min), the pressure amplitude will be slightly attenuated as it travels from the hub of the endotracheal tube to the alveoli. The alveoli will "see" a breath with a PIP of 22 and a PEEP of 8. Thus, the amplitude of the breath will have been *attenuated* from 20 cm H_2O to 14 cm H_2O.

      (3) At a higher frequency (e.g., 600 breaths/min), the attenuation is far more significant. A breath with an amplitude of 20 cm H_2O at the hub of the endotracheal tube may be attenuated to <5 cm H_2O at the alveoli.

    c. If everything else is constant, *decreasing frequency will increase alveolar amplitude*. Since amplitude has a greater impact on CO_2 exchange than does frequency, *decreasing frequency will increase CO_2 exchange*.

II. HFOV Has Two Theoretical Advantages Over Conventional Modes of Ventilation Which Deliver a Tidal Breath.

  A. With HFOV, the alveolus never deflates to the degree that it does with CV. Thus, surface forces are less likely to cause atelectasis. Preventing atelectasis is a key element in avoiding lung injury.

  B. With HFOV, the alveolus is never inflated with a typical tidal volume, so there is less chance of causing alveolar overdistension. Alveolar overdistension is a primary cause of both acute and chronic lung injury.

III. When to Use the SensorMedics 3100A

  A. HFOV is probably superior to CV for any lung disease characterized by severe, homogeneous decrease in compliance, and no airway involvement. The ideal HFOV patient is one with the "white out" of severe respiratory distress syndrome (RDS).

B. HFOV is probably better than CV for the patient with severe pulmonary interstitial emphysema (PIE) or bronchopleural fistula.

C. HFOV may be better than CV for term patients with severe nonhomogeneous disease like pneumonia or meconium aspiration syndrome (MAS).

D. HFOV may be superior to CV for most (or all) premature infants with lung disease. This has not been conclusively demonstrated, and there is at least one large trial in progress to test this hypothesis.

E. We prefer HFOV for most patients who meet one of the following criteria:

    1. FiO_2 >0.4–0.5

    2. PIP >25 cm H_2O

    3. Moderate or severe PIE or bronchopleural fistula (these patients may also be treated with high-frequency jet ventilaton).

IV. Mechanics of the SensorMedics 3100A: Only Six Parameters Can be Adjusted

A. Mean Paw, measured in cm H_2O

    1. Mean Paw is set by adjusting the pressure adjust knob.

    2. Increasing mean Paw recruits alveoli, leading to improved ventilation/perfusion matching, and improved oxygenation.

    3. Increasing mean Paw also leads to increased lung inflation, as seen on chest radiography.

    4. When placing a patient on HFOV, start with a mean Paw that is 2–3 cm H_2O above the mean Paw on CV.

    5. Follow chest radiographs closely to determine degree of lung inflation.

        a. In most patients, the lungs should be inflated so that the top of the right hemidiaphragm is between the 8th and 10th rib.

        b. Patients on HFOV should usually have chest radiographs ordered according to the following schedule *as a minimum*:

            (1) 30–60 minutes after starting HFOV

            (2) 2–4 hours after starting HFOV

            (3) 12 hours after starting HFOV

            (4) q 12 hours for the next 48 hours

            (5) q 24 hours until off HFOV

            (6) After any large change in mean Paw

    6. Changes in mean Paw

        a. Increase mean Paw if the lungs are underinflated and/or the patient is not oxygenating adequately.

   b. Decrease mean Paw if the lungs are overinflated and/or if the patient's oxygenation is improving.

   c. To cause a small change in lung inflation and/or oxygenation, change the mean Paw by 10–20%.

   d. To cause a larger change in lung inflation and/or oxygenation, change the mean Paw by 20–40%.

B. Amplitude is set by adjusting power (in arbitrary units) and is measured as delta pressure (ΔP).

   1. Increasing the power leads to an increase in the excursion of the ventilator diaphragm. This increases the amplitude of the pressure wave, and is reflected in an increased ΔP, which is measured at the hub of the endotracheal tube. Remember that this ΔP is markedly attenuated by the time it reaches the alveoli.

   2. Increasing the amplitude leads to an increase in chest movement ("chest wiggle") and a decrease in $PaCO_2$.

   3. Relatively small (10–20%) changes in amplitude will result in significant changes in $PaCO_2$.

   4. When placing a patient on HFOV, adjust the amplitude so that the patient is comfortable without much spontaneous respiratory effort, and so the "chest wiggle" looks appropriate (there is no way to learn this other than through experience). Follow $PaCO_2$ closely, and consider using a transcutaneous CO_2 monitor to help with initial adjustments in amplitude.

C. Frequency, measured in Hz (1 Hz = 1 breath/sec or 60 breaths/min). For neonatal patients, frequency is usually 6–15 Hz (360–900 breaths/min).

   1. Use higher frequencies for small babies with dense lung disease, and lower frequencies for large babies, babies with mild disease, and babies with nonuniform disease.

   2. Typical frequencies:

   a. Preterm infant with severe RDS: 12–15 Hz

   b. Preterm infant with mild RDS or early chronic changes: 10–12 Hz

   c. Term infant with severe pneumonia or meconium aspiration: 8 Hz

   3. In general, use a lower frequency for patients with nonhomogeneous lung disease, airway disease, or air trapping. If a patient has an unacceptable degree of air trapping (which does not respond to decreasing mean Paw), consider decreasing the frequency by at least 2 Hz.

D. Percent inspiratory time is almost always left at 33%, or an inspiratory: expiratory ratio of 1:2.

E. Flow, measured in liters per minute (LPM)

   1. As with other types of ventilator, more flow is needed for large patients than for small patients

   2. Although the ventilator is always calibrated and "set up" with a flow of 20 LPM, this should be decreased for premature infants. Typical flow settings:

    a. Premature infant <1,000 g: flow 6–8 LPM

    b. Premature infant 1,500–2,500 g: flow 10–12 LPM

    c. Term infant with severe meconium aspiration: flow 15–20 LPM

F. FiO_2. Adjustments in FiO_2 have the same impact on oxygenation for a patient on HFOV as they do for a patient on other forms of ventilation.

V. Weaning and Extubating from HFOV

A. Many patients can be extubated directly from HFOV, without changing back to another mode of ventilation.

    1. Decrease both mean Paw and amplitude as the patient improves.

    2. As the patient improves, and as amplitude decreases, the patient will do more spontaneous breathing. If the amplitude decreases sufficiently, the patient will essentially be on "oscillatory continuous positive airway pressure (CPAP)" rather than oscillatory ventilation.

    3. When the patient is achieving most of the CO_2 elimination with spontaneous breathing, and the mean Paw has been decreased sufficiently, the patient can be extubated.

    4. General guidelines for extubation:

        a. Patient <1,000 g: mean Paw <7 cm H_2O and FiO_2 <0.25

        b. Patient >1,000 g: mean Paw <8 cm H_2O and FiO_2 <0.3

B. Some clinicians prefer to wean patients from HFOV to another mode of ventilation before extubating. This is particularly useful in the institution that does not have many high-frequency ventilators available. In general, patients should not be weaned from HFOV until they have improved significantly. General guidelines for weaning from HFOV to another form of ventilation:

    1. FiO_2 <0.3–0.4

    2. Able to be ventilated with a PIP <25 cm H_2O

C. In some patients with chronic lung disease, HFOV may not be as effective as other forms of ventilation. If a patient is still on HFOV at 3–4 weeks of age with obvious chronic lung disease, it may be reasonable to give that patient a trial of CV do determine which mode is more effective.

Suggested Reading

Chang H: Mechanisms of gas transport during ventilation by high-frequency oscillation. J Appl Physiol 1984; 6:553–563.

Clark RH: High-frequency ventilation. J Pediatr 1994; 124:661–670.

SECTION IX

Management of Specific Respiratory Disorders

Chapter 40

Respiratory Distress Syndrome

Steven M. Donn, Sunil K. Sinha

I. **Description**

   A. Respiratory distress syndrome (RDS) is a primary pulmonary disorder that accompanies prematurity, which manifiests specifically as immaturity of the lungs and, to a lesser extent, the airways. It is a disease of progressive atelectasis, which in its most severe form can lead to severe respiratory failure and death.

   B. The incidence and severity of RDS is generally inversely related to gestational age. Approximate incidence:

      1. 24 weeks, >80%

      2. 28 weeks, 70%

      3. 32 weeks, 25%

      4. 36 weeks, 5%

II. **Pathophysiology**

   A. Biochemical abnormalities

      1. The major hallmark is a deficiency of surfactant, which leads to higher surface tension at the alveolar surface and interferes with the normal exchange of respiratory gases.

      2. The higher surface tension requires greater distending pressure to inflate the alveoli, according to LaPlace's law:

$$P = 2T/r$$

      where P is pressure, T is surface tension, and r is the radius.

      3. As the radius of the alveolus decreases (atelectasis), and as surface tension increases, the amount of pressure required to overcome these forces increases.

   B. Morphologic/anatomic abnormalities

      1. The number of functional alveoli (and thus the surface area available for gas exchange) increases with advancing gestational age.

      2. With extreme prematurity (23–25 weeks), the distance from the alveolus or terminal bronchiole to the nearest adjacent capillary

increases, thus increasing the diffusion barrier and interfering with oxygen transport from lung to blood.

    3. The airways of the preterm infant are incompletely formed and lack sufficient cartilage to remain patent. This can lead to collapse and increased airway resistance.

    4. The chest wall of the preterm newborn is more compliant than the lungs, tending to collapse when the infant attempts to increase negative intrathoracic pressure.

C. Functional abnormalities

    1. Decreased compliance

    2. Increased resistance

    3. Ventilation/perfusion abnormalities

    4. Impaired gas exchange

    5. Increased work of breathing

D. Histopathologic abnormalities

    1. The disorder was originally referred to as hyaline membrane disease (HMD) as a result of the typical postmortem findings in nonsurvivors.

    2. Macroscopic findings

        a. Decreased aeration

        b. Firm, rubbery, "liver-like" lungs

    3. Microscopic findings

        a. Air spaces filled with an eosinophilic staining exudate composed of a proteinaceous material, with and without inflammatory cells.

        b. Edema in the air spaces

        c. Alveolar collapse

        d. Squamous metaplasia of respiratory epithelium

        e. Distended lymphatics

        f. Thickening of pulmonary arterioles

III. **Clinical Manifestations of RDS**

A. Tachypnea. The affected infant breathes rapidly, attempting to compensate for small tidal volumes by increasing respiratory frequency.

B. Flaring of the ala nasi. This increases the cross-sectional area of the nasal passages and decreases upper airway resistance.

C. Grunting. This is an attempt by the infant to produce positive end-expiratory pressure (PEEP) by exhaling against a closed glottis. Its purpose is to maintain some degree of alveolar volume (distention) so that the radius of the alveolus is larger and the amount of work needed to expand it further is less than if the radius were smaller.

D. Retractions. The infant utilizes the accessory muscles of respiration, such as the intercostals, to help overcome the increased pressure required to inflate the lungs.

E. Cyanosis. This is a reflection of impaired oxygenation, in which there is more than 5 g/dL of deoxygenated hemoglobin.

IV. **Radiographic Findings**

A. The classic description is a "ground glass" or "reticulogranular" pattern with air bronchograms (see Chapter 6, Figure 18).

B. Severe cases with near total atelectasis may show complete opacification of the lung fields ("white out").

C. Extremely preterm infants with a minimal number of alveoli may actually have clear lung fields.

D. Most cases will show diminished lung volumes (unless positive pressure is being applied).

V. **Laboratory Abnormalities**

A. Arterial oxygen tension is usually decreased.

B. Arterial carbon dioxide tension may be initially normal if the infant is able to compensate (tachypnea), but it is usually increased.

C. Blood pH may reflect a respiratory acidosis (from hypercarbia), metabolic acidosis (from tissue hypoxia), or mixed acidosis.

VI. **Diagnosis**

A. Clinical evidence of respiratory distress

B. Radiographic findings

C. Laboratory abnormalities from impaired gas exchange

VII. **Differential Diagnoses**

A. Sepsis/pneumonia, especially group B streptococcal infection, which can produce a nearly identical radiographic picture

B. Transient tachypnea of the newborn

C. Pulmonary malformations (e.g., cystic adenomatoid malformation, congenital lobar emphysema, diaphragmatic hernia)

D. Extrapulmonary abnormalities (e.g., vascular ring, ascites, abdominal mass)

VIII. **Treatment**

A. Establish adequate gas exchange

1. If the infant is only mildly affected and has reasonable respiratory

effort and effective ventilation, only an increase in the FiO_2 may be necessary. This can be provided by an oxygen hood or nasal cannula.

2. If the infant is exhibiting evidence of alveolar hypoventilation ($PaCO_2$ >50 torr or 6.7 kPa), or hypoxemia (PaO_2 <50 torr or 6.7 kPa in FiO_2 ≥0.5), some form of positive pressure ventilation is indicated.

   a. Consider the use of continuous positive airway pressure (CPAP) if the infant has reasonable spontaneous respiratory effort and has only minimal hypercarbia (see Chapter 10). A level of 4–6 cm H_2O should be used.

   b. Consider endotracheal intubation and mechanical ventilation if:

     (1) Hypercarbia ($PaCO_2$ >60 torr or 8 kPa)

     (2) Hypoxemia (PaO_2 <50 torr or 6.7 kPa)

     (3) Decreased respiratory drive or apnea

     (4) Need to maintain airway patency

     (5) Plan to administer surfactant replacement therapy

   c. Mechanical ventilation

     (1) The goal is to achieve adequate pulmonary gas exchange while decreasing the patient's work of breathing.

     (2) Either conventional mechanical ventilation or high-frequency ventilation can be used.

     (3) RDS is a disorder of low lung volume, so the approach should be one that delivers an appropriate tidal volume while minimizing the risks of complications (see below).

B. Surfactant replacement therapy (see Chapter 71)

1. The development and use of surfactant replacement therapy has revolutionized the treatment of RDS.

2. Numerous preparations (natural, synthetic, and semisynthetic) are now available.

3. Types of intervention

   a. Prophylaxis – infant is immediately intubated and given surfactant as close to the first breath as possible

   b. Rescue – infant is not treated until the diagnosis is established

4. Dose and interval are different for each preparation.

5. Although there is little doubt as to efficacy, the treatment is still very expensive.

C. Adjunctive measures

1. Maintain adequate blood pressure (and hence pulmonary blood flow) with judicious use of blood volume expanders and pressors.

2. Maintain adequate oxygen carrying capacity in infants with a high oxygen (FiO_2 >0.4) requirement.

3. Maintain physiologic pH, but do not give sodium bicarbonate if hypercarbia is present.

4. Maintain adequate sedation/analgesia (see Chapters 53–55).

5. Provide adequate nutrition but avoid excessive nonnitrogen calories, which can increase CO_2 production and exacerbate hypercarbia.

6. Observe closely for signs of complications, especially infection.

IX. **Complications**

A. Respiratory

1. Airleaks

a. Pneumomediastinum

b. Pulmonary interstitial emphysema

c. Pneumothorax

d. Pneumopericardium

e. Pneumoperitoneum (transdiaphragmatic)

f. Subcutaneous emphysema

2. Airway injury (see Chapter 49)

3. Pulmonary hemorrhage (see Chapter 44)

4. Chronic lung disease (bronchopulmonary dysplasia; see Chapter 48).

B. Cardiac

1. Patent ductus arteriosus (see Chapter 50)

2. Congestive heart failure

3. Pulmonary hypertension

4. Cor pulmonale

C. Neurologic (see Chapter 51)

1. Relationship to intraventricular hemorrhage

2. Relationship to periventricular leukomalacia

3. Neurodevelopmental impact

D. Infectious

1. Nosocomial and acquired pneumonia

2. Sepsis

X. **Prenatal Treatments and Conditions Which Impact RDS**

A. Antenatal treatment of the mother with corticosteroids has been demonstrated to reduce the incidence and severity of RDS, particularly if given between 28–32 weeks' gestation.

1. Betamethasone

2. Dexamethasone

B. Other agents have been explored but results are thus far unconvincing.

1. Thyroid hormone

2. Thyrotropin

C. Accelerated pulmonary (i.e., surfactant system) maturation is seen in:
  1. Intrauterine growth retardation
  2. Infants of substance-abusing mothers
  3. Prolonged rupture of the membranes
D. Delayed pulmonary maturation is seen in:
  1. Infants of diabetic mothers
  2. Rh-sensitized fetuses
  3. Infants of hypothyroid mothers
  4. Infants who are hypothyroid

Suggested Reading

Cotton RB: Pathophysiology of hyaline membrane disease (excluding surfactant). In Polin RA, Fox WW (Eds.): *Fetal and Neonatal Physiology, 2nd Edition.* Philadelphia, W.B. Saunders, 1998, pp. 1165–1174.

Kattwinkel J: Surfactant: evolving issues. Clin Perinatol 1998; 25:17–32.

Martin GI, Sindel BD: Neonatal management of the very low birth weight infant: the use of surfactant. Clin Perinatol 1992; 19:461–468.

Nelson M, Becker MA, Donn SM: Basic neonatal respiratory disorders. In Donn SM (Ed.): *Neonatal and Pediatric Pulmonary Graphics: Principles and Clinical Applications.* Armonk, NY, Futura Publishing Co., 1998, pp. 253–278.

Robertson B, Halliday HL: Principles of surfactant replacement. Biochim Biophys Acta 1998; 1408:346–361.

Walsh MC, Carlo WA, Miller MJ: Respiratory diseases of the newborn. In Carlo WA, Chatburn RL (Eds.): *Neonatal Respiratory Care, 2nd Edition.* Chicago, Year Book Medical Publishers, 1988, pp. 260–288.

Chapter 41

Meconium Aspiration Syndrome

Thomas E. Wiswell

I. **Overview**
   A. Meconium-stained amniotic fluid (MSAF)
      1. Occurs in approximately 13% of all deliveries
      2. Meconium passage may be a marker of antepartum or intrapartum compromise (such as hypoxemia or umbilical cord compression)
      3. Passage of meconium may also be a maturational event. MSAF is rarely noted before 37 weeks gestation, but may occur in 35% or more of pregnancies ≥42 weeks gestation.
   B. Meconium aspiration syndrome (MAS)
      1. Definition: respiratory distress in an infant born through MSAF whose symptoms cannot be otherwise explained
      2. MAS occurs in approximately 6% of newborns born through MSAF.
      3. Aspiration may occur *in utero* or with the initial postnatal breaths.
      4. The thicker the MSAF consistency, the greater the likelihood of MAS.
      5. The more depressed a baby is (as reflected by the need for positive pressure ventilation or low Apgar scores), the greater the likelihood of MAS.
      6. Of those with MAS, 30–60% require mechanical ventilation, 10–25% develop pneumothoraces, and approximately 5% die.
      7. 50–70% of infants with persistent pulmonary hypertension of the newborn (PPHN) have MAS as an underlying disorder.

II. **Pathophysiology**
   A. Complex mechanisms involved (see Figure 67).
   B. At any given moment, several of these mechanisms may be influencing the degree of respiratory distress.

III. **Prevention of MAS**
   A. Amnioinfusion trials

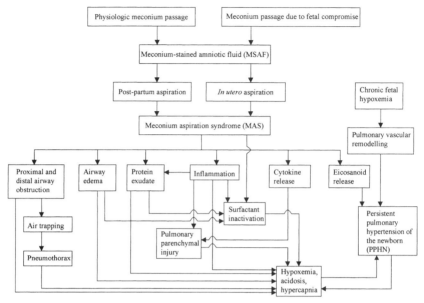

Figure 67. Pathophysiology of meconium aspiration syndrome.

1. Initial reports from the late 1980s and early 1990s indicated that amnioinfusion for thick consistency MSAF would improve Apgar scores and prevent MAS.
2. More recent reports from the mid-1990s have not found this therapy to be of benefit. In fact, amnioinfusion may be detrimental to both the mother and the fetus/newborn (uterine tetany, increased frequency of operative and instrument-assisted deliveries, more fetal heart rate abnormalities, increased maternal endometritis, and increased neonatal sepsis).

B. Oropharyngeal suctioning
   1. Performed before delivery of the infant's shoulders and trunk
   2. Removes MSAF from oropharynx before infant takes initial breaths
   3. Bulb syringe or a catheter attached to wall suctioning are equally efficacious.

C. Potentially dangerous maneuvers of no proven benefit
   1. Cricoid pressure: application of pressure to the infant's airway to prevent intratracheal meconium from descending into the lungs
   2. Epiglottal blockage: insertion of 1–3 fingers into the child's airway to manually "close" the epiglottis over the glottis to prevent aspiration
   3. Thorax compression: encircling the infant's chest and applying

pressure in an attempt to prevent deep inspiration prior to endo-tracheal cleansing

4. None of these maneuvers has ever been scientifically validated and all are potentially dangerous (trauma, vagal stimulation, or induction of deep inhalation with chest recoil upon removing encircling hands).

D. Endotracheal intubation and intratracheal suctioning in the delivery room

1. Widespread adoption of a philosophy of universal intubation and suctioning of meconium-stained infants led to a significantly de-creased incidence of MAS, as well as deaths from the disorder.

2. A recent large trial indicated that endotracheal intubation is of no benefit in the apparently vigorous infant born through any consis-tency MSAF. Apparent vigor was defined within the first 10–15 seconds of life by a heart rate >100 beats/min, spontaneous respi-rations, and reasonable tone.

3. Endotracheal intubation and suctioning should still be performed in infants born through MSAF if they are depressed, if they need positive pressure ventilation, or if they are initially apparently vigorous, but subsequently manifest any respiratory distress within the first minutes of life.

IV. Radiographic Findings

A. Varied roentgenographic findings among infants with MAS

1. Diffuse, patchy infiltrates
2. Consolidation
3. Atelectasis
4. Pleural effusions
5. Airleaks (pneumothorax, pneumomediastinum)
6. Hyperinflation
7. "Wet-lung" appearance similar to findings seen with transient tachypnea of the newborn
8. Hypovascularity
9. Apparently clear, virtually normal appearance

B. Correlation of radiographic findings with disease severity

1. One early study indicated direct correlation between severity of MAS and the degree of radiographic abnormalities.

2. Two more recent studies found no such correlation. Patients with minimal signs may have a horrible-appearing chest radiograph, while the sickest infant may have a virtually normal chest radiograph.

V. Conventional Management of MAS

A. Chest physiotherapy (CPT)

1. Objectives of CPT are to prevent accumulation of debris, improve mobilization of airway secretions, and improve oxygenation.

2. CPT consists of postural drainage, percussion, vibration, saline lavage, and suctioning (oropharyngeal and intratracheal).

3. Although commonly performed in both the delivery room and the neonatal intensive care unit (NICU), CPT for MAS has never been studied scientifically and its benefits are unproven.

B. Oxygen

1. The goal is to maintain acceptable systemic oxygenation. Generally, this consists of sustaining peripheral oxygen saturation levels between 92% and 97% or arterial partial pressure of oxygen (PaO_2) levels between 60 and 80 torr (8 and 10.7 kPa).

2. Because of the potential for air trapping and airleaks, some advocate increasing the fraction of inspired oxygen (FiO_2) to 1.0 before implementing more aggressive therapy (mechanical ventilation, etc.). Typically, however, once FiO_2 requirements exceed 0.60, more aggressive therapies are instituted.

3. Oxygen is also a pulmonary vasodilator. Since aberrant pulmonary vasoconstriction frequently accompanies MAS, clinicians often attempt to maintain higher than usual oxygenation levels early in the course of the disorder (peripheral oxygen saturation levels of 98–100% or PaO_2 levels between 100–120 torr or 13.3–16 kPa). The latter practice has not been validated in clinical trials.

4. Supplemental oxygen is used in conjunction with more aggressive therapy.

C. Continuous positive airway pressure (CPAP)

1. CPAP is often begun once FiO_2 requirements exceed 0.50–0.60 or if the patient exhibits substantial respiratory distress. Some clinicians, however, prefer to move directly to mechanical ventilation without a trial of CPAP.

2. CPAP is provided most commonly in newborns intranasally via prongs inserted into the nostrils. CPAP may also be administered via a facemask or via an endotracheal tube.

3. Major potential complications of CPAP are air trapping and increased functional residual capacity. These factors could contribute to airleaks or to decreased venous return to the heart, further compromising the infant.

4. There is limited published information concerning the use of CPAP in children with MAS.

D. Conventional mechanical ventilation

1. Typically provided with time-cycled, pressure-limited mechanical ventilators. Some clinicians avoid volume-limited ventilators because of an unsubstantiated fear of airleaks.

2. Multiple strategies have been advocated.

a. Use of any settings (pressure, rate, inspiratory:expiratory [I:E] ratio, FiO_2, etc.) that will maintain arterial blood gases within normal ranges

      b. Hyperventilation to achieve respiratory alkalosis in an attempt to attain pulmonary vasodilation. "Gentle" ventilation allows higher $PaCO_2$ levels and lower pH and PaO_2 levels in an attempt to prevent lung injury (from barotrauma or volutrauma) and potential side effects from hypocarbia and alkalosis.

    3. To date, there have been no prospective, randomized trials comparing any of the various mechanical ventilator strategies in the management of MAS. Hence, no single approach can be considered optimal.

  E. Other conventional therapies

    1. Sedation

    2. Paralysis

    3. Systemic alkalosis from parenteral administration of sodium bicarbonate

    4. Use of pressors (dopamine, dobutamine) or fluid boluses to maintain high systemic blood pressure

    5. None of these therapies have been rigorously investigated in infants with MAS.

VI. Nonconventional Management (Not the Standard of Care!)

  A. High-frequency ventilation.

    1. Includes both high-frequency jet ventilation and high-frequency oscillatory ventilation

    2. Trials in animal models of MAS have generally shown no benefit.

    3. Limited human anecdotal experience has been touted as indicating efficacy.

    4. To date, there are no published prospective human trials that have documented either form of high-frequency ventilation to be more efficacious than conventional ventilation in the management of MAS.

  B. Bolus exogenous surfactant

    1. Rationale

      a. Meconium produces a concentration-dependent direct inactivation of a newborn's endogenous surfactant.

      b. Meconium has a direct cytotoxic effect on the type II pneumocyte.

      c. Meconium causes decreased levels of surfactant proteins A and B.

    2. Studies in animal models of MAS in which bolus surfactant therapy was used demonstrate conflicting results. Some trials indicate efficacy, while others show no benefit.

    3. Anecdotal human data are similarly conflicting.

    4. In one multicenter trial of term-gestation infants with respiratory failure (51% had MAS), surfactant-treated infants with MAS had a decreased need for extracorporeal membrane oxygenation (ECMO). However, there were no differences in mortality, duration of mechanical ventilation or oxygen therapy, or total hospital days.

5. There has been only one small randomized, controlled trial assessing exogenous surfactant for MAS.

    a. 1½ times the standard dose of surfactant was used.

    b. Surfactant was not administered as a bolus, rather it was given via a continuous infusion over 20 minutes.

    c. Improved oxygenation only occurred 6–12 hours later, typically following subsequent doses.

6. Currently, no commercially available surfactant has been approved by the Food and Drug Administration (FDA) for use in MAS in the USA.

7. Further trials are necessary to assess this therapy.

C. Inhaled nitric oxide (see Chapter 77)

1. Results of several trials in neonates have been published (1996–1998). Approximately half of the babies in these trials had MAS.

2. Among MAS babies in the various nitric oxide studies, there have been no significant differences in the need for ECMO, mortality, length of hospitalization, or duration of mechanical ventilation.

3. Currently, inhaled nitric oxide remains an experimental agent and is not FDA-approved in the USA for use in MAS.

D. Liquid ventilation with perfluorochemicals (see Chapter 78)

1. Potential advantages include lowering of surface tension, improved oxygen transfer, recruitment of collapsed alveoli, and better ventilation/perfusion matching

2. Animal work is promising.

3. No published human data concerning its use for MAS

E. Steroid therapy

1. Rationale is the profound inflammation occurring within hours of aspiration.

2. Steroids could be administered either systemically or via the inhalation route.

3. Animal data are intriguing; human data are limited.

4. Clinical trials are warranted involving infants with substantial MAS who require mechanical ventilation.

F. ECMO (see Chapter 76)

1. ECMO is the therapy of last resort and is used when mortality is estimated to be >50–80%.

2. Of more than 11,000 newborns treated with ECMO since the mid-1980s, 35–40% had MAS as their underlying respiratory disorder.

3. Compared to ECMO-treated infants with other disorders, those with MAS have the shortest duration of cardiopulmonary bypass and the highest survival rates.

4. Venoarterial bypass is still most commonly used form of ECMO in infants with MAS. In most centers, this requires sacrifice of the right carotid artery and the right jugular vein.
5. ECMO survivors have morbidity rates of 20–40%. It is unknown how much of this morbidity is from preexisting conditions versus how much is from ECMO.

VII. Summary

A. MAS remains a common cause of respiratory distress among newborns.
B. Of the various therapies used in the management of MAS, few have been adequately investigated.
C. Further work to elucidate optimal management of MAS is sorely needed.

Suggested Reading

Cleary GM, Wiswell TE: Meconium-stained amniotic fluid and the meconium aspiration syndrome: an update. Pediatr Clin North Am 1998; 45:511–529.

Findlay RD, Taeusch HW, Walther FJ: Surfactant replacement therapy for meconium aspiration syndrome. Pediatrics 1996; 97:48–52.

Moses D, Holm B, Spitale P, et al: Inhibition of pulmonary surfactant function by meconium. Am J Obstet Gynecol 1991; 164:477–481.

The Neonatal Inhaled Nitric Oxide Study Group: Inhaled nitric oxide in full-term and nearly full-term infants with hypoxic respiratory failure. N Engl J Med 1997; 336:597–604.

Wiswell TE, Bent RC: Meconium staining and the meconium aspiration syndrome: unresolved issues. Pediatr Clin North Am 1993; 40:955–981.

Wiswell TE, Fuloria M. The meconium aspiration syndrome: the saga continues. Indian Pediatrics 1998; 35:1059–1062.

Wiswell TE, Tuggle JM, Turner BS: Meconium aspiration syndrome: have we made a difference? Pediatrics 1990; 85:715–721.

Chapter 42

Neonatal Pneumonia

Roger G. Faix

I. **Importance**

   A. Adequate lung function to support gas exchange is essential for survival.

   B. Frequently a marker of disseminated infection in this age group

   C. Frequency – reported rates vary, depending on definition of pneumonia used; most reports indicate rates of 5–50/1,000 liveborn infants. Of all neonatal deaths, pneumonia is a contributing factor in 10–25%.

   D. Diagnostic and therapeutic difficulties

   1. Nonspecificity of clinical presentations, radiographic, and laboratory findings

   2. Infection is not always the cause; many cases represent inflammation without infection (e.g., meconium or food aspiration), although infection may be superimposed on preexisting noninfectious inflammation.

   3. Frequent compromise of host defenses and dysregulation of inflammatory response in newborns

   4. Difficulty identifying invading pathogen (if any)

   5. Clinical response may not correlate with *in vitro* antimicrobial efficacy, even if a pathogen is identified.

   6. Often adversely impacts myocardial performance via effect on right ventricular afterload; interferes with delivery of oxygen and removal of CO_2 for every organ in the body

   E. The possibility of effective intervention with advances in cardiopulmonary support techniques is promising, but still limited.

II. **Pathogenesis**

   A. Histopathology – inflammation (with or without infection) of lower respiratory tract

   1. Inflammatory cells in alveoli and airways

   2. Alveolar exudates/hyaline material

   3. Interstitial infiltrates

4. Intraluminal exudate/mucosal injury in conducting airways
5. Multifocal hemorrhage/petechiae
6. Pleural effusions/empyema
7. Vasculitis and vascular congestion
8. Multifocal necrosis
9. Abscesses (unusual)
10. Superimposed injury attributable to oxygen, volutrauma, pressure-related injury, and other changes induced by therapeutic support techniques

B. Pathophysiology
   1. Pathogen-related damage
      a. Direct invasion by organisms with attendant disruption and/or destruction of normal (often fragile) tissues
      b. Indirect injury mediated by production of toxins by organisms (e.g., endotoxin, leukocidin, toxic shock syndrome toxin-1) that may have adverse effects on metabolism, synthetic machinery, local perfusion, delivery/removal of oxygen, nutrients, waste products
   2. Host inflammatory response – a two-edged sword
      a. Facilitates ingestion and killing of invaders *but* often poorly targeted, with significant injury to "innocent bystander" host tissues
      b. Release or activation of mediators by inflammatory cells (e.g., cytokines, reactive oxygen metabolites, complement) that trigger pathways/cascades which adversely impact:
         (1) Endothelial and epithelial integrity
         (2) Vasomotor tone
         (3) Coagulation and thrombolysis
         (4) Activation of phagocytes
      c. Airway obstruction (partial or complete) caused by inflammatory debris, edema, mucus, with resultant air trapping, atelectasis, and increased dead space
      d. Surfactant-related abnormalities – altered composition and reduced function

C. Lung host defenses – many features compromised in newborn infants
   1. Ciliary escalator – conducts foreign material up and out of the airways; may be partially circumvented if endotracheal tube in place
   2. Secretions – provide lubrication, barrier, and nonspecific antimicrobial properties (e.g., surfactant, mucus, defensins). Quality and quantity of components often compromised, especially in premature infants.
   3. Mucosal antibodies – usually not present until several weeks of age

274

4. Circulating factors – usually serve to amplify and target inflammatory response
   a. Antibodies – transplacental delivery of maternal immunoglobin G antibodies after second trimester; active synthesis of endogenous antibodies and creation of corresponding memory cells usually takes several weeks after exposure
   b. Complement – at term, both classical (activation dependent on antigen-specific antibody) and alternate (independent of specific antibody) pathways have 50% or less of adult activity
   c. Granulocytes – migrate to involved inflammatory sites; ingest and kill invading organisms, release toxic contents of granules into local microenvironment. Ingestion often less efficient than adults; generation of chemokines to attract these and other phagocytes less well developed and bone marrow reserve smaller than in older individuals.
   d. Lymphocytes – elaboration and regulation of cytokines that support activation, antigen processing, proliferation, development of memory, killer, suppressor, other functions of these cells less well developed than in older individuals

III. **Clinical Syndromes**
   A. Congenital pneumonia – already present at birth
      1. Hematogenous transplacental infection
      2. Ascending transamniotic infection
      3. Aspiration of infected or inflamed amniotic fluid
   B. Intrapartum pneumonia – acquired during birth process
      1. Hematogenous infection
      2. Aspiration of infected or inflamed fluid
      3. Aspiration of meconium, amniotic fluid, others
   C. Acquired/postnatal pneumonia – arising in infant well after birth
      1. Hematogenous
      2. Mucosal colonization, disruption, and invasion; via lymphatics or blood: organisms in the neonatal intensive care unit often resistant to multiple antibiotics because of selection pressure from frequent use
      3. Aspiration of gastric contents
         a. Gastroesophageal reflux
         b. Upper alimentary and/or airway anomalies
      4. Nosocomial – respiratory equipment, caretakers, endotracheal tubes, suctioning, disruption of usual lung defenses
      5. Immune deficiency states – congenital or acquired (e.g., long-term glucocorticoid therapy for chronic lung disease)

IV. **Clinical Manifestations – Often Protean and Nonspecific**

 A. Respiratory
  1. Tachypnea
  2. Accessory muscle recruitment – flaring, retractions
  3. Grunting
  4. Change in secretions – quantity and/or quality
  5. Increasing respiratory support requirements
  6. Cyanosis
  7. Rales/rhonchi – less frequent and specific than in older patients
  8. Cough – less frequent and specific than in older patients
  9. Others
 B. Systemic manifestations
  1. Temperature instability
  2. Impaired perfusion
  3. Other signs suggestive of sepsis
 C. Suggestive localized findings
  1. Conjunctivitis
  2. Vesicles, other skin lesions
  3. Nasal secretions
  4. Others

V. **Diagnosis – often difficult given the myriad of other conditions that may mimic pneumonia; may be superimposed on other underlying conditions (e.g., respiratory distress syndrome [RDS])**

 A. History
  1. Maternal – fever, prolonged (>18 hr) rupture of membranes, fetal distress, meconium-stained amniotic fluid, uterine tenderness, foul-smelling amniotic fluid, maternal birth canal infection, premature onset of labor, venereal disease research laboratory (VDRL) and other antenatal screening tests
  2. Infant – late-onset or persistent tachypnea, other features as noted above
 B. Physical examination – breath sounds, percussive changes, thoracic symmetry, retractions, grunting, flaring, cyanosis, perfusion, heart rate, blood pressure, organomegaly, others
 C. Chest radiography – anterposterior and lateral (other views as needed). Often nonspecific or indistinguishable from RDS, transient tachypnea of the newborn (TTNB), other common respiratory diagnoses. Common findings include:
  1. Frank lobar infiltrates (e.g., *Klebsiella*)
  2. Patchy, irregular infiltrates
  3. Air bronchograms

4. Obscuring of cardiothymic margins
5. Effusions/empyema
6. Miliary patterns (e.g., *Listeria*)
7. Generalized hyperinflation
8. Irregular inflation
9. Pneumatoceles (e.g., *S. aureus*)

D. Microbiology – it is likely that organisms vary with route and timing of acquisition of the infection. It may not be possible to identify specific organism for a variety of reasons, including the fact that not all pneumonia is infectious in etiology.

1. Congenital pneumonia
   a. Chronic pathogens – cytomegalovirus, *Toxoplasma, T. pallidum, Ureaplasma*
   b. Acute hematogenous – group B streptococcus, untypable *Hemophilus influenzae, E. coli, Listeria,* others
   c. Nonspecific

2. Intrapartum – inhabitants of maternal birth canal; maternal bacteremia As with congenital pneumonia plus other gram-negative bacteria, *Staphylococcus aureus,* herpes simplex, *Mycoplasma, Ureaplasma, Trichomonas*

3. Acquired/postnatal
   a. Nosocomial – *Staphylococcus* species, *Candida* species, *Enterococcus, Serratia, Pseudomonas* species, other gram-negative organisms (other "water bugs")
   b. *Chlamydia,* especially after 2 weeks
   c. Other agents – respiratory syncytial virus, parainfluenza, adenovirus, mycoplasma, herpes simplex virus

E. Cultures – bacterial, fungal, viral, *Ureaplasma,* and others as clinically dictated by history and circumstances

1. Blood (cerebrospinal fluid if infant sufficiently stable)
2. Endotracheal aspirate – most helpful in newborn freshly intubated after birth; in most other settings it is difficult to distinguish colonizers from invaders, although pure growth of a single pathogen may be helpful
3. Pleural fluid if present, including gram stain
4. Bronchoscopic specimen (using available techniques to minimize oral/nasal contamination)
5. Lung aspirate/biopsy, including appropriate stains (be cautious regarding postprocedure pneumothorax, other airleak)
6. Conjunctival, vesicular, other associated specimens if abnormal on physical examination

F. Selected other tests for detection of microorganisms

1. Antigen detection – latex agglutination, fluorescent antibodies, others
2. Nucleic acid probes, e.g., *Chlamydia*

3. Polymerase chain reaction
4. Serology
   a. VDRL/FTA (fluorescent treponemal antibody)
   b. Conventional acute/convalescent sera for selected agents
   c. Occasionally used method employing patient's own endotracheal bacteria to assess antibody response in acute and convalescent sera in an attempt to distinguish invasive pathogens from commensals. Often facilitates diagnosis only retrospectively, but may be helpful in cases refractory to initial antimicrobial therapy or for infection control purposes. Controversial specificity for distinguishing invasion from colonization

G. Complete blood count with differential – extremely limited utility with poor diagnostic specificity, although may be useful to assess resolution of inflammatory process during treatment. Other acute phase reactants, such as quantitative C-reactive protein (CRP) and interleukin-6 (IL-6) are reportedly more specific but still plagued with variable positive predictive value.

H. Differential diagnosis during acute presentation is **broad**: may have concurrent diseases superimposed or underlying, e.g., RDS, TTNB, congestive heart failure, lung anomalies, atelectasis, inspissated secretions, inadequate gas humidification

VI. Treatment

A. Problematic. In cases caused by infection, killing or preventing further replication of the invading organism is important, but not the whole answer; pathologic processes initiated by structural and metabolic constituents of organisms may persist or even be exacerbated by lysis of the organism.

B. Antimicrobial therapy
   1. Antibiotics
      a. Selected by sensitivity patterns of likely pathogens tempered by knowledge of delivery of drug to infected site within lung (parenchyma, bronchial lumen, intraphagocytic), and intrapulmonary confounding factors
      b. Aminoglycosides reach bronchial lumen marginally when given by systemic route, although alveolar delivery is adequate. Endotracheal treatment in adults has been reported to be helpful with borderline sensitive organisms. Alternative agents (e.g., cefotaxime) may be preferable if bronchial involvement is suspected or if the patient fails to respond.
      c. If gram-negative pneumonia is suspected, continuous exposure to concentration greater than mean inhibitory concentration may be more important than peak concentration; tracheal delivery, intramuscular route, or intravenous treatment with more frequent dosing interval but same total daily dose may be

advantageous if patient fails to respond to conventional administration.

    d. If empyema is present, may need to directly instill antimicrobial agent via thoracostomy tube

  2. Documentation of efficacy – decreasing respiratory support requirements, resolving radiographic changes, clinical appearance, sterilization of any infected normally sterile site/body fluid

  3. If culture of normally sterile site yields a specific pathogen, alter antibiotic therapy accordingly.

  4. Surveillance for complications that may require change in antibiotic selection, surgical drainage, other interventions

  5. Duration of therapy variable – usually 7–10 days, assuming rapid resolution of clinical abnormalities; 7–10 days following sterilization of normally sterile site if cultures are initially positive; may need longer periods (2–6 weeks) for sequestered infections such as empyema, abscess

C. Supportive therapy

  1. Hemodynamic support

    a. Volume expansion/pressor/afterload reduction support as needed to assure adequate systemic and pulmonary perfusion

    b. Packed erythrocytes as needed to assure adequate oxygen carrying capacity (hematocrit 40–60%); prefer adult erythrocytes for better oxygen-tissue delivery characteristics of adult hemoglobin

  2. Respiratory support

    a. Airway patency

      (1) Judicious suctioning

      (2) Vibration/percussion to mobilize secretions – concern raised by recent reports of association with brain injury in premature infants <1,500 gm

      (3) Place or replace endotracheal tube as needed to assure airway patency; tracheostomy may be warranted if infection involves epiglottis, other parts of upper airway

    b. Supplemental oxygen, as needed

    c. Positive airway pressure

      (1) Avoid high pressures that interfere with myocardial performance, venous return

      (2) No data to assess relative efficacy of synchronized, patient-triggered, or volume-cycled ventilation versus time-cycled, pressure-limited ventilation for pneumonia in newborns

    d. Drainage of effusions, if interfering with ventilation

    e. Adjunctive respiratory rescue treatments, if respiratory failure refractory to above maneuvers; limited controlled human data regarding efficacy in neonatal pneumonia are available.

(1) Exogenous surfactant

(2) High-frequency ventilation

(3) Inhaled nitric oxide, if associated pulmonary hypertension or severe V̇/Q̇ mismatch

(4) Extracorporeal membrane oxygenation (ECMO) – mortality rates higher than with most other noninfectious diseases that require ECMO (with exception of congenital diaphragmatic hernia) as of 1997 registry date (International Extracorporeal Life Support Organization, Ann Arbor, MI, USA)

Suggested Reading

Bone RC, Grodzin CJ, Balk RA: Sepsis: a new hypothesis for pathogenesis of the disease process. Chest 1997; 112:235–243.

Braude AC, Hornstein A, Klein M, et al: Pulmonary disposition of tobramycin. Am Rev Resp Dis 1983; 127:563–565.

Doellner H, Arntzen KJ, Haereid PE, et al: Interleukin-6 concentration in neonates evaluated for sepsis. J Pediatr 1998; 132:295–259.

Giacoia G, Neter E, Ogra P: Respiratory infection in infants on mechanical ventilation: the immune response as a diagnostic aid. J Pediatr 1981; 98:691–695.

Gunther A, Siebert C, Schmidt R, et al: Surfactant alterations in severe pneumonia, acute respiratory distress syndrome, and cardiogenic lung edema. Am J Physiol Crit Care Med 1996; 153:176–184.

Harding JE, Miles FKI, Becroft DMO, et al: Chest physiotherapy may be associated with brain damage in extremely premature infants. J Pediatr 1998; 132:440–444.

Herting E, Sun B, Jarstrand C, et al: Surfactant improves lung function and mitigates bacterial growth in immature ventilated rabbits with experimentally induced neonatal group B streptococcal pneumonia. Arch Dis Child 1997; 76F:3–8.

Marks MI, Klein JO. Bacterial infections of the respiratory tract. In Remington JS, Klein JO (Eds.): *Infectious Diseases of the Fetus and Newborn Infant, 4th Edition*. Philadelphia, W.B. Saunders Co., 1995, pp. 898–908.

Pennington JE: Penetration of antibiotics into respiratory secretions. Rev Infect Dis 1981; 3:67–73.

Chapter 43

Persistent Pulmonary Hypertension of the Newborn

Robert E. Schumacher, Steven M. Donn

I. **Description**

   A. Persistent pulmonary hypertension of the newborn (PPHN) is a condition that results from a failure of the normal postbirth decrease in pulmonary vascular resistance, leading to a variable degree of right-to-left shunting through persistent fetal channels, the foramen ovale and ductus arteriosus, and severe hypoxemia.

   B. Although the disorder is also referred to as persistent fetal circulation (PFC), this is a misnomer because the fetal organ of respiration, the placenta, has been removed, and the infant is dependent on the lungs for gas exchange.

II. **Pulmonary Vascular Development**

   A. Alveolar development is primarily a postbirth event. Intra-acinar vascular development is thus also a postbirth phenomenon. At birth, there is a decreased cross-sectional area available for pulmonary blood flow which causes high vascular resistance.

   B. Vascular smooth muscle development does not generally extend to the level of the alveolus. If present, it can result in medial thickening. Increased muscularization occurs at the end of gestation, and thus true PPHN is uncommon in the preterm infant.

   C. At term, pulmonary vascular resistance is high and pulmonary artery pressure is near systemic levels.

   D. A number of factors may significantly impact pulmonary vascular reactivity and pressure, including arterial oxygen and CO_2 tensions and pH. Hypoxia, hypercarbia, and acidosis cause vasoconstriction and elevate pulmonary artery pressure, and their presence may lead to maladaptation from fetal to neonatal (adult-type) circulation.

III. **Pathogenesis**

   A. Normal pulmonary vascular morphology/myocardial dysfunction or increased vascular reactivity from vasoconstrictive stimuli

1. Associated with asphyxia
   a. Vasoconstrictive effects of hypoxia, hypercarbia, acidosis
   b. Myocardial dysfunction (especially left ventricle) leading to pulmonary venous hypertension and subsequent PPHN with right-to-left shunting through the ductus arteriosus
2. Associated with meconium aspiration syndrome (MAS)
   a. Alveolar hypoxia results in vasoconstriction.
   b. Gas trapping and lung overdistention contribute to increased pulmonary vascular resistance.
   c. Concomitant effects of severe parenchymal lung disease
   d. Some infants will also have morphological changes in pulmonary vasculature (see below).
3. Sepsis/pneumonia
   a. Infection initiates an inflammatory response.
   b. Release of cytokines and other vascular mediators increases pulmonary vascular resistance.
   c. Severe parenchymal lung disease aggravates hypoxemia.
4. Thrombus or microthrombus formation with release of vasoactive mediators
5. Hyperviscosity syndrome

B. Morphologically abnormal pulmonary vasculature
   1. Abnormal extension of vascular smooth muscle, with thickening and increased resistance deeper into the pulmonary vascular tree. May be related to chronic intrauterine hypoxia.
      a. Some cases of MAS
      b. *In utero* closure of the ductus arteriosus
      c. Idiopathic PPHN
   2. Abnormally small lungs with decreased cross-sectional area of the pulmonary vascular bed and muscular thickening and distal extension
      a. Pulmonary hypoplasia (either primary or secondary)
      b. Congenital diaphragmatic hernia
      c. Cystic adenomatoid malformation

C. Structurally abnormal heart disease
   1. Left ventricular outflow tract obstruction
   2. Anomalous pulmonary venous return
   3. Ebstein's anomaly
   4. Left ventricular cardiomyopathy
   5. Any structural abnormality which results in a obligatory right-to-left shunt

IV. Diagnosis

A. Differential diagnoses of hypoxemia in the term or near-term infant

    1. Primary pulmonary disease
    2. Cyanotic congenital heart disease (CHD)
    3. PPHN, with or without lung disease
  B. Initial work-up
    1. History
      a. Evidence of infection
      b. Meconium-stained amniotic fluid
      c. Intrauterine growth retardation
      d. Postdatism
      e. Maternal aspirin use
    2. Physical examination (findings are nonspecific, but may help to suggest etiologic considerations)
      a. Murmur
      b. Abnormal breath sounds
      c. Inequality of pulses
      d. Scaphoid abdomen
      e. Potter's facies
    3. Chest radiograph (again, nonspecific, but may suggest or exclude associated conditions)
    4. Arterial blood gas determination. Attempt to correct ventilation and acid-base abnormalities before attributing hypoxemia to PPHN.
  C. The hyperoxia test
    1. Expose infant to 1.0 FiO_2 for 10–15 minutes.
    2. Expected responses:
      a. Parenchymal lung disease – PaO_2 should rise
      b. Cyanotic CHD – no change in PaO_2
      c. PPHN – PaO_2 may rise slightly, but usually does not
  D. Simultaneous evaluation of pre- and postductal oxygenation
    1. Obtain simultaneous arterial blood gas samples from pre- (right radial artery) and postductal (umbilical or posterior tibial artery) sites.
    2. If there is a gradient (20 torr or 2.7 kPa higher in the preductal PaO_2), a right-to-left ductal shunt may be inferred. Low values from both sites does not rule out PPHN; shunting may still be occurring at the level of the foramen ovale. If both values are high and essentially equal, PPHN is unlikely to be present.
    3. Double site (e.g., right arm and a leg) monitoring, using either transcutaneous oxygen electrodes or pulse oximetry can also be used to detect the presence of a ductal shunt.
  E. The hyperoxia-hyperventilation test
    1. Hypoxemia and acidosis augment pulmonary vasoconstriction.
    2. Alkalosis and hyperoxia decrease pulmonary vascular resistance.

3. Method
   a. Hyperventilate infant (either mechanically or manually) using 1.0 FiO_2 for 10–15 minutes.
   b. Attempt to decrease $PaCO_2$ (usually to the range of 25–30 torr or 3.3–4.0 kPa), and increase pH to 7.5–7.7 range.
   c. Obtain arterial blood gas
4. Result
   a. A dramatic response (increase in PaO_2) along with marked lability generally suggest PPHN.
   b. Must differentiate whether increase in PaO_2 came from induced alkalosis and hyperoxia vs. increased mean airway pressure during test
F. Echocardiography
   1. Will rule out CHD
   2. Evaluates myocardial function
   3. May enable direct visualization of shunting (Doppler blood flow)
   4. Estimates pulmonary artery pressure from regurgitant tricuspid jet (see Chapter 10)

V. **Treatment**

A. Prenatal
   1. Pregnancies found to be complicated by conditions associated with PPHN (e.g., congenital diaphragmatic hernia, prolonged oligohydramnios) should be referred to a high-risk center capable of caring for the infant following delivery.
   2. Identification and appropriate obstetrical management of other at-risk pregnancies (e.g., meconium-staining, chorioamnionitis, postdatism)
B. Postnatal
   1. Adequate resuscitation
   2. Avoidance of hypothermia, hypovolemia, hypoglycemia
   3. Avoidance of acidosis, hypoxia, and hypercarbia
   4. Prompt treatment of suspected sepsis, hypotension, or other problems
C. Establish the diagnosis.
D. General supportive measures
   1. Use an appropriate ventilatory strategy and mode.
   2. Assure adequate systemic blood pressure.
   3. Maintain adequate oxygen carrying capacity (hemoglobin >15 mg/dL)
   4. Treat the underlying disorder.
      a. Surfactant replacement for respiratory distress syndrome

      b. Antibiotics, if indicated

      c. Correct mechanical problems (e.g., ascites, pleural effusions, pneumothorax).

E. Mechanical ventilation

  1. Initial approach should be to establish adequate normal ventilation while correcting the underlying pulmonary disease if present. Both conventional mechanical ventilation and high-frequency ventilation have been utilized.

  2. There is a paucity of literature to define an optimal approach to the ventilatory management of PPHN. Two diametrically opposite approaches have been suggested, but have not been compared by adequate clinical investigation.

      a. Hyperventilation and alkalosis. This approach attempts to take advantage of the vasodilatory effects of alkalosis and hypocarbia on the pulmonary vasculature. Decrease the $PaCO_2$ to the "critical" value, below which there is a sharp rise in PaO_2. Alkalosis can be augmented by infusion of sodium bicarbonate. pH levels are usually kept above 7.5. Skeletal muscle relaxants are also frequently used. Ventilator changes and decrease in adjunctive support is done very slowly.

      b. Conservative ventilation uses the least amount of support possible to achieve gas exchange and pH which is marginally acceptable. The philosophy is to decrease the level of ventilatory support to the lowest possible, so that lung hyperexpansion (which contributes to pulmonary vascular resistance) and barotrauma are avoided. PaO_2 levels of 40–45 torr (5.7–6.0 kPa), $PaCO_2$ levels of 55–60 torr (7.7–8.0 kPa), and pH levels of 7.25 are tolerated. The use of sedatives and skeletal muscle relaxants is discouraged.

      c. Many clinicians prefer a "middle of the road" approach, where physiologically normal blood gases and pH are targeted by using ventilator support that is somewhere in between those approaches described above.

  3. No matter which approach is chosen, remember that infants with PPHN demonstrate extreme lability. It is usually better to attempt several small ventilator/FiO_2 changes than one large one.

  4. A transitional phase of PPHN occurs at 3–5 days of age. Vascular reactivity diminishes and support can be decreased at a faster rate.

F. Pharmacotherapy

  1. Maintain adequate cardiac output and systemic blood pressure. The degree of right-to-left shunting depends on the pulmonary-to-systemic gradient. Avoidance of systemic hypotension is critical. Central venous pressure monitoring may be of benefit.

      a. Correct hypovolemia by administering volume expanders.

      b. Cardiotonic agents (e.g., dopamine, dobutamine)

  2. Alkalinizing agents

   a. Sodium bicarbonate – may be given as a bolus (1–3 mEq/kg) or as a continuous infusion ($\leq$1.0 mEq/h). Avoid hypernatremia; assure adequate ventilation.

   b. Tris-hydroxyaminomethane (THAM, 0.3 M). Can be given even if $PaCO_2$ is elevated. Dose is 4–8 mL/kg. Observe for hypokalemia, hypoglycemia, and respiratory depression.

3. Pulmonary vasodilating agents

   a. Tolazoline. Nonselective vasodilator with variable responsiveness in PPHN.

     (1) Make sure blood pressure is adequate before using, and be prepared to treat sudden hypotension after it is given. Prepare 10–20 mL/kg colloid.

     (2) Give a test dose of 1–2 mg/kg through a vein that drains to the superior vena cava. This minimizes the delivery of drug across the foramen ovale into the systemic circulation, where it can cause severe hypotension.

     (3) A positive response is indicated by a bright, red skin blush *and* a rapid increase in oxygenation (PaO_2, $TcPO_2$, or SaO_2). If no response, stop the drug.

     (4) For responders, initiate continuous infusion at 1–2 mg/kg/h. Start to wean slowly when FiO_2 <0.4.

     (5) Side effects include hypotension, renal failure, and gastrointestinal bleeding.

     (6) DO NOT use this agent as a "last ditch" effort just prior to transporting an infant to a higher level center.

   b. Other intravenous agents which have been tried

     (1) Chlorpromazine

     (2) Magnesium sulfate

   c. Inhaled nitric oxide (see Chapter 77). Still investigational, inhaled nitric oxide has been promising in the treatment of PPHN. Given by inhalational route at doses up to 80 ppm. Potential toxicities include methemoglobinemia and lung injury from metabolites formed during the oxidation of nitric oxide.

G. Extracorporeal membrane oxygenation (see Chapter 76)

1. Rescue modality generally used when predicted mortality from PPHN approaches 80%

2. Overall survival exceeds 80% and is dependent upon underlying disease; lower rates for congenital diaphragmatic hernia and pulmonary hypoplasia.

3. Long-term sequelae in about 20%, which is equivalent to that reported in infants surviving PPHN treated by conventional means.

Suggested Reading

Deluga KS: Persistent pulmonary hypertension of the newborn. In Donn SM, Faix RG (Eds.): *Neonatal Emergencies.* Armonk, NY, Futura Publishing Co., 1991, pp. 279–296.

Donn SM: Alternatives to ECMO. Arch Dis Child 1994; 70:F81–F84.

Drummond WH, Gregory GA, Heyman MA, et al: The independent effects of hyperventilation, tolazoline, and dopamine on infants with persistent pulmonary hypertension. J Pediatr 1981; 98:603–609.

Kinsella JP, Shaffer E, Neish SR, et al: Low-dose inhalational nitric oxide in persistent pulmonary hypertension of the newborn. Lancet 1992; 340:818–822.

Peckham GJ, Fox WW: Physiological factors affecting pulmonary artery pressures in infants with persistent pulmonary hypertension. J Pediatr 1978; 93:1005–1110.

Roberts JD, Polaner DM, Lang P, et al: Inhaled nitric oxide in persistent pulmonary hypertension of the newborn. Lancet 1992; 340:818–821.

Wung JT, James LS, Kilchevsky E, et al: Management of infants with severe respiratory failure and persistence of the fetal circulation, without hyperventilation. Pediatrics 1985; 76:488–493.

Chapter 44

Neonatal Pulmonary Hemorrhage

Tonse N. K. Raju

I. **Description**
Pulmonary hemorrhage is an acute disorder in which there is bleeding into the lungs and airways, leading to marked clinical deterioration and poor long-term outcome.

II. **Infants at Risk**

A. Host factors
  1. <28 weeks gestation and/or <1,000 gm birthweight
  2. Small for gestational age
  3. Twin

B. Etiology and underlying clinical considerations
  1. Respiratory distress syndrome (RDS), especially following treatment with either synthetic or natural exogenous surfactant
  2. Patent ductus arteriosus (PDA)
  3. Pulmonary interstitial emphysema (PIE) and/or pneumothorax
  4. Systemic or pulmonary infections: bacterial, viral, or fungal (*Listeria* and *Hemophilus influenzae* are notorious)
  5. Severe metabolic acidosis during the first week of life
  6. Hypothermia, hypoglycemia, and shock during the first week of life
  7. Extracorporeal membrane oxygenation (ECMO) – severe pulmonary hemorrhage might develop even after decannulation
  8. Disseminated intravascular coagulation (DIC) from any cause
  9. Trauma to the vocal cords, trachea, or other laryngeal and oropharyngeal structures (difficult and/or traumatic intubation)
  10. In experimental animals, inhaled nitric oxide (NO) at concentrations of 80 ppm has been shown to cause pulmonary hemorrhage because of increased production of nitrogen dioxide (1 ppm).

C. Incidence
  1. The reported incidence varies depending upon the definition, diligence of monitoring and reporting, and patient characteristics.

2. Inversely related to the gestational age between 23–30 weeks

3. 1.4% of all infants admitted to a neonatal intensive care unit had pulmonary hemorrhage; 80% of them had RDS.

4. A meta-analysis of trials using surfactants for RDS found the mean pulmonary hemorrhage incidence to be 3% (range 1–7%) in surfactant-treated infants, and 2% (range 0.1–4%) in controls with a relative risk of 1.47 (47% increase with surfactant use).

5. The mean incidence is 6% among ECMO-treated infants (range 5–10%)

6. The incidence with inhaled NO therapy is unknown.

D. Pathophysiology

    1. Poorly understood. Three sets of related factors might be involved:

        a. Local hemodynamic factors. Pulmonary hemorrhage may be an exaggerated hemorrhagic pulmonary edema brought about by an acute increase in pulmonary blood flow from multiple, but related factors. The normally occurring postnatal reduction in the pulmonary vascular resistance and improving pulmonary compliance (from surfactant therapy or absorption of lung fluid) sets the stage for enhancing pulmonary vascular flow. A left-to-right shunt via the normally patent and large ductus arteriosus in preterm infants further aggravates the pulmonary blood flow leading to hemorrhagic pulmonary edema.

        b. Hematological factors. Sepsis-induced DIC results in coagulation abnormalities causing hemorrhage in multiple sites. DIC, shock, or infection may also alter local vascular integrity (from tissue necrotic factors), leading to capillary leak or rupture.

        c. Surfactant. Exogenous surfactants have been shown to increase red blood cell toxicity and hemolysis in *in vivo* experiments. Red blood cell toxicity was seen with all commercial surfactants tested, although its intensity varied.

E. Pathology. Autopsy findings depend upon the severity of the pulmonary hemorrhage and the interval between the episode and death. The most dramatic changes are seen in infants dying within a short time after the hemorrhage (Figure 68).

    1. Macroscopic. The lung weight is increased from the blood; its lobar borders are obliterated, and frank blood may be found in the large airways, trachea, and pleural space.

    2. Microscopic. Varying amounts of frank blood may be found bilaterally; the blood is seen in the pulmonary interstitial and pleural spaces obliterating areas of gas exchange. Reactive leukocytosis superimposed upon RDS, bronchopulmonary dysplasia (BPD), or pneumonia may be found, depending upon the underlying cause. There may be evidence of bleeding in the bowel, kidney, and brain. In one study based on autopsy cases, the distribution of pulmonary hemorrhage was found to be predominantly alveolar in those infants who had received exogenous surfactant, while the hemor-

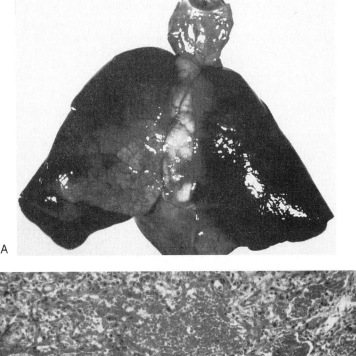

A

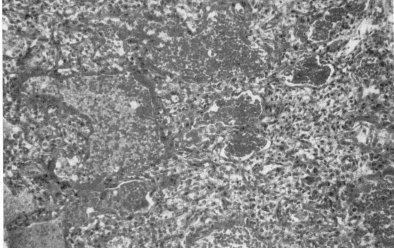

B

Figure 68. Gross appearance of the lungs in an infant who died of massive pulmonary hemorrhage **(A).** Microscopic findings of lung section in the same infant shows large quantities of blood in the alveolar spaces and scattered bleeding sites in the interstitial spaces. Generalized features of hyaline membrane formation and widespread inflammatory reaction are seen **(B).** Two other cases are shown. (*continued*)

290

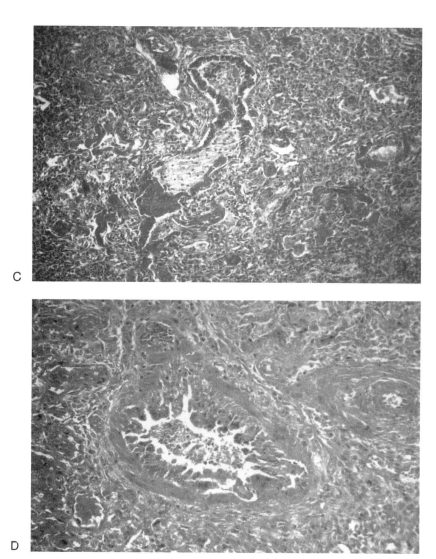

Figure 68 (*continued*). **(C)** Massive pulmonary hemorrhage occurred 2 weeks prior to death. **(D)** Infant died at 4 weeks of age from respiratory failure secondary to bronchopulmonary dysplasia; there was no clinical evidence of pulmonary hemorrhage. Scattered areas of bleeding can be identified. Both infants show varying degrees of chronic changes in the lungs.

rhage was predominantly interstitial in those who had not. This suggests that exogenous surfactant therapy may simply alter the *distribution* of the bleeding sites (predominantly alveolar) rather than increasing the risk for pulmonary hemorrhage.

F. Clinical features. The clinical manifestations result from: worsening of pulmonary compliance from blood in the lung tissue; excessive consumption (or inhibition) of endogenous surfactant; reduced gas exchange; irritation from blood leading to inflammation and later, infection of the lungs; mechanical effects from blocking of the airways by blood and clots; and anemia, acidosis, shock, and cardiac failure. The magnitude and severity of signs will depend upon the magnitude of hemorrhage and the severity of the underlying disease.

1. Suspect pulmonary hemorrhage when an otherwise "stable" infant suddenly deteriorates. Hypoxia, hypercapnia, and mixed acidosis with an increase in ventilator setting requirements are common; grossly bloody or blood-tinged tracheal and oropharyngeal effluent and shock may also accompany. Pulmonary mechanics tests will show deteriorating lung compliance and increasing airway resistance.

2. In the presence of systemic shock and sudden deterioration, consider pulmonary hemorrhage *even in the absence of blood or blood-tinged orotracheal effluent,* since the bleeding may be interstitial.

3. Localized, small, pulmonary hemorrhage may cause a gradual evolution of signs. In those cases, the diagnosis of pulmonary hemorrhage is established by exclusion of other causes.

4. A reduction in hematocrit and platelet counts may occur hours later.

5. Cardiac murmur and/or other signs of PDA may be found.

6. Other causes of left-to-right shunting and of pulmonary edema must be evaluated, such as congestive cardiac failure (ventricular septal defect, atrial septal defect, or cerebral arteriovenous malformations).

G. Investigations – should depend upon the clinical presentation.

1. Chest radiograph. There are no specific diagnostic features in chest radiographs. Diffusely scattered haziness, consolidation, fluffy radio-densities and features of the underlying disease (RDS, BPD, or PIE) should suggest pulmonary hemorrhage. Cardiomegaly may or may not be present, depending upon the underlying cause of pulmonary hemorrhage (Figures 69 and 70).

2. Evaluating the PDA. Suspect a significant PDA in an infant with pulmonary hemorrhage, *even in the absence of a typical "PDA murmur";* other signs of PDA (a wide pulse pressure, heaving precordium) may be present. An echocardiogram is recommended.

3. Blood tests and work-up for sepsis. Blood gas and acid-base status, hemoglobin and hematocrit, platelet, and a total and differential white blood cell count are done as standard tests. Bacterial culture

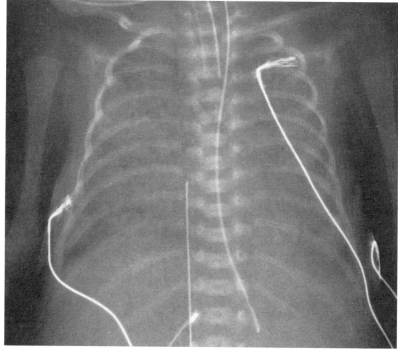

A

Figure 69. Evolution of pulmonary hemorrhage in an infant with respiratory distress syndrome. Chest radiographs show typical features of severe pulmonary interstitial emphysema on the 5th day **(A),** and severe pulmonary hemorrhage on the 7th day. (*continued*)

from blood and urine should be considered and, if other signs indicate, viral and fungal cultures may be obtained. Tests for DIC (prothrombin time, partial thromboplastin time, fibrin split products, etc.) are optional.

4. For bleeding in other organs. Urinalysis to rule out major bleeding in the kidney and a cranial ultrasound examination to rule out intracranial hemorrhage is recommended depending upon other findings.

H. Treatment is supportive.

1. Intensive care and antishock measures. Transfuse with blood, plasma, or platelets as indicated; correct metabolic acidosis with infusions of alkali, and support systemic blood pressure with inotropic agents.

2. Ventilatory care. Increase the ventilatory settings to provide a higher rate, positive end-expiratory pressure (PEEP), and mean airway pressure (Pāw). The use of high-frequency ventilation for this disorder is not yet approved, remains controversial, is not clinically proven, and is potentially dangerous.

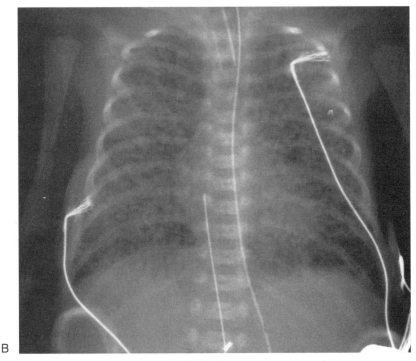

B

Figure 69 (*continued*). **(B)** Heart size is normal.

3. Treat the PDA. Unless there is severe thrombocytopenia, indomethacin therapy can be used in proven or suspected pulmonary hemorrhage, even if it was given before.

4. Exogenous surfactant. Although paradoxical, exogenous surfactant has been shown to improve the respiratory status in infants with pulmonary hemorrhage. The administered surfactant replenishes the endogenous surfactant pool depleted either from an inhibition or inactivation from blood and plasma in the alveoli.

5. Treatment of infection. Antibiotics most likely to be effective against common bacterial pathogens are used: ampicillin (or vancomycin), along with a drug for gram-negative coverage may be given until a specific etiologic agent, if any, is identified.

6. Measures to stop pulmonary hemorrhage. Nebulized epinephrine with or without 4% cocaine has been found to temporize massive bleeding. Experience using these drugs is limited in the newborn.

I. Outcome
   1. Mortality: average 50%; range 30–90%
   2. Morbidity: 50–75% of survivors develop BPD of varying severity

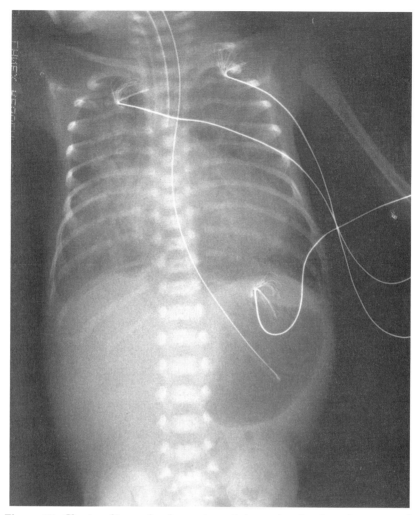

Figure 70. Chest radiograph of a preterm infant who developed severe pulmonary hemorrhage on the 6th day secondary to a large, florid patent ductus arteriosus and signs of congestive heart failure. Pulmonary hemorrhage was accompanied by respiratory deterioration. Scattered radio-opaque densities, mostly in both lower lobes can be seen, and there is moderate cardiomegaly.

J. Prevention

1. Monitoring for PDA. Vigilant monitoring for the signs of PDA in extremely small preterm infants with RDS requiring assisted ventilation is prudent. It is felt that reducing PDA incidence might reduce pulmonary hemorrhage.

2. Antenatal corticosteroid enhances lung maturity, and most likely, reduces pulmonary hemorrhage through its effect on the lungs and on blood vessels and capillaries.

Suggested Reading

Findlay RD, Taeusch HW, David WR, Walther FJ: Lysis of blood cells and alveolar epithelial toxicity by therapeutic pulmonary surfactants. Pediatr Res 1995; 37:26–30.

Goretksy MJ, Martinasek D, Warner BW: Pulmonary hemorrhage: a novel complication after extracorporeal life support. J Pediatr Surg 1996; 31: 1276–1281.

Long W, Corbet A, Allen A, et al: Retrospective search for bleeding diathesis among premature newborn infants with pulmonary hemorrhage after synthetic surfactant treatment. J Pediatr 1992; 120:S45–S48.

Pandit PB, Dunn MS, Colucci EA: Surfactant therapy in neonates with respiratory deterioration due to pulmonary hemorrhage. Pediatrics 1995; 95: 32–36.

Pappin A, Shenker N, Jack M, Redline RW: Extensive intraalveolar pulmonary hemorrhage in infants dying after surfactant therapy. J Pediatr 1994; 124: 621–626.

Raju TNK, Langenberg P: Pulmonary hemorrhage and exogenous surfactant therapy: a meta-analysis. J Pediatr 1993; 123:603–610.

Rao KVS, Michalski L: Intrauterine pulmonary hemorrhage secondary to antenatal Coxsackie B-2 infection. Pediatr Res 1997; 41:265A.

van Houten J, Long W, Mullett M, et al: Pulmonary hemorrhage in premature infants after surfactant treatment with synthetic surfactant: an autopsy study. J Pediatr 1992; 120:S40–S44.

Chapter 45

Thoracic Airleaks

Kim K. Tekkanat, Steven M. Donn

I. **Description**
Thoracic airleak refers to a collection of gas outside the pulmonary space. A variety of disorders are included in this category including pneumothorax, pneumomediastinum, pneumopericardium, pulmonary interstitial emphysema, pneumoperitoneum, and subcutaneous emphysema.

II. **Incidence and Risk Factors**
Estimates for the overall incidence of airleak in normal term infants range from 0.07–1%.

   A. The incidence of airleak varies depending on:
   1. Degree of perinatal hypoxemia
   2. Technique of resuscitation
   3. Concomitant respiratory disease
   4. Type and style of assisted ventilation
   5. Quality of radiographs and their interpretation
   B. The likelihood of pneumothorax being symptomatic without underlying lung disease is small and many go undetected.
   C. Several disease states increase the risk of pulmonary airleaks
   1. Respiratory distress syndrome (RDS), incidence 5–20%
   2. Meconium aspiration syndrome (MAS), incidence 20–50%
   3. Pulmonary hypoplasia
   4. Pulmonary interstitial emphysema (PIE)

III. **Pathophysiology**
Airleak syndromes arise by a common pathway that involves damage of the respiratory epithelium, usually by high transpulmonary pressures. Damaged epithelium allows air to enter the interstitium causing pulmonary interstitial emphysema. With continued high transpulmonary pressures, air dissects toward the visceral pleura and/or hilum via peribronchial or perivascular spaces.

A. Pneumothorax results when the pleural surface is ruptured with air leaking into the pleural space.

B. Pneumomediastinum results when air, following the path of least resistance enters the mediastinum.

C. Pneumopericardium results as above when air dissects into the pericardium.

D. Subcutaneous emphysema occurs when air from the mediastinum egresses into the fascial planes of the neck and skin.

E. Pneumoperitoneum results from the dissection of retroperitoneal air, from pneumomediastinal decompression, into the peritoneum. (It can also occur from a ruptured abdominal viscus.)

IV. Airleak Syndromes

A. Pneumothorax often results from high inspiratory pressures and uneven ventilation.

   1. Etiology

      a. Spontaneous pneumothoraces (seen in up to 1% of normal term infants around the time of birth; only about 10% of these are symptomatic)

      b. Lung diseases such as meconium aspiration syndrome, congenital bullae, and pulmonary hypoplasia which result in uneven lung compliance and alveolar overdistention

      c. Direct injury by suctioning through the endotracheal tube is a rare cause of pneumothorax

      d. Respiratory support

         (1) Prolonged inspiratory time (inspiratory:expiratory [I:E] ratio ≥1:1)

         (2) High mean airway pressure (≥12 cm H_2O)

         (3) Low inspired gas temperature (<36.5°C). This is especially true for infants weighing <1,500 gm and is thought to result from decreased mucociliary clearance precipitating airway obstruction at lower temperatures and lower humidity.

         (4) Poor patient-ventilator interaction (dyssynchrony, i.e., infants who actively expire during part or all of the positive pressure plateau)

   2. Diagnosis is made using the combination of clinical signs, physical examination, arterial blood gases, transillumination, and radiography.

      a. Clinical signs of pneumothorax include that of respiratory distress, e.g., tachypnea, grunting, flaring, and retractions. Cyanosis, decreased breath sounds over the affected side, chest asymmetry, episodes of apnea and bradycardia, shift in cardiac point of maximum impluse, and hypotension also occur.

    b. Arterial blood gases may show respiratory or mixed acidosis and hypoxemia.

    c. Transillumination may reveal an increased transmission of light on the involved side.

    d. Chest radiography remains the gold standard for diagnosis of pneumothorax.

  3. Treatment of pneumothorax is discussed in Chapter 67.

  4. Prevention

    a. Fast rate ventilation (>60 bpm) may reduce active expiration, a precursor of pneumothorax. This is done in an attempt to provoke more synchronous respiration. If this fails, the patient may require sedation and/or paralysis to reduce active expiration. High-frequency ventilation may also provide better ventilation and oxygenation while decreasing the incidence of pneumothorax.

    b. Patient-triggered ventilation reduces the incidence of airleak by synchronizing respiration. Using this mode of ventilation, the infant's respiratory efforts trigger the delivery of the positive pressure inflation. When synchronous respiration is achieved, the development of pneumothorax is lessened. Flow-cycling enables complete synchronization, even in expiration.

    c. Suppression of respiratory activity by patient paralysis may be an important means of preventing pneumothoraces in patients who are actively exhaling or "fighting" the ventilator.

B. PIE occurs most often in ventilated, preterm infants with RDS. Interstitial air can be localized or widespread throughout one or both lungs. PIE alters pulmonary mechanics by decreasing compliance, increasing residual volume and dead space, and increasing $\dot{V}/\dot{Q}$ mismatch. It also impedes pulmonary blood flow.

  1. Diagnosis is made using a combination of clinical signs, transillumination and chest radiography.

    a. Clinical signs of PIE include profound respiratory acidosis and hypoxemia. Because air is interstitial instead of intra-alveolar, proper gas exchange does not occur, decreasing ventilation. Trapped gas reduces pulmonary perfusion by compression of blood vessels resulting in hypoxemia.

    b. Transillumination of a chest with diffuse and widespread PIE will result in increased transmission of light, similar to that seen in a pneumothorax.

    c. Chest radiography may reveal a characteristic cystic appearance or may be more subtle with rounded, nonconfluent microradiolucencies in earlier stages. In later stages of PIE, there may be large bullae formation with hyperinflation in the involved portions of lung.

  2. Management

    a. Generalized PIE management is focused on reducing or preventing further barotrauma to the lung.

(1) Decreasing peak inspiratory pressure to the minimum required to attain acceptable arterial blood gases (PaO_2 45–50 torr or 6–6.7 kPa, and $PaCO_2$ <60 torr or 8 kPa).

(2) Reduction in positive end-expiratory pressure (PEEP) may also help decrease PIE.

(3) High-frequency jet ventilation is a successful means of ventilation for infants with PIE. This mode results in improved ventilation at lower peak and mean airway pressures with more rapid resolution of PIE.

b. Localized PIE may resolve spontaneously or persist for several weeks with a sudden enlargement and deterioration in the infant's condition. Progressive overdistension of the affected area can cause compression of the adjacent normal lung parenchyma.

Suggested Reading

Alpan G, Goder K, Glick F, et al: Pneumopericardium during continuous positive airway pressure in respiratory distress syndrome. Crit Care Med 1984; 37:511–515.

Douglas-Jones J, Bustamante S, Mirza M: Pneumopericardium in a newborn. J Pediatr Surg 1981; 16:75–78.

Keszler M, Donn SM, Bucciarelli RL, et al: Controlled multicenter trial of high frequency jet ventilation vs. conventional ventilation in newborns with pulmonary interstitial emphysema. J Pediatr 1991; 119:85–93.

Madansky DL, Lawson EE, Chernick V, et al: Pneumothorax and other forms of pulmonary air leak in newborns. Am Rev Respir Dis 1979; 120:729–733.

Zak LK, Donn SM: Thoracic air leaks. In Donn SM, Faix RG (Eds.): *Neonatal Emergencies.* Mount Kisco, NY, Futura Publishing Co., 1991, pp. 311–325.

Chapter 46

Congenital Diaphragmatic Hernia

David J. Field

I. **Background**
  A. Embryology. Failure of normal development of the diaphragm during the first trimester. Four types:
    1. Complete absence of the diaphragm, rare, most severe, worst prognosis
    2. Failure of normal development of the diaphragm anteriorly – only 2% of cases
    3. Failure of the diaphragm to close posteriorly – most common (approximately 1 in 5,000 births) – 85% left sided, 10% right sided, 5% bilateral
    4. Eventration – not a true hernia – results from a failure of muscle development in the primitive diaphragm (not considered further here)
  B. Can be part of a syndrome (e.g., Fryns) or associated with a chromosomal anomaly (e.g., trisomy 13 or 18) – prognosis is worse in such cases.
  C. Pathophysiology
    1. Compression of both lungs during pregnancy results in hypoplasia especially in the ipsilateral lung.
    2. In most severe cases, cardiac function can also be compromised *in utero.*
    3. After delivery, gaseous distension of gut in the chest results in further cardiorespiratory compromise.
    4. Pulmonary hypoplasia and poor oxygenation following delivery commonly result in severe persistent pulmonary hypertension of the newborn.
    5. In mild cases cardiopulmonary development and function may be sufficient to enable normal extrauterine adaptation with presentation at a later stage.

II. **Presentation and Diagnosis**
  A. Antenatal
    1. Easily detected on routine maternal sonographic scan during second

301

or third trimester; herniated abdominal viscera and mediastinal shift are readily identifiable.

2. Right-sided lesions more difficult to detect because of the similar echogenicity of lung and liver.

3. Polyhydramnios commonly seen

4. Various other anomalies have been noted in association with diaphragmatic hernia.

B. Postnatal. Where not suspected antenatally, presentation may be:

1. At delivery with failure to respond to normal resuscitative measures – in such cases a barrel chest and scaphoid abdomen may be noted

2. Within the first 48 hours of life with respiratory distress

3. In later childhood, where signs can be various and may be respiratory and or gastroenterological in nature. Currently, <5% of cases present in this way.

C. Differential diagnosis. Cystic lesions of the lung (most commonly cystic adenomatoid malformation) and growths or effusions which render one hemithorax opaque can cause confusion.

D. Investigations. Antenatal ultrasound findings or clinical presentation alone may strongly suggest the diagnosis. Useful additional investigations:

1. Chest radiograph – essential

2. Contrast studies – used to confirm presence of stomach/gut in the chest – rarely necessary

3. Ultrasound or isotope study to document position of the liver

4. Rarely, computed tomography scan

III. Predicting Outcome

Rationale. Diaphragmatic hernia produces a spectrum of pathology from very mild (causing minimal compromise) to severe (incompatible with life). Significant numbers fall into this latter category. If they can be identified, pointless exposure to surgery and intensive care can be avoided. A variety of techniques have been used; none are uniformly successful. Suggested indicators of poor prognosis that are still commonly attempted include:

A. Antenatal sonographic scans (polyhydramnios, reduced chest circumference, significant mediastinal shift, reduced fetal breathing)

B. Postnatal chest radiograph (intrathoracic stomach, estimated degree of pulmonary hypoplasia)

C. Postnatal lung function (lung volumes, pulmonary compliance)

D. Echocardiography (ventricular thickness)

IV. Management

A. Antenatal. Once a diagnosis is made, families should be counseled by the obstetrician, neonatologist, and neonatal surgeon regarding available options

1. Termination (criteria and regulations vary markedly between countries)
2. Continuing the pregnancy and performing postnatal repair
3. Antenatal surgery – practiced in only a few centers around the world. Current results are poor. Repair often induces premature delivery.

B. At delivery in cases diagnosed antenatally
   1. **Avoid gaseous distension of the gut.**
      a. Paralyze, intubate, and ventilate as soon as possible (i.e., in the delivery room). Do not use positive pressure ventilation via a mask or airway; this will cause gaseous distension of the gut.
      b. Pass a nasogastric tube in the delivery room, ensure it is left on free drainage – aspirate every 30 minutes. Alternatively, insert a Replogle tube and use continuous suction.
   2. **Minimize factors that could precipitate pulmonary hypertension.**
      a. Use adequate sedation.
      b. Try to ensure adequate ventilation.

C. In the neonatal intensive care unit (NICU) – preoperatively
   1. Where infants are not diagnosed antenatally but present soon after delivery with respiratory distress, avoidance of gaseous distension of the bowel and efforts to minimize pulmonary hypertension remain essential.
   2. Establish continuous monitoring. Invasive blood pressure/arterial access is essential (remember that samples obtained from sites other than the right arm will be affected by right-to-left shunting). Central venous pressure monitoring, if available via the umbilical vein, is of great help in fluid management.
   3. Ensure adequate systemic blood pressure (maintains tissue perfusion and minimizes right-to-left shunting). May require infusion of both colloid and inotropes. Take care not to induce fluid overload.
   4. Provide adequate ventilatory support. Local policy usually governs the first choice. Both conventional and oscillatory ventilation can be used with success. Aim to provide stability as a minimum (i e , sufficient oxygenation to prevent metabolic acidosis, sufficient control of CO_2 elimination to prevent respiratory acidosis). If this cannot be achieved despite maximum support (including extracorporeal membrane oxygenation [ECMO]) the child should be considered nonviable. The clinical condition of babies who stabilize should be optimized prior to surgery. Local guidelines often govern the timing of operation; however, evidence to support these more specific criteria is weak.
   5. Introduce pulmonary vasodilators as indicated. Pulmonary hyper-

tension is a common and major complication of diaphragmatic hernia. Nitric oxide appears to be the agent of choice, but is still investigational with unproven efficacy.

   6. Surfactant – no clear role for surfactant use has been established

D. Operation is clearly essential, but should occur only when the child is stable. It may be performed through the abdomen (allows correction of association malrotation at the same time) or chest (large defect may require use of a patch).

E. In the NICU – postoperatively
   Essentially the same pattern of management is recommended. Failure to be able to wean respiratory support in the days following operation may indicate pulmonary hypoplasia that is incompatible with life.

F. ECMO is clearly able to provide stability and control pulmonary hypertension; however, no evidence of long-term benefit over other forms of care has been demonstrated.

V. Outcome

A. Short term. Almost all published results are difficult to interpret since they are hospital-based and therefore:

   1. Contain referral bias

   2. Do not make clear the effect of antenatal counseling

   3. May exclude high-risk groups, such as those with associated anomalies. 50–60% survival beyond the neonatal period would represent good results.

B. Medium term. A proportion of infants who survive the neonatal period will die within the first 2 years of life as a result of pulmonary hypertension/hypoplasia.

C. Long term. Respiratory outcome reflects the severity of the initial lesion and the amount and type of respiratory support required. Survivors are also at significant risk of neurodevelopmental delay, presumably secondary to problems in the perinatal period and other medical problems (e.g., volvulus, gastroesophageal reflux, chronic lung disease).

VI. New Approaches Under Development

A. Tracheal occlusion *in utero* can raise intrapulmonary pressure and clear gut from the chest. It can also produce secondary problems (e.g., hydrops).

B. Liquid ventilation (see Chapter 68) may be able to maintain gas exchange while encouraging increased lung volume. It remains investigational.

Suggested Reading

Cannon C, Dildy GA, Ward R, et al: A population-based study of congenital diaphragmatic hernia in Utah: 1988–1994. Obstet Gynecol 1996; 87:959–963.

Graf JL, Gibbs DL, Adzick NS, et al: Fetal hydrops after in utero tracheal occlusion. J Pediatr Surg 1997; 32:214–215.

Kinsella JP, Truog WE, Walsh WF, et al: Randomized, multicenter trial of inhaled nitric oxide and high-frequency oscillatory ventilation in severe, persistent pulmonary hypertension of the newborn. J Pediatr 1997; 131: 55–62.

Nio M, Haase G, Kennaugh J, et al: A prospective randomized trial of delayed versus immediate repair of congenital diaphragmatic hernia. J Pediatr Surg 1994; 29:618–621.

Nobuhara KK, Lund DP, Mitchell J, et al: Long-term outlook for survivors of congenital diaphragmatic hernia. Clin Perinatol 1996; 23:873–887.

Pranikoff T, Gauger PG, Hirschl RB: Partial liquid ventilation in newborn patients with congenital diaphragmatic hernia. J Pediatr Surg 1996; 31: 613–618.

Chapter 47

Pulmonary Hypoplasia

David J. Field

I. **Classification**

A. Pulmonary

1. Agenesis – can be isolated or part of syndrome. Failure of one or both lung buds to develop at the very beginning of lung development. Bilateral agenesis is always fatal. Unilateral defect may be asymptomatic.

2. Hypoplasia (structural)

   a. Primary – rare defect, may be associated with other congenital anomalies

   b. Secondary – consequence of any lesion that impairs normal development (Table 27)

3. Hypoplasia (biochemical), primary. A handful of cases have been identified which present with features of pulmonary hypoplasia but structurally normal lungs. Abnormalities of surfactant have been identified, in particular absence of surfactant protein B.

B. Vascular

1. Macroscopic. Atresia of the main pulmonary trunk can disrupt normal pulmonary vascular development; however, pulmonary function is normally satisfactory. Presentation is with severe cyanosis, which can be remedied by improving pulmonary blood flow.

2. Microscopic. Pulmonary vasculature can be disrupted at the alveolar level and result in severely reduced gas exchange. Dysplasia is rare, but a small number of patterns have been recognized to date (e.g., malalignment of the pulmonary veins, alveolar capillary dysplasia).

II. **Pathophysiology**

The exact pathophysiology varies with the underlying mechanism.

A. Reduced lung capacity (secondary to thoracic dystrophy)

B. Structural immaturity (secondary to oligohydramnios)

C. Diffusion deficit (secondary to malalignment of the pulmonary veins). Functional problem in all pulmonary insufficiency. Main clinical problem tends to be oxygen transfer.

Table 27
Factors That Can Impair Lung Growth *in Utero*

- Compression of chest (e.g., oligohydramnios – all causes)
- Compression of lung (e.g., effusion, diaphragmatic hernia)
- Reduction in fetal breathing (e.g., neuromuscular disorder)

III. **Diagnosis**

A. Antenatal – diagnosis may be anticipated on the basis of maternal antenatal ultrasound scan (e.g., severe oligohydramnios, small fetal chest cavity).

B. Postnatal diagnosis may be apparent immediately after birth if hypoplasia is severe (i.e., cannot be resuscitated, or severe respiratory distress from birth), or is part of recognizable syndrome (e.g., Potter's). Diagnosis may be delayed; the infant may present with mild to moderate respiratory distress; no dysmorphic features and no other etiological features may be detectable. This includes exclusion of rare infectious agents. In all cases where hypoplasia is the possible diagnosis, the following should be considered:

1. Genetics consultation
2. Measurement of lung volumes
3. Measurement of pulmonary compliance
4. Examination of surfactant genotype
5. Lung biopsy
   The choice of investigation will vary with severity of the child's problem. In severe respiratory failure, lung biopsy may be performed as a terminal event to permit diagnosis and counseling for future pregnancies (see below). If more minor respiratory problems (e.g., unexplained persistent tachypnea) are present, assessment of pulmonary mechanics is appropriate.

IV. **Management**

A. Antenatal. If a diagnosis of pulmonary hypoplasia is made *in utero*, families should be counseled by the obstetrician, neonatologist, clinical geneticist, and surgeon (if appropriate). Potential options will vary according to:

1. Diagnosis and prognosis
2. Degree of diagnostic certainty resulting from the evaluation. Essentially, parents must decide between:

   a. Termination of pregnancy (criteria and regulations vary markedly among countries)
   b. Continuing the pregnancy with postnatal intervention and "treatment"

307

    c. Antenatal intervention – practiced only in relation to certain conditions (e.g., bilateral pleural effusions). Results vary with both the nature and severity of underlying problem.

B. At delivery, standard resuscitation should take place. Where antenatal scans indicate, special measures (e.g., draining pleural effusions) should be performed. Vigorous resuscitation of infants with small volume lungs often results in pneumothorax. If dysmorphic features in the child indicate a lethal syndrome, or if oxygenation proves impossible, intensive care can be withdrawn.

C. In the neonatal intensive care unit

1. Establish routine monitoring. Invasive blood pressure/arterial access is essential in the severest cases; central venous pressure, if available via the umbilical vein, is of great help in fluid management.

2. Ensure adequate systemic blood pressure (maintain tissue perfusion and minimize right-to-left shunting). May require both infusion of colloid and inotropes. Take care not to induce fluid overload.

3. Provide adequate respiratory support. Infants with mild hypoplasia may not require ventilation. For those requiring invasive support, local policy usually governs the first choice; both conventional and high-frequency ventilation can be used with success. Aim to provide stability of blood gases (i.e., sufficient oxygenation to prevent metabolic acidosis). More aggressive ventilation may induce pulmonary damage and further impair lung function. If blood gas control proves impossible despite maximum support, the child should be considered nonviable.

4. Introduce pulmonary vasodilators as indicated; pulmonary hypertension is often a complication. Doppler studies may help confirm the diagnosis. Inhaled nitric oxide appears to be the agent of choice but remains experimental and unproven.

5. Surfactant. There is no clear role for surfactant use in this setting.

6. Extracorporeal membrane oxygenation (ECMO) is clearly able to provide stability, but there is no evidence of benefit over other forms of care in pulmonary hypoplasia.

7. A role for the use of partial liquid ventilation is not established.

8. Investigate to establish the diagnosis. Where there are no clear features to support a diagnosis of pulmonary hypoplasia, routine tests should exclude all other causes of respiratory distress.

V. Outcome

Pulmonary hypoplasia results from a large number of different conditions. The prognosis is governed mainly by the etiology and any associated anomalies.

A. Mild cases often become asymptomatic with growth. Abnormalities of function can still be measured in later childhood.

B. Infants with moderate hypoplasia can survive with intensive care but often need long-term respiratory support. The effect of growth is uncertain and death in later childhood can occur.

C. Severely affected babies die despite full support. No current intervention is known to help in such cases.

VI. Counseling About Future Pregnancies

Some infants will be affected by conditions that can recur in future pregnancies. A proportion of severely affected cases cannot be diagnosed without examination of lung tissue. Lung biopsy may be impossible to perform safely while the child is alive. Postmortem study should be obtained whenever possible. If permission for postmortem examination is not obtained, an open or needle biopsy of the lung obtained soon after death may still allow a tissue diagnosis (in many areas, consent to do so is required).

Suggested Reading

Aiton NR, Fox GF, Hannam S, et al: Pulmonary hypoplasia presenting as persistent tachypnea in the first few months of life. BMJ 1996; 312:1149–1150.

DiFiore JW, Wilson JM. Lung development. Semin Pediatr Surg 1994; 3:221–232.

Kilbride HW, Yeast J, Thibeault DW: Defining limits of survival: lethal pulmonary hypoplasia after midtrimester premature rupture of membranes. Am J Obstet Gynecol 1996; 175:675–681.

Major D, Cadenas M, Cloutier R, et al: Morphometrics of normal and hypoplastic lungs in preterm lambs with gas and partial liquid ventilation. Pediatr Surg Int 1997; 12:121–125.

McIntosh N, Harrison A: Prolonged premature rupture of membranes in the preterm infant: a 7 year study. Eur J Obstet Gynecol Reprod Biol 1994; 47:1–6.

Sirkin W, O'Hara BP, Cox PN, et al: Alveolar capillary dysplasia: lung biopsy diagnosis, nitric oxide responsiveness, and bronchial generation count. Pediatr Pathol Lab Med 1997; 17:125–132.

Chapter 48

Bronchopulmonary Dysplasia

Jonathan M. Davis

I. **Introduction**

Bronchopulmonary dysplasia (BPD) is the chronic lung disease that develops in newborns treated with oxygen and mechanical ventilation for a primary lung disorder. Approximately 7,500 new cases occur yearly in the USA with 10–15% of these infants subsequently dying in the first year of life. BPD has become the most common form of chronic lung disease in infants.

II. **Definition**

The exact definition of BPD has become complicated since the nature of BPD has changed with exogenous surfactant and other therapeutic interventions. BPD may be defined as oxygen dependency at 28 days of age accompanied by an abnormal chest radiograph, or alternatively as oxygen dependency at 36 weeks postconceptual age (for premature infants).

III. **Incidence**

Incidence will depend on the definition used and the population studied. While surfactant treatment has improved overall survival for premature infants, the incidence of BPD in these babies remains approximately 30–40%. Incidence is lower in full-term infants.

IV. **Pathogenesis**

    A. Barotrauma: initial injury is the result of the primary disease process (e.g., respiratory distress syndrome [RDS]). Superimposed mechanical ventilation adds to the lung injury. Inflammatory cascade is then activated, leading to injury and chronic lung disease.

    B. Oxygen/antioxidants: balance exists between the production of oxygen free radicals (molecules with extra electrons in their outer ring which are toxic to tissues, causing direct damage to growth factors, antiproteases, cell membranes and nucleic acids) and antioxidant defenses (Table 28). Balance may be disturbed by increased free radical production under conditions of hyperoxia, ischemia/reperfu-

Table 28
Free Radicals and Antioxidant Quenchers

Radical	*Symbol*	*Antioxidant*
Superoxide anion	O_2^-	Superoxide dismutase, uric acid, vitamin E
Singlet oxygen	$^1O_2$	β-carotene, uric acid, vitamin E
Hydrogen peroxide	H_2O_2	Catalase, glutathione peroxidase, glutathione
Hydroxyl radical	OH*	Vitamins C, E
Peroxide radical	LOO^O (L = lipid)	Vitamins C, E
Hydroperoxyl radical	LOOH (L = lipid)	Glutathione transferase, glutathione peroxidase
Peroxynitrite	$ONOO^-$	Superoxide dismutase

sion, or inflammation. The premature newborn may be more susceptible to free radical damage since the concentration of these enzymes (which develop at a rate similar to pulmonary surfactant) may be inadequate.

C. Inflammation: plays an important role in the pathogenesis of BPD and permits a unifying hypothesis. Early elevations (by 12 h of age) of cytokines (IL-6, IL-8), followed by neutrophil/mononuclear cell influx leading to increased elastase activity and protease/antiprotease imbalance. This leads to decreased epithelial/endothelial cell integrity, pulmonary edema, and exudate.

D. Infection: group B streptococcus, gram negative rods, and *Ureaplasma urealyticum* implicated as cause of chorioamnionitis, prematurity, and BPD.

E. Nutrition: inadequate calories, essential nutrients (vital components for immunological and antioxidant defenses), vitamin deficiencies (vitamin A), decreased polyunsaturated fatty acids (PUFA).

F. Fluids/patent ductus arteriosus (PDA): PDA and BPD have been associated with increased fluid administration. Early closure of the PDA (indomethacin or surgical ligation) has not substantially affected the incidence of BPD.

G. Genetics: strong family history of atopy and asthma and HLA_2.

V. Pathophysiologic changes

A. Clinical assessment: clinical scoring system (Toce)

B. Radiographic aspects: abnormalities first described by Northway no longer usually seen; new radiographic classification

C. Cardiovascular changes: abnormal pulmonary circulation (endothelial cell degeneration and proliferation; medial muscle hypertrophy;

peripheral extension of smooth muscle; and vascular obliteration), increased pulmonary vascular resistance; and the development of cor pulmonale.

D. Pulmonary mechanics

    1. Initially an increase in pulmonary resistance and airway reactivity. Later expiratory flow limitation may become more significant.

    2. Increased resistance causes increased work of breathing and $\dot{V}/\dot{Q}$ mismatch.

    3. Functional residual capacity can be reduced initially because of atelectasis, but can be increased in later stages from air trapping and hyperinflation.

    4. Reduction of lung compliance

E. Pathologic changes

    1. Airways – large upper airways (trachea, main bronchi)

        a. Earliest histologic changes: patchy loss of cilia from columnar epithelial cells. Mucosal edema and/or necrosis (focal or diffuse), which may lead to frank ulcerations.

        b. Infiltration of inflammatory cells and granulation tissue (area of the endotracheal tube tip)

        c. Mucosal cells regenerate or are replaced by stratified squamous or metaplastic epithelium.

    2. Terminal bronchioles and alveolar ducts: necrotizing bronchiolitis and fibroblast proliferation and activation may lead to peribronchial fibrosis and obliterative fibroproliferative bronchiolitis.

    3. Alveoli

        a. Earliest findings involve interstitial and/or alveolar edema.

        b. Later, areas of atelectasis, inflammation, exudate, and fibroblast proliferation

        c. Finally, areas of atelectasis alternating with areas of marked hyperinflation

F. Management: multidisciplinary approach to improve the complex pathophysiology.

    1. Mechanical ventilation: the benefits from continued ventilation should outweigh the risks of continued progression of chronic lung damage.

    2. Oxygen: in BPD, chronic hypoxia will result in pulmonary vasoconstriction, pulmonary hypertension, and cor pulmonale. PaO_2 should be maintained between 55–70 torr (7.3–9.3 kPa) and SaO_2 between 90–95% to reduce pulmonary pressures. Oxygen should be withdrawn gradually and may be required for months.

    3. Nutrition

        a. Maximize calories for tissue repair and growth (120–140 kcal/kg/day)

    b. Adequate calcium and phosphorus (especially if receiving furosemide)

    c. Vitamins and trace elements

  4. Medication: commonly used medications in BPD

    a. Diuretics (furosemide, chlorothiazide, hydrochlorothiazide, spirono-lactone)

    b. Inhaled agents (albuterol, ipratropium, beclomethasone)

    c. Systemic agents (aminophylline, caffeine, dexamethasone, nifedipine)

    d. In infants with RDS who are at high risk for developing BPD, early dexamethasone improves pulmonary mechanics, and promotes weaning from oxygen and mechanical ventilation, but may increase mortality. In infants with documented BPD, dexamethasone acutely reduces tracheal inflammatory markers, improves pulmonary mechanics and clinical pulmonary status, and facilitates weaning from ventilation. Dexamethasone did not result in significant improvements in survival, duration of oxygen treatment, or total length of hospital stay in any study of infants with BPD. Concerns exist about multiple side effects and adverse neurodevelopmental outcomes in treated infants. At present, systemic steroids should be reserved for ventilator-dependent infants with moderate to severe BPD who are resistant to more conventional treatments in the first 4 weeks of life.

    e. Antibiotics – with respiratory decompensation from possible infection, appropriate broad spectrum antibiotics should be used initially. More specific coverage is determined once specific organisms are isolated. Beware of fungal sepsis.

    f. Physical therapy – results are controversial

VI. Outcome

  A. Most infants with BPD ultimately achieve normal lung function and thrive. They are at higher risk for death in the 1st year of life and for long-term complications.

  B. In childhood, respiratory problems (e.g., reactive airway disease) and abnormal neurologic development may occur.

  C. Cardiac function: cor pulmonale may develop

  D. Infection: increased susceptibility to viral infections (respiratory syncytial virus, influenza).

  E. Growth failure and neurodevelopmental abnormalities are increased. In contrast, severity of BPD is not a major predictor of neurologic outcome.

VII. Prevention

  A. Antenatal steroids for mothers delivering prematurely may reduce the severity and incidence of BPD.

B. Early use of nasal continuous positive airway pressure (CPAP) in RDS may eliminate the need for mechanical ventilation or facilitate earlier extubation.

C. Exogenous surfactant reduces mortality and the severity of BPD, although the total number of survivors with BPD will increase.

D. Treatment of symptomatic PDA (fluid restriction, diuretics, indomethacin, or surgery)

E. Ventilator pressures and FiO_2 should be reduced as low and as soon as possible.

F. Nutritional support – vitamins (A, C, E); minerals (Se, Cu, Zn, Mn).

G. Prophylactic human recombinant antioxidant enzymes – superoxide dismutase (SOD – Cu/Zn, intra- and extracellular; Mn – in mitochondria), catalase and glutathione peroxidase.

   1. Cell culture studies demonstrating prevention of cell damage from hyperoxia with the addition of antioxidant enzymes (AOE) to the media.

   2. Variety of animal models show reduction in acute hyperoxic lung injury by intravenous, intraperitoneal, or intratracheal administration of AOE. Studies in newborn piglets showed that intratracheal administration of rhCu/ZnSOD prevents the inflammatory changes and acute lung injury from hyperoxia and mechanical ventilation. The rhSOD is rapidly incorporated into a variety of cell types in the lung following intratracheal administration. The rhSOD remains active for 48-72 hours. Genetically engineered mice with overexpressed SOD have improved survival, while mice with disrupted SOD genes die sooner when exposed to prolonged hyperoxia compared to diploid controls. Human trials in premature infants at highest risk for the development of BPD have been performed. Preliminary studies in premature infants have shown that instillation of rhSOD increases the concentration and activity of the enzyme in the tracheal aspirate fluid, serum, and urine and is associated with a significant decrease in inflammation in the lung. Multicenter trials examining the ability of rhSOD administration to prevent acute and chronic lung injury in infants are ongoing. Gene therapy studies with known antioxidant and other novel genes (virus, liposome vectors) are also currently being performed in animals.

Suggested Reading

Bancalari E, Sosenko I: Pathogenesis and prevention of neonatal chronic lung disease: recent developments. Pediatr Pulmonol 1990; 8:109–116.

Davis JM, Dickerson B, Metlay L, Penney DP: Differential effects of oxygen and barotrauma on lung injury in the neonatal piglet. Pediatr Pulmonol 1991; 10:157–163.

Davis JM, Rosenfeld WN, Sanders RJ, Gonenne A: The prophylactic effects of human recombinant superoxide dismutase in neonatal lung injury. J Appl Physiol 1993; 74:22–34.

Davis JM, Rosenfeld W: Chronic lung disease in the newborn. In Avery GB, Fletcher MA, MacDonald MG (Eds): *Textbook of Neonatology, 4th Edition.* Philadelphia, JB Lippincott Company, 1994, pp. 453–477.

Davis JM, Sinkin RA, Aranda JV. Drug therapy for bronchopulmonary dysplasia. Pediatr Pulmonol 1990; 8:117–125.

Frank L, Groseclose EE: Preparation of birth into an O_2 rich environment: the antioxidant enzymes in the developing rabbit lung. Pediatr Res 1984; 18:240–244.

Merritt TA, Cochrane CG, Holcomb K, et al: Elastase and α_1-proteinase inhibitor activity in tracheal aspirates during respiratory distress syndrome: role of inflammation in the pathogenesis of bronchopulmonary dysplasia. J Clin Invest 1983; 72:656–666.

Northway WH Jr, Rosan C, Porter DY: Pulmonary disease following respiratory therapy of hyaline-membrane disease. N Engl J Med 1967; 76:357–368.

Pitkanen OM, Hallman M, Andersson SM: Correlation of free oxygen radical-induced lipid peroxidation with outcome in very low birth weight infants. J Pediatr 1990; 116:760–764.

Rojas MA, Gonzalez A, Bancalari E, et al: Changing trends in the epidemiology and pathogenesis of neonatal chronic lung disease. J Pediatr 1995; 126: 605–610.

Rosenfeld WN, Davis JM, Parton L, et al: Safety and pharmacokinetics of recombinant human superoxide dismutase administered intratracheally to premature neonates with respiratory distress syndrome. Pediatrics 1996; 97:811–817.

Toce SS, Farrell PM, Leavitt, LA, et al: Clinical and radiographic scoring systems for assessing bronchopulmonary dysplasia. Am J Dis Child 1984; 138:581–585.

Yoder MC Jr, Chua R, Tepper R: Effect of dexamethasone on pulmonary inflammation and pulmonary function of ventilator-dependent infants with bronchopulmonary dysplasia. Am Rev Respir Dis 1991; 143:1044–1048.

SECTION X

Complications of Mechanical Ventilation

Chapter 49

Airway and Respiratory Complications of Mechanical Ventilation

Steven M. Donn, Sunil K. Sinha

I. **Airway Complications Associated with Endotracheal Intubation**
  A. Vocal cord injury
    1. Unilateral – dysphonia
    2. Bilateral – aphonia
  B. Tracheomalacia
    1. Stridor, usually inspiratory
    2. Dyspnea
  C. Subglottic edema
    1. Generally transient following extubation
    2. May respond to sympathomimetics or corticosteroids
  D. Subglottic stenosis
    1. Idiosyncratic response; specific etiology unknown
    2. May be related to duration of intubation or multiplicity of intubations
    3. May require surgical intervention
      a. Tracheostomy
      b. Cricoid split
  E. Increased airway resistance
  F. Nasal septum damage (nasotracheal tubes)
  G. Acquired palatal groove (orotracheal tubes)
  H. Esophageal perforation
  I. Obstruction of endotracheal tube (ETT)
  J. Malpositioned or dislodged ETT

II. **Pulmonary Complications of Positive Pressure Ventilation**
  A. Gas trapping

B. Airleaks
   1. Pneumomediastinum
   2. Pneumothorax
   3. Pulmonary interstitial emphysema
   4. Pneumopericardium
   5. Pneumoperitoneum (transdiaphragmatic)
   6. Subcutaneous emphysema
   7. Air embolus
C. Pneumonia
D. Barotrauma (excessive pressure)
E. Volutrauma (excessive volume)
F. Imposed work of breathing
   1. ETT
   2. Ventilator circuit
   3. Demand valve
G. Chronic lung disease (bronchopulmonary dysplasia)
H. Reactive airways disease
I. Pulmonary hypertension
J. Cor pulmonale

Suggested Reading

Bancalari E, Sosenko I: Pathogenesis and prevention of neonatal chronic lung disease: recent developments. Pediatr Pulmonol 1990; 8:109–116.

Dreyfuss D, Saumon G. Ventilator-induced injury. In Tobin MJ (Ed.): Principles and Practice of Mechanical Ventilation. New York. McGraw-Hill, Inc., 1994, pp. 793–811.

Martin RJ, Fanaroff AA: Complications of neonatal respiratory care. In Carlo WA, Chatburn RL (Eds.): *Neonatal Respiratory Care, 2nd Edition.* Chicago, Year Book Medical Publishers, 1988, pp. 347–365.

Strong RM, Passy V. Endotracheal intubation: complications in neonates. Arch Otolaryngol 1977; 103:329–335.

Chapter 50

Patent Ductus Arteriosus

Jonathan P. Wyllie

I. **Incidence**

   A. Most common cardiac problem in preterm newborns

   B. Varies inversely with gestational age

   1. Up to 20% at >32 weeks
   2. 20–40% between 28–32 weeks
   3. 60% at <28 weeks

II. **Fetal Circulation**

   A. Derived from sixth aortic arch

   B. May be absent in association with congenital heart disease involving severe right outflow tract obstruction (rare)

   C. Carries most of right ventricular output (50–60%) from 6th to 7th week on; caliber equal to descending aorta

   D. Patency both passive (from high blood flow) and active (locally derived prostaglandin E_2 [PGE_2])

III. **Postnatal Closure**

   A. Mechanisms mature after 35 weeks.

   B. Initiated by spiral medial muscle layer starting at pulmonary end

   C. Duct shortens and thickens with functional closure at 12–72 hours.

   D. Factors promoting closure

   1. Low ductal flow (increased pulmonary flow)
   2. Reduced sensitivity to PGE_2
   3. Decreased production of PGE_2
   4. Increased arterial oxygen tension

IV. **Persistent Ductal Patency**

   A. Isolated patent ductus arteriosus (PDA) accounts for 3.5% of congenital heart disease presenting in infancy. It occurs despite ductal constriction and has a different pathogenesis from that in the preterm infant.

B. Preterm PDA is related to:
   1. Immature closure mechanism
   2. Decreased sensitivity to constrictors such as oxygen tension
   3. Increased sensitivity to PGE_2
   4. Other associated factors
      a. Acidosis
      b. Severe lung disease
      c. Exogenous surfactant use
      d. Phototherapy
      e. Furosemide use
      f. Excessive fluid administration

V.   Physiologic Effects of the PDA
   A. Left-to-right shunt
      1. Exacerbation of respiratory disease
      2. Altered pulmonary mechanics
      3. Increased cardiac workload
   B. Diastolic steal
      1. Altered perfusion of brain, systemic organs
      2. Risk of necrotizing enterocolitis

VI.   Clinical Effects of PDA
   A. Left-to-right shunt
      1. Increased oxygen requirement
      2. Increased ventilatory requirement
      3. Apnea
      4. Bronchopulmonary dysplasia
      5. Impaired weight gain
      6. Congestive heart failure
   B. Pulmonary hemorrhage

VII. Clinical Features
   A. Occurs after fall in pulmonary resistance
   B. Onset related to severity of lung disease and size of baby
   C. In very low birthweight (VLBW) infant, most common manifestation is after 4 days of age, earlier in LBW.
   D. Signs
      1. Failure of respiratory distress syndrome to improve (or deterioration) at 2–7 days

2. Increased FiO_2/ventilator settings
3. Acidosis
4. Apnea
5. Hyperdynamic precordium (95%)
6. Bounding pulses (85%)
7. Murmur (80%)
   a. Normally silent until day 4
   b. Systolic
   c. Upper left sternal border
   d. Variable

VIII. Diagnosis

A. Chest radiograph
   1. Cardiac enlargement
   2. Pulmonary engorgement (hyperemia)
   3. Absence of pulmonary explanation for deterioration
B. Electrocardiogram not usually helpful unless attempting to rule out other condition
C. Echocardiogram
   1. Ductal patency
   2. Flow velocity/pattern
   3. Left atrial volume load (left atrial:aortic ratio >1.3)
   4. Left ventricular end-diastolic dimension:aortic ratio >2.0
   5. Left ventricular output
   6. Left ventricular function
   7. Reversed diastolic flow in descending aorta

IX. Treatment

A. Fluid restriction
B. Diuretics
   1. Furosemide
   2. Chlorothiazide
C. Ventilation
   1. Increase mean airway pressure (peak inspiratory pressure)
   2. Increase positve end-expiratory pressure (PEEP)
D. Indomethacin
   1. Less than 2–3 weeks old
   2. Reasonable renal function (serum creatinine <1.3 mg/dL)
   3. No thrombocytopenia (platelets >50,000/mm^3)
   4. No significant hyperbilirubinemia

5. Dosage regimens:
   a. 0.2 mg/kg × 2–3 doses
   b. 0.1 mg/kg/d × 6 doses
E. Surgical ligation

Suggested Reading

Negegme RA, O'Connor TZ, Lister G, Bracken MB: Patent ductus arteriosus. In Sinclair JC, Bracken MB (Eds.): *Effective Care of the Newborn Infant.* Oxford, Oxford University Press, 1992, pp. 281–324.

Chapter 51

Neurologic Complications of Mechanical Ventilation

Jeffrey M. Perlman

I. Background

The developing brain of the newborn and, in particular, the premature infant is at increased risk for hemorrhagic and/or ischemic injury (Table 29). The most frequent lesions noted are periventricular-intraventricular hemorrhage (PV-IVH) and periventricular leukomalacia (PVL). These lesions are most likely to occur in the premature infant with respiratory distress syndrome (RDS) requiring mechanical ventilation. Although the etiology of both lesions is likely multifactorial, perturbations in cerebral blood flow (CBF) are considered to be of paramount importance. This becomes highly relevant because, in the sick newborn infant, the cerebral circulation appears to be pressure-passive, i.e., changes in CBF directly reflect similar changes in systemic blood pressure. This increases the potential for cerebral injury during periods of systemic hypotension or hypertension. The cerebral circulation is also exquisitely sensitive to changes in $PaCO_2$ and, to a lesser extent, pH. Mechanical ventilation of the sick newborn infant can directly or indirectly affect CBF via systemic vascular or acid-base changes and thus increase the risk for cerebral injury. These potential mechanisms of injury are discussed below.

II. Mechanical Ventilation and Potential Brain Injury

A. Direct effects

1. Infants breathing out of synchrony with the ventilator.

The sick infant with RDS may exhibit beat-to-beat fluctuations in arterial blood pressure. The arterial fluctuations which affect both the systolic and diastolic components of the waveform appear to be related to the infant's own respiratory effort, which invariably is out of synchrony with the ventilator breaths. Thus, the fluctuations are increased with increasing respiratory effort and are minimized when respiratory effort is absent (Figure 71). The arterial blood pressure fluctuations are associated with similar beat-to-beat fluctuations in the cerebral circulation consistent with a pressure-passive state. The cerebral fluctuations, if persistent, have been associated with subse-

---

Table 29
Risk Factors for Cerebral Injury in Sick Premature Infants Requiring Mechanical Ventilation

---

Cerebral
- Vulnerable capillary beds, e.g., germinal matrix, periventricular white matter
- Pressure-passive cerebral circulation

Respiratory
- Respiratory distress syndrome
- Pneumothorax/pulmonary interstitial emphysema

Vascular
- Pertubations in systemic hemodynamics: e.g., hypotension, hypertension, fluctuations in systemic blood pressure

Consequences of mechanical ventilation
- High mean airway pressure
- Hypocarbia

---

quent PV-IVH. Minimizing the fluctuation is associated with a reduction in hemorrhage. The fluctuations can be minimized by: increasing ventilator support; use of synchronized mechanical ventilation; sedation; or muscle paralysis.

2. Impedance of venous return.
   Increase in mean airway pressure (Pāw) may impede venous return to the heart with two consequences: (a) an increase in central venous pressure and, as a result, an increase in intracranial venous pressure; and (b) a decrease in cardiac output. A combination of an elevated venous pressure and a concomitant decrease in cardiac output markedly increases the risk for cerebral hypoperfusion within vulnerable regions of brain (i.e., periventricular white matter). High mean Paw's are often utilized with either conventional or high-frequency ventilation in the sick infant with respiratory failure. An association between the use of high-frequency ventilation and PVL has been observed. Close monitoring of the vascular system is critical in the sick infant requiring high mean Paw to support respiratory function.

3. Effects of $PaCO_2$
   The cerebral circulation is exquisitely sensitive to changes in $PaCO_2$, (i.e., hypocarbia decreases CBF, and hypercarbia increases CBF). This relationship appears to be intact in the sick newborn infant. Hyperventilation with a reduction in $PaCO_2$ has been utilized as a strategy to augment pulmonary blood flow. The resultant hypocarbia may significantly reduce CBF. Several studies report the association of hypocarbia and PVL, as well as subsequent neurodevelopmental defects. Conversely, hypercarbia with an increase in CBF has been associated with an increased risk for PV-IVH.

B. Indirect effects – complications of RDS

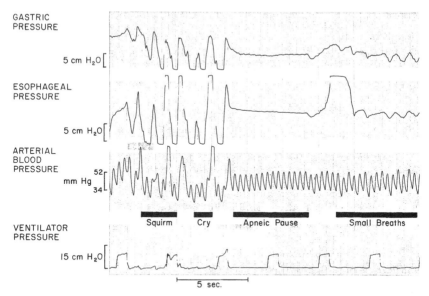

Figure 71. Tracing obtained from an infant depicting the temporal association between blood pressure fluctuations and gastric, esophageal, and respiratory pressure changes. Note the marked continuous fluctuations in arterial blood pressure affecting both systolic and diastolic blood pressures during "squirm-like" activity. Note immediate stabilization of arterial blood pressure associated with a brief variety of respiratory activity. Variability in blood pressure is again seen in association with small breaths at the end of the tracing.

Ventilated infants with RDS are at increased risk for airleaks, (i.e., pneumothorax and/or pulmonary interstitial emphysema). There is a strong association between pneumothorax and subsequent PV-IVH. The potential mechanisms that link these two conditions are likely multifactorial and include: an impediment of venous return; a decrease in cardiac output; an increase in $PaCO_2$; and hemodynamic changes that accompany evacuation of pleural air.

C. Other associations

  1. Sensorineural hearing loss
     Term infants with pulmonary hypertension subjected to hyperventilation are at increased risk for sensorineural hearing loss. The mechanism of such injury remains unclear.

  2. Intracerebellar hemorrhage
     Intracerebellar hemorrhage was noted in a series of infants who had received positive pressure ventilation via a facemask attached by a band across the occiput. It is presumed that the band induced occipital molding that resulted in distortion and obstruction of the major venous sinuses.

D. Potential therapeutic strategies
  1. Reduce fluctuations in systemic hemodynamics
    Strategy:
    a. Synchronized ventilation
    b. Sedation
    c. Paralysis
  2. Avoid systemic hypotension and/or hypertension
    Strategy:
    a. Consider inotropic support
    b. Consider volume expansion
  3. Avoid impedance of venous return
    Strategy: Lower mean Paw (if feasible)
  4. Avoid hypocarbia
    Strategy:
    a. Decrease ventilator rate and/or pressure
    b. "Permissive hypercapnia" (controversial)
  5. Avoid pneumothorax
    Strategy:
    a. Surfactant administration for RDS
    b. Synchronized ventilation
    c. Wean rapidly as tolerated

Suggested Reading

Fujimoto S, Togari H, Yamaguchi N, et al: Hypocarbia and cystic periventricular leukomalacia in premature infants. Arch Dis Child 1994; 71:F107–F110.

Greisen G, Munck H, Lou H: Severe hypocarbia in preterm infants and neurodevelopmental deficit. Acta Pediatr Scand 1987; 76:401–404.

Hendricks-Munoz KD, Walter JP: Hearing loss in infants with persistent fetal circulation. Pediatrics 1988; 81:650–656.

Hill A, Perlman JM, Volpe J: Relationship of pneumothorax to the occurrence of intraventricular hemorrhage in the premature newborn. Pediatrics 1982; 69:144–149.

Mirro R, Busija D, Green R, Leffler CB: Relationship between mean airway pressure, cardiac output and organ blood flow with normal and decreased respiratory compliance. J Pediatr 1987; 111:101–106.

Pape KE, Armstrong DL, Fitzhardinge PM: Central venous system pathology associated with mask ventilation in the very low birth weight infant: a new etiology for intracerebellar hemorrhage. Pediatrics 1976; 58:473–483.

Perlman JM, McMenamin JB, Volpe JJ: Fluctuating cerebral blood flow velocity in respiratory distress syndrome: relationship to subsequent development of intraventricular hemorrhage. N Engl J Med 1983; 309:204–209.

Perlman JM, Goodman S, Kreusser KL, Volpe JJ: Reduction in intraventricular hemorrhage by elimination of fluctuating cerebral blood flow velocity in preterm infants with respiratory distress syndrome. N Engl J Med 1985; 312:1353–1357.

Perlman JM, Volpe JJ: Are venous circulatory changes important in the pathogenesis of hemorrhagic and/or ischemic cerebral injury? Pediatrics 1987; 80:705–711.

Perlman JM, Volpe JJ: Episodes of apnea and bradycardia in the preterm newborn: impact on cerebral circulation. Pediatrics 1985; 76:333–338.

Perlman JM: Intraventricular hemorrhage. Pediatrics 1989; 84:913–915.

Pryds O, Greisen G, Lou H, Friis-Hansen B: Heterogeneity of cerebral vasoreactivity in preterm infants supported by mechanical ventilation. J Pediatr 1989; 115:638–645.

Wiswell TE, Graziani LJ, Kornhauser MS: Effects of hypocarbia on the development of cystic periventricular leukomalacia in premature infants treated with high frequency jet ventilation. Pediatrics 1996; 98:918–924.

Chapter 52

Retinopathy of Prematurity

Alistair R. Fielder

I. **Introduction**

    A. Retinopathy of prematurity (ROP) affects only the developing retinal vasculature.

    B. It has early and late phases, which are classified according to the International Classification of ROP (Table 30).

    C. Early phase (acute) ROP has five stages.

        1. Mild disease – ROP which reaches a maximum of stages 1 and 2 (this resolves fully)

        2. Severe ROP – stages 3–5 which frequently have severe visual sequelae

        3. Severe ROP – achieving threshold severity (Table 31) requires treatment that significantly improves the outcome for many babies

II. **Prophylaxis**

    A. Standard of care is still critical in keeping severe disease to a minimum, although it is recognized that despite meticulous neonatal care, ROP is not entirely preventable.

    B. The major risk factor is the degree of prematurity, but many other associations and complications of preterm birth have also been implicated.

        1. Oxygen

            a. Hyperoxia, hypoxia, and fluctuations of arterial oxygen tension even within the normal range have all been implicated as etiological factors.

            b. Keep arterial oxygen tensions within the recommended range. Avoid fluctuations of arterial oxygen levels when possible.

        2. Steroids

            a. Steroids administered antenatally have been shown to reduce the incidence of severe ROP.

            b. Postnatal steroids to treat respiratory distress syndrome may be associated with more severe ROP, but it is not known whether this is a causal relation.

Table 30
International Classification of Retinopathy of Prematurity

Stage	Severity
1	**Demarcation line** Thin white line, lying within the plane of the retina and separating avascular from vascular retinal regions.
2	**Ridge** The line of stage 1 has increased in volume to extend out of the plane of the retina. Isolated vascular tufts may be seen posterior to the ridge at this stage.
3	**Ridge with extraretinal fibrovascular proliferation** This may: • Be continuous with the posterior edge of the ridge • Be posterior, but disconnected, from the ridge • Extend into the vitreous
4	**Retinal detachment – subtotal** 4A Extrafoveal 4B Involving the fovea
5	**Retinal detachment – total** The detached retina is funnel-shaped and may be open or closed along all or part of its extent.

3. Surfactant treatment does not affect ROP incidence.

4. Light reduction – lowering the ambient illumination of the neonatal unit may reduce the incidence or severity of ROP.

5. Many other risk factors have been suggested including vitamin E deficiency, exchange transfusions, necrotizing enterocolitis, treatment for patent ductus arteriosus, and other complications of prematurity.

Table 31
Threshold Retinopathy of Prematurity

• The retinopathy of prematurity (ROP) stage at which the risk of blindness, if untreated, is about 50%.

• Definition: stage 3 ROP extending over 5 or more continuous, or 8 or more cumulative, clock hours of the retinal circumference, with "plus" disease.

• "Plus" disease: an indicator of ROP activity. In order of increasing severity: engorgement and tortuosity of the posterior pole retinal vessels; iris vessel engorgement; pupil rigidity and vitreous haze.

III. **Screening**

A. Purpose – to identify severe ROP that might require treatment, and even if it does not, is associated with a high incidence of visually important sequelae

B. Which babies to examine?

1. ROP incidence and severity both rise with increasing immaturity.
2. UK guidelines: all babies <1,500 g birthweight **and** ≤31 weeks gestational age, regardless of clinical condition
3. USA guidelines: all babies <1,500 g birthweight **or** ≤28 weeks gestational age, as well as heavier babies considered by the neonatologist to be at high risk
4. Larger babies may be at risk in countries with more variable standards of neonatal care (e.g., Latin America, Eastern Europe). This emphasizes the need for local protocols.

IV. **Examination Protocol**

A. Principles

1. Age of ROP onset and rate of progression are determined mainly by postconceptional (PCA) or postmenstrual age (PMA) rather than neonatal events.
2. The time available for treatment is short – within 2–3 days of the diagnosis of threshold ROP (usually between 34–40 weeks PCA).
3. PCA and PMA are used synonymously to describe gestational age at birth plus postnatal age.
   a. Initial examination should be between 4–6 weeks (USA guidelines) or between 6–7 weeks (UK guidelines) postnatal age.
   b. Subsequent examinations
      (1) Every 2 weeks, or
      (2) Every week – this minimizes loss to follow-up and ensures that almost all screening is completed while the baby is in the hospital
      (3) Babies for transfer to another hospital prior to completion of the screening program – ensure that the receiving hospital is alerted to screening requirements
      (4) Babies for discharge to home – ensure a follow-up appointment until screening is completed
   c. Completion of screening
      (1) Vascularization that has proceeded into zone III (peripheral most portion of the temporal retina) – without ROP
      (2) The development of ROP, at which point examinations are dictated by clinical criteria
   d. Screening examination
      (1) To be carried out by an ophthalmologist following pupillary dilatation

331

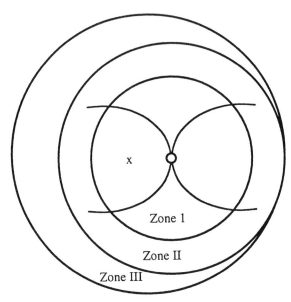

Figure 72. International classification zones for retinopathy of prematurity. See text for description; x indicates macula.

(2) ROP is recorded (Figure 72) as:
  (a) Severity by stages: 1 to 5
  (b) Location by zone: I–III; the closer to zone I (i.e., posterior) the greater the propensity to become severe
  (c) Extent by clock hour involvement
  (d) Presence of "Plus" disease

V. Responsibilities and Organization

A. Effective and efficient screening for ROP and its subsequent management requires multidisciplinary teamwork.
B. National guidelines form the basis of protocols, which should be developed locally and jointly by the neonatal and ophthalmic teams.
C. Identification of babies requiring screening is the responsibility of the neonatal team.
D. Arrangement for postexamination follow-up is the responsibility of the ophthalmologist.

VI. Information for Parents

A. Most babies do not develop severe ROP, so conversations and literature need to convey this sense.

   B. For babies with, or close to, stage 3 ROP, a personal discussion between the ophthalmologist and parents is important and should also involve a member of the neonatal team.

VII. Management of ROP

   A. Once ROP has been diagnosed, the baby leaves the screening program and is managed according to standard ophthalmic practice.

   B. While most of these babies require examination every 2 weeks, ROP in zone I or that which is close to, or at, stage 3 requires more frequent examination as indicated.

VIII. Treatment

   Once "threshold" ROP has been diagnosed, treatment by cryotherapy or laser should be performed within 2–3 days.

IX. Long-Term Follow-Up

   A. All stage 3 ROP requires ophthalmic follow-up, at least to 5 years of age because of the risk of reduced vision, myopia, and strabismus.

   B. The follow-up of very low birthweight babies who did not develop severe ROP is less well defined, but the likelihood of developing myopia and strabismus in childhood is much higher than in full-term counterparts.

Suggested Reading

American Academy of Pediatrics Section on Ophthalmology, Retinopathy of Prematurity Subcommittee: Screening examination of premature infants for retinopathy of prematurity. Pediatrics 1997; 100:273.

Fielder AR: Retinopathy of prematurity. In Taylor D (Ed.): *Paediatric Ophthalmology, 2nd Edition.* London, Blackwell Scientific Ltd., 1997, pp. 537–556.

Higgins RD, Mendelsohn AL, DeFeo MJ, et al: Antenatal dexamethasone and decreased severity of retinopathy of prematurity. Arch Ophthalmol 1998; 116:601–605.

Palmer EA, Robertson JE: Treatment of ROP by peripheral retinal ablation. In Isenberg SJ (Ed.): *The Eye in Infancy.* St. Louis, Mosby, 1994, pp. 437–447.

Phelps DL: Retinopathy of prematurity: a neonatologist's perspective. In Isenberg SJ (Ed.): *The Eye in Infancy.* St. Louis, Mosby, 1994, pp. 437–447.

Report of a joint working party: Retinopathy of prematurity: guidelines for screening and treatment. Royal College of Ophthalmologists and British Association of Perinatal Medicine, 1995. Early Hum Dev 1996; 46:239–258.

Reynolds JD, Hardy RJ, Kennedy KA, et al: Lack of efficacy of light reduction in preventing retinopathy of prematurity. N Engl J Med 1998; 338:1572–1576.

Urrea PT, Rosenbaum AL: Retinopathy of prematurity: ophthalmologist's perspective. In Isenberg SJ (Ed.): *The Eye in Infancy.* St. Louis, Mosby, 1994, pp. 448–470.

SECTION XI

Sedation and Control of Pain

Chapter 53

Assessment of Pain and Sedation

Susan Kidd, Neil McIntosh

I. **Definitions**

    A. Stress – spectrum of physiologic responses normally generated by certain external stimuli

        1. Adaptive, probably not harmful

        2. There may be no conscious awareness and, thus, no associated suffering.

    B. Distress – suffering resulting from emotional effects of excessive stress

        1. Harmful

        2. Requires higher consciousness for recognition

        3. Often affected by comparison with past experiences

        4. In the newborn, it is inferred by an observer from behavioral cues.

    C. Pain – particular form of distress, easily related in the adult as a hurtful experience or emotion

    D. Nociception – the effects (e.g., metabolic, neurobehavioral, etc.) of a noxious stimulus independent of any judgment of higher consciousness, memory, or possible emotional effects or suffering, i.e., neonatal "pain" (Table 32)

II. **Ways of Assessing Pain and Distress (Table 33)**

    A. Premature Infant Pain Profile

    B. Acute distress – based largely on behavioral or physiologic measures

    C. Subacute distress – difficult to assess

        1. Thrashing or wiggling

        2. "Frozen" or withdrawn behavior

III. **Indices Used in Pain Assessment**

    A. Behavior

        1. Cry (not applicable to intubated infants)

        2. Facial expression (brow bulge, eye squint, nasolabial furrowing,

Table 32
Causes of Distress in the Newborn Infant

Ventilation
  Presence of endotracheal tube and fixation devices
  Distress of mandatory ventilator breaths
  Restriction of movement and posture required for ventilation
Repeated acute invasive procedures
  Endotracheal suctioning
  Arterial/venous/capillary blood sampling
  Venipuncture
Minor surgical procedures
  Chest drain insertion
  Suprapubic aspiration of urine
  Lumbar puncture
  Ventricular tap
Coexisting infective/inflammatory conditions
  Necrotizing enterocolitis
  Osteomyelitis
  Meningitis
  Generalized sepsis
Complications of necessary procedures
  Cellulitis or abscess from infiltrated intravenous infusion
  Cutaneous probe burns
Postoperative following major surgery
  Patent ductus arteriosus ligation
  Laser therapy for retinopathy of prematurity
  Bowel repair/resection following perforation or necrotizing enterocolitis
Disruptive handling
  Positioning for radiographs
  Ultrasound scans
  General caregiving procedures
Environmental stress
  Excessive light, either daylight or from phototherapy
  Excessive and distressing sound from monitor alarms, banging incubator
    doors, etc.
  Unfamiliar tactile environment without containment or fluidity
Physiologic stress
  Drug withdrawal
  Respiratory insufficiency/air hunger
  Nutritional, i.e., hunger
Repeated relatively noninvasive procedures
  Transcutaneous gas monitoring probe changes
  Bolus feeds
  Drug administration
  Blood pressure measurement using inflatable cuffs

Table 33
Validated Pain Assessment Scores for Use in the Newborn

Neonatal Facial Coding System: (NFCS)

Facial response to heel-stick (i.e., acute and obvious pain) in different sleep-wake states.
10 features scored:
1. Brow bulge
2. Eye squint
3. Nasolabial furrow
4. Open lips
5. Vertical stretch mouth
6. Horizontal mouth
7. Lip purse
8. Tongue taut
9. Chin quiver
10. Tone exaggeration with startling or twitching

    mouth or lip purse, tongue tautness, chin quiver, tone exaggeration with startling or twitching)
3. Changes in tone (general diffuse increase in activity, flexion of trunk and extremities, "fetal" posturing or arching, leg extension, finger splaying, or fisting)
4. Sleep cycle disturbances accompanied by twitches, sounds, jerks, irregular respirations, whimpers, or grimaces
5. Observed self-regulatory or comforting behaviors such as lowered state, posture changes, hand-to-mouth movements, sucking, gasping, or an expression of "focused alertness"
B. Physiologic
  1. Increased heart rate
  2. Respiratory rate increases, except in immediate acute pain, where it decreases
  3. Increases in blood pressure
  4. Variable oxygenation changes
  5. Fluctuations in skin color/temperature
  6. Galvanic skin response (increased palmar sweating after 37 weeks)
  7. Swings in cerebral circulation and intracranial pressure
  8. Gastrointestinal disturbances (e.g., hiccups, gagging, grunting, straining)
C. Research tools
  1. Neuroendocrine markers (cortisol, adrenaline, endorphins)
  2. Metabolic-biochemical markers of catabolism (3-methylhistidine)
  3. Computerized analysis of physiologic data (e.g., vagal tone changes)

IV. Problems in the Ventilated or Preterm Infant

    A. True cry not possible

    B. Endotracheal tube and tape alter facial expression.

    C. Posture/movement altered by restraints, leads, infusions, etc.

    D. Prematurity impacts behavioral responses.

    E. Much stress is subacute and habituates.

    F. Medical compromise alters or blunts response to distress.

    G. Arousal state modifies responses.

    H. Environmental modulators (e.g., light, noise, temperature, physical containment)

    I. Agitation/distress may be secondary to respiratory insufficiency, drug withdrawal, or something other than pain, *per se.*

Suggested Reading

Grunau RV, Johnston CC, Craig KD: Neonatal facial and cry responses to invasive and non-invasive procedures. Pain 1990; 42:295–305.

Johnston CC, Stevens B, Craig KD: Developmental changes in pain expression in premature, full-term, two and four month old infants. Pain 1993; 52:201–208.

Stevens B, Johnston C, Petryshen P, Taddio A: The premature infant pain profile: development and initial validation. Clin J Pain 1996; 12:13–32.

Chapter 54

Pharmacologic Intervention

Gopi Menon, Christine A. Walker, Neil McIntosh

I. **Drugs Available for Pain Relief**

   A. Opioids

     1. Reduce endocrine stress response

     2. Reduce asynchronous respiration during ventilation (sedative effect)

     3. Produce physiologic stability

     4. Side effects

       a. Respiratory depression

       b. Hypotension

       c. Bronchospasm (theoretical)

       d. Decreased gut motility

       e. Chest wall rigidity (caused by stimulation of excitatory pathways in spinal cord; give boluses slowly)

       f. Withdrawal. Wean gradually if given >5 days. Late rebound respiratory depression from enterohepatic recirculation or release from fat stores may occur.

     5. Specific agents

       a. Morphine

         (1) Most widely used

         (2) Loading dose: 100–150 μg/kg IV over 30 minutes

         (3) Maintenance: 10–20 μg/kg/h

         (4) Dose for procedures: 50–100 μg/kg over 30 minutes

       b. Fentanyl

         (1) Less histaminic effect

         (2) Tends to reduce pulmonary vascular resistance; may be preferable in persistent pulmonary hypertension of the newborn, congenital diaphragmatic hernia, bronchopulmonary dysplasia, during extracorporeal membrane oxygenation.

         (3) Large doses tolerated without adverse hemodynamic effects

         (4) Chest wall rigidity if given quickly

         (5) Bolus dose: 10–15 μg/kg

B. Nonopioids

1. Acetaminophen (paracetamol)

   a. Analgesic and antipyretic. Analgesia is additive to opioid effect

   b. Newborn relatively resistant to liver toxicity with no respiratory or cardiovascular depression, gastrointestinal irritation, or platelet dysfunction

   c. Useful in inflammatory pain

   d. Dose

      (1) Oral: 10–15 mg/kg q4–6 h

      (2) Rectal: 20–25 mg/kg q4–6 h (maximum daily dose, 60 mg/kg)

2. Ibuprofen – recommended dose same as for ductal closure (no information available regarding analgesic dose): 10 mg IV/PO, then 5–10 mg q24 h

C. Sedative drugs

1. Adjuvants to analgesic, but no pain relief

2. Useful for long-term ventilation

3. Useful when tolerance to opioids develops

4. May allow weaning from opioids

5. May help older babies with severe bronchopulmonary dysplasia

6. Specific agents

   a. Midazolam

      (1) Benzodiazepine

      (2) IV bolus for procedures, infusion for background sedation

      (3) Respiratory depression and hypotension; synergistic with opioids

      (4) Withdrawal (agitation, abnormal movements, depressed sensorium) after prolonged use

      (5) Dose

         (a) Loading: 0.2 mg/kg over 30 minutes

         (b) Maintenance: 0.4 μg/kg/h

   b. Chloral hydrate

      (1) Causes generalized neuronal depression

      (2) Does not appear to produce respiratory depression

      (3) May be given orally or rectally

      (4) Onset of action in 30 minutes, duration 2–4 hours

      (5) Slow development of tolerance

      (6) Dose

         (a) Sedation: 25–50 mg/kg

         (b) Hypnosis: up to 100 mg/kg

D. Local anesthetics

1. Lidocaine

   a. Infiltrate skin/mucous membranes

Table 34
Use of Analgesics and Sedatives

Relatively Minor Procedures

Procedure	Comment	Suggested Approach
Heel prick	Affected by technique and heel perfusion EMLA vasoconstricts	Automated lances Avoid EMLA
Vein and arterial puncture		EMLA
Suprapubic urine aspiration		EMLA
Insertion of nasogastric tube	Discomfort with gag Vagal reflex	Insert slowly
Handling for radiography		Opiate–slow bolus for ventilated babies or use sedative

(continued)

Table 34
Use of Analgesics and Sedatives (*continued*)

Moderate/Major Procedures

Procedure	Issues	Suggested Approach
Lumbar puncture	Pain of skin puncture Stress of restraint	EMLA Correct positioning/technique Lidocaine infiltration of skin (avoid deep infiltration as risk of spinal injection) Opiate or midazolam if ventilated
Chest drain (insertion)	Skin, muscle, pleural pain	Opiate slow bolus. Lidocaine infiltration of skin and pleura–if time Consider electively
Chest drain (*in situ*)		Opiate infusion
Ventricular tap	Pain of skin penetration	EMLA, opiate, or midazolam if ventilated
Elective intubation	Discomfort Gag/cough Vagal reflex	Opiate or midazolam slow bolus
Endotracheal tube suctioning	Discomfort Gag/cough Vagal reflex	Opiate or midazolam slow bolus
Laser/cryotherapy for retinopathy of prematurity	Discomfort/restraint Eyeball pain Vagal reflex (Reestablish full monitoring before procedure)	Ventilation Oxybuprocaine eye drops Topical anesthesia Opiate loading and infusion or inhaled anesthetic before intubation Muscle relaxant to abolish eye and other movements (after intubation) Atropine to prevent bradycardia (intubation, oculocardiac reflex)

b. 0.5% solution, maximum dose 1.0 mL/kg

c. With overdosage, systemic absorption may cause sedation, cardiac arrhythmia, cardiac arrest, seizures

2. EMLA cream (eutectic mixture of Lidocaine and Prilocaine as 5% cream)

    a. Vasoconstrictor

    b. Risk of methemoglobinemia minimal

    c. Apply pea-sized amount with occlusive dressing 30–60 minutes before procedure.

II. Clinical Use

A. Pain and stress may be episodic or related to medical/surgical procedures.

B. Aims of treatment

    1. Sedation

    2. Analgesia

    3. Reduce ventilator asynchrony

    4. Produce physiologic stability

C. "Background" treatment for ventilated infants

    1. Morphine sulfate

        a. Loading dose: 150 μg/kg over 30 minutes

        b. Maintenance: 10 μg/kg/h. May increase up to 20 μg/kg/h

        c. Weaning

            (1) Depends on duration of treatment

            (2) Signs of withdrawal

                (a) Irritability

                (b) Inconsolable cry

                (c) Tachypnea

                (d) Jitteriness

                (e) Hypertonicity

                (f) Vomiting

                (g) Diarrhea

                (h) Sweating

                (i) Skin abrasions

                (j) Seizures

                (k) Yawning

                (l) Nasal stuffiness

                (m) Sneezing

                (n) Hiccups

            (3) If treatment <3 days, stop or reduce by 50%

            (4) If 3–7 days, reduce by 25–50% of maintenance dose daily

            (5) If >7 days, reduce by 10% every 6–12 hours as tolerated

2. Fentanyl
   a. For situations enumerated above
   b. Loading dose: 10–15 μg/kg over 30 minutes
   c. Maintenance: 1–5 μg/kg/h
   d. Wean as for morphine
D. Painful conditions
   1. Necrotizing enterocolitis
      a. Low threshold for analgesia
      b. Intravenous treatment needed; suggest opiates
      c. Nonsteroidal anti-inflammatory agents contraindicated (gastrointestinal side effects)
   2. Meningitis/osteomyelitis
      a. Consider morphine if distressed
      b. Acetaminophen/paracetamol to relieve pain, fever
   3. Medical/surgical procedures (Table 34)

Suggested Reading

Anand KJS, Shapiro BS, Berde CB: Pharmacotherapy with systemic analgesics. In Anand KJS, McGrath PJ (Eds.): *Pain Research and Clinical Management, Vol. 5.* Limerick, Ireland, Elsevier Science Publishers BV, 1993, pp. 155–198.

Chapter 55

Effects of Inadequate Analgesia or Sedation

Jan Reiss, Neil McIntosh

I. **Pain Experience**

   A. Experience of pain in the preterm infant

      1. Increased sensitivity to pain (reduced pain threshold)

      2. The development of hypersensitivity as a result of repeated tissue damage

      3. The spinal cord of the preterm infant has more pain neurotransmitters present and delayed expression of inhibitory neurotransmitters resulting in hyperalgesia.

      4. Higher plasma concentrations of analgesics and anesthetics are required to obtain clinical effects, compared with older age groups.

      5. This sometimes results in ordinarily nonpainful handling (e.g., caregiving) activating pain pathways and being experienced as chronic pain.

   B. Short-term consequences of pain and inadequate analgesia

      1. Acute pain causes physiologic and behavioral changes designed to limit the duration of painful experience by "protest." They involve great energy expenditure.

         a. Behavioral changes

            (1) Withdrawal of affected limb

            (2) Kicking of other limb

            (3) Writhing body movements

            (4) High-pitched cry

            (5) Specific facial expression with furrowed forehead, increased nasolabial folds, wide mouth

         b. Physiologic changes

            (1) Increased heart rate

            (2) Blood pressure increase

            (3) Heart rate variability

            (4) Respiratory variability

(5) Intracranial pressure changes

(6) Decreased arterial oxygen saturation

(7) Skin blood flow

(8) Alterations in intracranial blood volume and cerebral blood flow

2. With continuing (i.e., chronic) pain, these changes do not persist as the body reorients its expression of pain with the purpose of conserving energy and expresses "despair."

   a. Behavioral changes

   (1) Passivity

   (2) Little or no body movement

   (3) Expressionless face

   b. Physiologic changes

   (1) Decreased heart rate variability and respiratory variability

   (2) Decreased oxygen consumption

II. Clinical Implications of Pain or Inadequate Analgesia

A. Short-term consequences

   1. Any of the above may be extreme enough to have an adverse effect on clinical state. Some experimental evidence:

   a. Frequent invasive procedures soon after birth (e.g., endotracheal suctioning, heelstick sampling) in the extremely immature infant cause physiologic changes sufficient to cause reperfusion injury and venous congestion that contributes to intraventricular hemorrhage and periventricular leukomalacia with profound later neurodevelopmental consequences.

   b. Cardiac surgery – extreme metabolic responses and clinical outcome can be improved by analgesia (reduced incidence of postoperative sepsis, metabolic acidosis, disseminated intravascular coagulation, death).

   c. Circumcision without analgesia in full-term boys causes increased irritability, decreased attentiveness and orientation, poor regulation of behavioral state and motor patterns, altered patterns of feeding and sleeping – some lasting 2–7 days.

   d. A study comparing a group of babies born at 28 weeks gestation at 4 weeks of age with a group of babies born at 32 weeks gestation found reduced behavioral and increased cardiovascular responsiveness in the babies born at 28 weeks, with the magnitude of the changes correlating with the total number of invasive procedures experienced.

B. Long-term consequences

   1. Neonatal circumcision results in increased behavioral responses to vaccination at 4–6 months, which can be attenuated by the use of anesthetics.

2. Stressful conditions at birth are associated with an increased cortisol response to vaccination at 4–6 months.
3. Increased behavioral reactivity to heelstick sampling in term newborns correlates with increased distress to immunizations at 6 months.
4. Ex-preterm infants show increased somatization at 4½ years, the strongest predictor of which was the duration of stay in neonatal intensive care.

C. Therapeutic interventions and outcome
1. Analgesia – acute physiologic and behavioral changes can be attenuated with opioid analgesia. Trials thus far have not been of sufficient size to show whether this results in better clinical outcome, but do suggest this to be the case.
2. Individualized developmental care to minimize stress and pain and support neurobehavioral development is associated with a reduced incidence of intraventricular hemorrhage and improved developmental outcomes.

D. Conclusion
Pain and stress contribute to causes of early neurologic injury and thus adverse outcomes. They can result in long-term increased behavioral responses to pain.

Suggested Reading

Anand KJS, McIntosh N, Lagercrantz H, et al: Analgesia and sedation in preterm neonates who require ventilatory support: results from the NOPAIN trial. Neonatal Outcome and Prolonged Analgesia in Neonates. Arch Pediatr Adolesc Med 1999; 153:331–338.

SECTION XII

Weaning from Mechanical Ventilation

Chapter 56

Essentials of Weaning

Steven M. Donn, Sunil K. Sinha

I. **Weaning**
   A. Process of shifting work of breathing from ventilator to patient by decreasing level of support
   B. Generally heralded by:
      1. Improvement in gas exchange
      2. Improving spontaneous drive
      3. Greater assumption of work of breathing by patient

II. **Imposed Work of Breathing**
   A. Endotracheal tube resistance
   B. Ventilator circuit
   C. Demand valve
   D. Estimated to require tidal volume (V_T) of 4 mL/kg to overcome imposed work of breathing

III. **Physiologic Essentials for Weaning**
   A. Respiratory drive
      1. Must be adequate to sustain alveolar ventilation
      2. Assessment
         a. Observation
         b. Measurement of V_T
         c. Trial
            (1) Low intermittent mandatory ventilation (IMV) rate
            (2) Endotracheal tube continuous positive airway pressure (ETCPAP)
            (3) Minute ventilation (see below)
   B. Reduced respiratory system load
      1. Respiratory system load – forces required to overcome the elastic and resistive properties of lung and airways
      2. Part of total pressure generated by respiratory muscles must overcome elasticity to change lung volume while the remainder must overcome resistive properties in order to generate gas flow.

    3. Time constant
        a. Product of compliance and resistance
        b. Describes how quickly gas moves in and out of lung
        c. Determines whether there is adequate time to empty lung and avoid gas trapping and inadvertent positive end-expiratory pressure (PEEP)

C. Maintenance of Minute Ventilation
    1. Product of V_T and rate
    2. Normal range 240–360 mL/kg/min
    3. Inadequate alveolar ventilation can result from inadequate V_T, rate, or both.

IV. Elements of Weaning

  A. V_T determinants
    1. Amplitude (ΔP) – the difference between peak inspiratory pressure (PIP) and PEEP
    2. Inspiratory time (T_I)
    3. Gas flow rate
    4. Compliance

  B. Frequency (rate)
    1. Impacts CO_2 removal
    2. If too rapid, may lead to hypocarbia and decreased spontaneous drive

  C. Minute ventilation
    1. Measure V_T and rate
    2. Assess spontaneous vs. mechanical components

  D. Work of breathing
    1. Force or pressure necessary to overcome forces which oppose volume expansion and gas flow during respiration
    2. Product of pressure and volume, or the integral of the pressure-volume loop
    3. Proportional to compliance
    4. Additional components
        a. Imposed work
        b. Elevated resistance
    5. Indirect measure is energy expenditure (oxygen consumption)

  E. Nutritional aspects
    1. Inadequate calories may preclude successful weaning by not providing sufficient energy.
    2. Prevent catabolism
    3. Avoid excess non-nitrogen calories, which increase CO_2 production.

Chapter 57

Weaning Strategies

Steven M. Donn, Sunil K. Sinha

I. **General Principles**
   A. Decrease the most potentially harmful parameter first.
   B. Limit changes to one parameter at a time.
   C. Avoid changes of a large magnitude.
   D. Document the patient's response to all changes.

II. **Oxygenation**
   A. Primary determinants
      1. FiO_2
      2. Mean airway pressure
         a. Peak inspiratory pressure (PIP)
         b. Positive end-expiratory pressure (PEEP)
         c. Inspiratory time (T_I)
   B. Sequence
      1. Try to decrease FiO_2 to ≤ 0.4
      2. If PaO_2 is high and $PaCO_2$ is normal, decrease PIP, PIP and PEEP, or T_I.
      3. If PaO_2 is high and $PaCO_2$ is low, decrease PIP and rate (if intermittent mandatory ventilation [IMV]).
      4. If PaO_2 and $PaCO_2$ are both high, decrease PEEP or T_I, and/or increase rate.
   C. Practical hints
      1. If FiO_2 is >0.4, maintain Hgb >15 g/dL.
      2. Weaning is facilitated by continuous pulse oximetry.
      3. Avoid "flip-flop" by making small FiO_2 changes early in the disease course.
      4. Avoid a mean airway pressure that is too low to maintain adequate alveolar volume.

III. **Ventilation**
   A. Primary determinants

    1. Amplitude (ΔP) = PIP – PEEP

    2. Rate (frequency, f)

    3. Minute ventilation = $V_T \times f$

    4. Expiratory time (T_E) (or inspiratory:expiratory [I:E] ratio)

B. Sequence

    1. If $PaCO_2$ is low and PaO_2 is high, decrease PIP or rate (if IMV).

    2. If $PaCO_2$ is low and PaO_2 is normal, decrease rate (if IMV), or T_E.

    3. If $PaCO_2$ and PaO_2 are both low, increase PEEP or decrease T_E (longer I:E ratio), or decrease rate (if IMV).

C. Practical hints

    1. Try to maintain normal minute ventilation.

    2. Keep V_T in 4–8 mL/kg range.

    3. Avoid overdistention but maintain adequate lung volumes.

    4. Low $PaCO_2$ diminishes spontaneous respiratory drive.

    5. Avoid pre-extubation fatigue caused by weaning below an adequate level of support to overcome the imposed work or breathing.

IV. Specific Modes of Ventilation

A. Assist/control

    1. Decrease PIP (decreases in rate have no effect if spontaneous rate is above control rate)

    2. Maintain sufficient ΔP to achieve adequate ventilation.

    3. Provide adequate V_T to avoid tachypnea.

    4. Alternative strategy: slowly increase assist sensitivity to increase patient effort and condition respiratory musculature

    5. Extubate from assist/control or consider switching to synchronized intermittent mandatory ventilation (SIMV).

B. SIMV

    1. Decrease SIMV rate.

    2. Decrease PIP.

    3. Maintain minute ventilation.

    4. Alternative: increase assist sensitivity.

C. IMV

    1. Decrease PIP (lower mean airway pressure) for O_2.

    2. Decrease rate for CO_2.

    3. Maintain minute ventilation and adequate V_T.

D. SIMV/pressure support

    1. Decrease SIMV rate.

    2. Decrease pressure support level.

    3. Extubate when $V_T \leq 4$ mL/kg.

E. High-frequency ventilation (see Chapters 36–39)

Chapter 58

Adjunctive Treatments for Weaning

Steven M. Donn, Sunil K. Sinha

I. **Methylxanthines (theophylline, aminophylline, caffeine)**
   A. Mechanisms of action
      1. Increase diaphragmatic contractility and decrease fatigability
      2. Direct stimulant of respiratory center
      3. Reset CO_2 responsiveness
      4. Diuretic effect
   B. Indications
      1. Periextubation support
      2. Apnea or periodic breathing
   C. Complications
      1. Gastric irritation, vomiting
      2. Tachycardia
      3. Central nervous system irritation, seizures
   D. Comments
      1. Follow serum concentrations.
      2. Periextubation support usually discontinued 48-72 hours post-extubation

II. **Diuretics**
   A. Mechanism of action – treat pulmonary edema
   B. Indications
      1. Pulmonary edema
      2. Patent ductus arteriosus
      3. Chronic lung disease
   C. Complications
      1. Electrolyte disturbances
      2. Contraction alkalosis
      3. Nephrolithiasis/nephrocalcinosis (furosemide)
   D. Comments

    1. Follow serum electrolytes

    2. May need supplemental Na, K, Cl

    3. Long-term furosemide therapy not advised; spironolactone and chlorothiazide preferred

III. Bronchodilators

    A. Mechanism of action – relaxation of bronchial smooth muscle

    B. Indication – bronchospasm or reactive airways leading to increased airway resistance

    C. Complications

        1. Tachyphylaxis

        2. Tachycardia

        3. Hypertension

    D. Comments

        1. Document efficacy before continuing

        2. May be given systemically or by inhalation

        3. If inhalational route, use spacer

IV. Corticosteroids

    A. Mechanisms of action

        1. Anti-inflammatory

        2. Decrease edema

    B. Indications

        1. Upper airway edema

        2. Pulmonary edema

        3. Chronic lung disease

    C. Complications

        1. Hypertension

        2. Hyperglycemia

        3. Increased risk of infection

        4. Gastric bleeding

        5. Myocardial hypertrophy (long-term use)

        6. Decreased growth velocity (long-term use)

    D. Comments

        1. Multiple dosing regimens have been suggested.

        2. Must be tapered

        3. Be aware of need for stress doses for infection, surgery, etc.

        4. Inhalational route **may** be effective.

        5. May wish to administer concomitant histamine-2 blocker such as ranitidine

Chapter 59

Impediments to Weaning

Steven M. Donn, Sunil K. Sinha

I.   **Infection (especially pulmonary)**
   A. Increased caloric expenditure
   B. Inflammation
   C. Edema
   D. Decreased pulmonary blood flow
   E. Myocardial depression

II. **Neurologic Dysfunction or Neuromuscular Disease**
   A. Decreased respiratory drive
   B. Neuromuscular incompetence
   C. Alveolar hypoventilation
   D. Examples
      1. Significant intraventricular hemorrhage
      2. Posthemorrhagic hydrocephalus
      3. Periventricular leukomalacia

III. **Electrolyte Disturbances**
   A. Chronic diuretic therapy
   B. Renal tubular dysfunction
   C. Excess free water intake
   D. Total parenteral nutrition

IV. **Metabolic Alkalosis**
   A. Infant may hyperventilate
   B. Correct underlying abnormality

V. Congestive Heart Failure

   A. Pulmonary edema

   B. Impaired gas exchange

   C. Organ hypoperfusion

   D. May require high positive end-expiratory pressure (PEEP)

VI. Anemia

   A. Decreased oxygen carrying capacity

   B. High circulatory demands and excessive energy expenditure

   C. Apnea

VII. Pharmacologic Agents

   A. Sedatives may depress respiratory drive.

   B. Prolonged use of paralytics may lead to atrophy of respiratory musculture.

VIII. Nutritional

   A. Inadequate caloric intake

   B. Too many non-nitrogen calories, resulting in excess CO_2 production

Chapter 60

Extubation and Postextubation Care

Steven M. Donn, Sunil K. Sinha

I. Extubation

A. Assessment

   1. Reliable respiratory drive and ability to maintain adequate alveolar ventilation

   2. Low ventilatory support

   3. No contraindications

B. Extubation

   1. The stomach should be empty. If infant has recently been fed, aspirate stomach contents.

   2. Suction endotracheal tube and nasopharynx.

   3. When heart rate and SaO_2 are normal, quickly remove endotracheal tube.

   4. Provide FiO_2 as needed.

II. Postextubation Care

A. Nasal continuous positive airway pressure (CPAP) (see Chapter 18)

   1. Clinical trials show mixed results. Some clinicians prefer to extubate directly to nasal CPAP to maintain continuous distending pressure and decrease work of breathing.

   2. Use 4–6 cm H_2O.

   3. May also be useful to maintain upper airway patency in infants with stridor

B. Nasal cannula

   1. Can provide necessary FiO_2

   2. Can provide gas flow to help overcome nasal resistance

   3. Allows most patient freedom

C. Oxygen hood

   1. Can provide necessary FiO_2

2. More confining than nasal cannula, but easier to regulate specific FiO_2

D. Prone positioning

   1. Stabilizes chest wall
   2. Improves diaphragmatic excursion by allowing abdominal viscera to fall away from diaphragm and thus decreases work of breathing
   3. Umbilical catheters should be removed

E. Stridor

   1. May result from subglottic edema or laryngotracheomalacia
   2. Treatment options
      a. FiO_2/humidity
      b. CPAP
      c. Inhalational sympathomimetics (e.g., racemic epinephrine)
      d. Corticosteroids
   3. If persistent, consider reintubation or airway evaluation (see Chapter 69)
   4. Subglottic stenosis may require tracheostomy

F. Methylxanthines

   1. Some studies have suggested efficacy in the periextubation setting.
   2. Duration of treatment 24–96 hours (longer if respiratory control irregularities occur)
   3. Recommended serum theophylline concentration 8–12 μg/mL.

G. Ongoing assessments

   1. Blood gas assessment. Assure adequate gas exchange.
   2. Chest radiograph. Not routinely necessary unless clinical evidence of respiratory distress.
   3. Weight gain. If inadequate, may indicate excessive caloric expenditure for respiratory work.

Suggested Reading (Chapters 56–60)

Balsan MJ, Jones JG, Watchko JF, Guthrie RD: Measurements of pulmonary mechanics prior to the elective extubation of neonates. Pediatr Pulmonol 1990; 9:238–243.

Barrington KJ, Finer NN: A randomized, controlled trial of aminophylline in ventilatory weaning of premature infants. Crit Care Med 1993; 21:846–850.

Baumeister BL, El-Khatib M, Smith PG, Blumer JL: Evaluation of predictors of weaning from mechanical ventilation in pediatric patients. Pediatr Pulmonol 1997; 24:344–352.

Bernstein G, Mannino FL, Heldt GP, et al: Randomized multicenter trial comparing synchronized and conventional intermittent mandatory ventilation in neonates. J Pediatr 1996; 128:453–463.

Chan V, Greenough A: Comparison of weaning by patient triggered ventilation or synchronous intermittent mandatory ventilation in preterm infants. Acta Paediatr 1994; 83:335–337.

Davis P, Jankow R, Doyle L, Henschke P: Randomised, controlled trial of nasal continuous positive pressure in the extubation of infants weighing 600 to 1250 g. Arch Dis Child 1998; 79:F54–F57.

Dimitriou G, Greenough A, Laubscher B: Lung volume measurements immediately after extubation by prediction of "extubation failure" in premature infants. Pediatr Pulmonol 1996; 21:250–254.

Donn SM, Nicks JJ: Special ventilatory techniques and modalities I: patient-triggered ventilation. In Goldsmith JP, Karotkin EH (Eds.): *Assisted Ventilation of the Neonate, 3rd Edition.* Philadelphia, W.B. Saunders Co., 1996, pp. 215–228.

Donn SM, Nicks JJ, Becker MA: Flow-synchronized ventilation of preterm infants with respiratory distress syndrome. J Perinatol 1994; 14:90–94.

Donn SM, Sinha SK: Controversies in patient-triggered ventilation. Clin Perinatol 1998; 25:49–61.

El-Khatib MF, Baumeister B, Smith PG, et al: Inspiratory pressure/maximal inspiratory pressure: does it predict successful extubation in critically ill infants and children? Intens Care Med 1996; 22:264–268.

Fiastro JF, Habib MP, Quan SF: Pressure support compensation for inspiratory work due to endotracheal tubes and demand continuous positive airway pressure. Chest 1988; 93:499–505.

McIntyre NR, Leatherman NE: Mechanical loads on the ventilatory muscles. Am Rev Respir Dis 1989; 139:968–972.

Piotrowski A, Sobala W, Kawczynski P: Patient-initiated, pressure-regulated, volume-controlled ventilation compared with intermittent mandatory ventilation in neonates: a prospective randomised study. Intens Care Med 1997; 9:975–981.

Robertson NJ, Hamilton PA: Randomised trial of elective continuous positive airway pressure (CPAP) compared with rescue CPAP after extubation. Arch Dis Child 1998; 79:F58–F60.

Rutledge ML, Hawkins EP, Langston C: Clinical and laboratory observations: skeletal muscle growth failure induced in premature newborn infants by prolonged pancuronium treatment. J Pediatr 1986; 109:883–886.

Sheth RD, Pryse-Phillips WEM, Riggs JE, Bodensteiner JB. Critical illness neuromuscular disease in children manifested as ventilator dependence. J Pediatr 1995; 126:259–261.

Sillos EM, Veber M, Schulman M, et al: Characteristics associated with successful weaning in ventilator-dependent preterm infants. Am J Perinatol 1992; 9:374–377.

Sinha SK, Donn SM: Advances in neonatal conventional ventilation. Arch Dis Child 1996; 75:F135–140.

Sinha SK, Donn SM, Gavey J, McCarty M: A randomised trial of volume-controlled versus time-cycled, pressure-limited ventilation in preterm infants with respiratory distress syndrome. Arch Dis Child 1997; 77:F202–F205.

Strong RM, Passy V: Endotracheal intubation: complications in neonates. Arch Ototaryngol 1977;103:329–335.

Tapia JL, Cancalari A, Gonzales A, Mercado ME: Does continuous positive airway pressure (CPAP) during weaning from intermittent mandatory ventilation in very low birth weight infants have risks or benefits? A controlled trial. Pediatr Pulmonol 1995; 19:269–274.

Venegas JG, Fredberg JJ: Understanding the pressure cost of ventilation. Why does high-frequency ventilation work? Crit Care Med 1994; 22:S49–S54.

Veness-Meehan, Richter S, Davis JM: Pulmonary function testing prior to extubation in infants with respiratory distress syndrome. Pediatr Pulmonol 1990; 9:2–6.

Wilson BJ Jr, Becker MA, Linton ME, Donn SM: Spontaneous minute ventilation predicts readiness for extubation in mechanically ventilated preterm infants. J Perinatol 1998; 18:436–439.

SECTION XIII

Nursing Care

Chapter 61

Nursing Documentation

Mary E. Linton

Documentation of an assessment of the infant's tolerance of any procedure makes the team approach to neonatal care more effective. Clear and precise communication, both written and verbal, between disciplines allows each team member to have a clear picture of the infant and how well he/she is able to sustain the current baseline status during times of stress. The following is an example of appropriate documentation of the suctioning procedure.

I.   Record baseline vital signs and oxygenation saturation.

II.   Auscultate to assess the need for suctioning and document data.

III.   Monitor for any physiologic changes that occur during suctioning and record the type and duration.

IV.   Make a note of the infant's tolerance of the procedure as well as any need to increase oxygen or ventilatory support during suctioning.

V.   Record the degree of hypoxia, if any, based on pulse oximeter monitoring or transcutaneous oxygen monitoring as well as the time it takes to regain baseline settings.

VI.   Report the type, character, and amount of secretions obtained.

VII.   Evaluate and record the effectiveness of the suctioning procedure by auscultating the chest.

VIII.   Reevaluate the clinical status of the infant and document how long it takes to return to baseline settings.

Suggested Reading

Driscoll KM: Legal aspects of perinatal care. In Kenner C, Lott JW, Flander-meyer AA (Eds.): *Comprehensive Neonatal Nursing. A Physiologic Perspective, 2nd Edition.* Philadelphia, W.B. Saunders, 1998, pp. 32–45.

Hodge D: Endotracheal suctioning and the infant: a nursing care protocol to decrease complications. Neonatal Network 1991; 5:7–14.

Chapter 62

Chest Physiotherapy/
Postural Drainage

Jill M. Neubert

I. **Methods of Chest Physiotherapy (CPT)**

A. Dependent on the particular institution. Not all neonatal intensive care units have respiratory therapists trained in chest percussion techniques. In some institutions, bedside nurses institute chest percussion if needed.

1. Consists of postural drainage, percussion, vibration, and suctioning

2. May be inconsistent therapy because of intolerance of individual infants

3. Postural drainage, particularly head down position, is not routinely used in preterm infants, because of unknown effects on autoregulation of cerebral blood flow.

4. Uses vary widely between institutions regarding routine, patient population, and timing.

5. Believed to alter pressure in the airways to help dislodge mucus, to improve mucociliary clearance, release chemical mediators in the airways, prevent pooling of secretions, and help propel mucus from the smaller bronchi to the larger airways

6. Infants are not routinely placed in the prone position if they have umbilical artery catheters, abdominal wall defects, or if they have undergone abdominal surgery.

B. Benefits

1. Removes secretions and prevents atelectasis in recently extubated infants

2. Increased oxygenation after CPT

3. In one recent study, neurologic complications were no more frequent in infants who had CPT versus infants not treated with CPT.

C. Complications

1. Decrease in oxygenation with CPT

2. Bradycardia and decreased lung compliance after CPT and suctioning

3. Rib fractures and subperiosteal hemorrhage have been associated with CPT.

4. Increased risk of intraventricular hemorrhage may be associated with CPT.
5. Adrenaline and noradrenaline levels are higher after CPT.
6. Encephaloclastic porencephaly is associated with number of CPT treatments in the first month of life, hypotension in the first week of life, and breech presentation. With discontinuation of CPT, no further cases were seen according to one study.

D. Recommendations
1. Although CPT is widely used, there is conflicting evidence supporting its use.
2. Reappraisal of CPT indicates that it should be reserved for use in infants with respiratory disorders in which there is increased mucus production, such as meconium aspiration, pneumonia, and segmental atelectasis.

II. Respiratory Assessment

A. Landmarks and structure
1. Chest cavity, sternum, twelfth thoracic vertebra
2. Lower boundary of the thorax is formed by the diaphragm
3. Suprasternal notch is found in the upper aspect of the sternum
4. Xiphoid process protrudes below the sternum
5. Clavicles and scapulae

B. Reference lines
1. Midsternal line: bisects the suprasternal notch
2. Midclavicular line: vertical line drawn through the clavicle
3. Anterior axillary line: extends from the anterior axillary fold

C. Observation
1. Color
2. Rate of respiration
3. Presence of oral or nasal secretions
4. Symmetry and synchrony
5. Grunting – increases end-expiratory pressure, increases air exchange
6. Retractions – indicate ineffective respiration; infant compensates by using accessory muscles to help compensate for poor alveolar ventilation
   a. Suprasternal
   b. Intercostal
   c. Substernal
   d. Subcostal
   e. Subxiphoid
7. Nasal flaring – flaring nostrils is an effort to decrease upper airway resistance

8. Gasping – ominous sign of respiratory failure, usually when infant is profoundly acidotic

9. Apnea – cessation of breathing for 20 seconds or longer, may be accompanied by bradycardia and oxygen desaturation

D. Auscultation – compare and contrast both sides of the chest and back for equality of breath sounds

   1. Normal

      a. Vesicular – more audible on inspiration, found over the entire chest except the manubrium and trachea

      b. Bronchial – seldom heard in newborns

      c. Bronchovesicular – heard on inspiration and expiration, found over the manubrium and interscapular regions

   2. Abnormal

      a. Crackles. Fine – may sound like rubbing together strands of hair, heard frequently after birth, with pulmonary edema, with respiratory distress syndrome, and with bronchopulmonary dysplasia. Medium – sounds louder, like the fizzing of soda water, heard with pneumonia, transient tachypnea of the newborn, and pulmonary edema. Coarse – sounds loud and bubbly, heard with much edema and mucus in the airways.

      b. Wheezing – inspiratory and/or expiratory – secondary to narrowing of airways, bronchospasm, airway edema

      c. Rhonchi – deeper, coarser snoring sounds, usually with large amounts of mucus or debris in the larger airways

      d. Stridor – hoarse sound on inspiration or expiration, usually indicates partial obstruction of the airways

      e. Decreased – the presence of secretions, pleural space contains fluid or air, hyperinflation, atelectasis, obstruction

      f. Peristaltic sounds – diaphragmatic hernia

      g. Mouth breathing with agitation may indicate nasal obstruction

E. Palpation

   1. Clavicles-crepitus or swelling could indicate fracture

   2. Chest, sternum and ribs-crepitus, masses, swelling, edema

Suggested Reading

Al-Alaiyan S, Dyer D, Khan B: Chest physiotherapy and post-extubation atelectasis in infants. Pediatr Pulmonol 1996; 21:227–230.

Askin DF: Chest and lung assessment. In Tappero EP, Honeyfield ME (Eds.): *Physical Assessment of the Newborn.* Petaluma, CA, NICU INK Book Publishers, 1993, pp. 55–65.

Greisen G, Frederiksen PS, Hertel J, Christensen NJ: Catecholamine response to chest physiotherapy and endotracheal suctioning in preterm infants. Acta Paediatr Scand 1985; 74:525–529.

Harding JE, Miles FK, Becroft DM, et al: Chest physiotherapy may be associated with brain damage in extremely premature infants. J Pediatr 1998; 132:440–444.

Quinn W, Sandifer L, Goldsmith JP: Pulmonary care. In Goldsmith JP, Karotkin EH (Eds.): *Assisted Ventilation of the Neonate, 3rd Edition.* Philadelphia, W.B. Saunders Co., 1996, pp. 101–123.

Raval D, Yeh TF, Mora A, et al: Chest physiotherapy in preterm infants with RDS in the first 24 hours of life. J Perinatol 1987; 7:301–304.

Spitzer AR, Stefano J: Respiratory distress syndrome. In Polin RA, Yoder MC, Burg FD (Eds.): *Workbook in Practical Neonatology.* Philadelphia, W.B. Saunders Co., 1993, pp. 151–187.

Sutton P: Chest physiotherapy: time for reappraisal. Br J Dis Chest 1988; 82:127–135.

Turner BS: Nursing procedures. In Nugent J (Ed.): *Acute Respiratory Care of the Neonate.* Petaluma, CA, Neonatal Network, 1991, pp. 75–98.

Vivian-Beresford A, King C, Macauley H: Neonatal post-extubation complications: the preventative role of physiotherapy. Physiother Canada 1987; 39:184–190.

Chapter 63

Endotracheal Tube Suctioning

Mary E. Linton

I. **Introduction**
Endotracheal suctioning is a common practice in neonatal intensive care units to maintain a patent airway in intubated infants. There does not seem to be a consensus among institutions regarding protocols for endotracheal suctioning, and most are not based on scientific investigation. There is an abundance of research related to suctioning, but the outcomes are inconsistent and have not resulted in procedures for minimizing adverse side effects. Endotracheal intubation impairs the infant's ability to clear secretions because the endotracheal tube (ETT) results in an open glottis, preventing the cough reflex, and interferes with normal mucociliary function. With this in mind, the goal of endotracheal suctioning should be the removal of secretions without adverse effects on the infant.

II. **Complications of Endotracheal Suctioning**
   A. Bacteremia
   B. Atelectasis
   C. Hypoxemia
   D. Pneumothorax
   E. Tachycardia
   F. Bradycardia
   G. Mucosal trauma
   H. Systemic hypertension
   I. Increase in intracranial pressure
   J. Increased cerebral blood flow velocity

III. **Frequency of endotracheal suctioning is somewhat controversial but most practitioners agree that suctioning should not be performed on a routine basis.**

   A. The need to suction is based on the quantity of secretions, gestational age, type of lung disease, clinical condition, and the infant's past response to the procedure.

B. Occurrence of suctioning depends on the need of the individual infant and can be determined by changes in breath sounds, irritability, fluctuations in oxygenation, or rising $PaCO_2$ levels.

IV. Irrigation by instillation of normal saline prior to endotracheal suctioning is thought to thin secretions and aid in their removal. However, there is no scientific evidence to support this practice when compared to suctioning alone. Therefore, it is recommended that instillation of normal saline should be reserved for those infants who have thick tenacious secretions. Generally, 0.25–0.5 mL of normal saline used during suctioning is thought to be acceptable for use in the neonatal population.

V. Outer-to-inner diameter ratio should be considered when choosing the size of the suction catheter.

A. The safest ratio to prevent excessive negative pressure exerted to the lungs and avoid atelectasis is thought to be when the outer diameter of the suction catheter does not exceed half the size of the inner diameter of the ETT.

B. A customary guideline is: 2.5 ETT = 5 French suction catheter, 3.0–3.5 ETT = 6.5 French suction catheter, and 4.0–4.5 ETT = 8 French suction catheter.

VI. Depth of suctioning should be determined by the length of the ETT with an additional length for the adapter (usually 15 mm). It is helpful if this information is recorded on a card at the infant's bedside. To avoid injury to the mucosa it is essential that suctioning be performed just to the end of the ETT and should never exceed more than 1 cm beyond the end of the tube.

VII. Amount of negative pressure should be determined by the weight of the infant. In general the amount of negative pressure ranges from –60 mm Hg to –100 mm Hg.

VIII. Duration of negative pressure should be <10 seconds to avoid hypoxemia. Negative pressure should only be applied when the suction catheter is being withdrawn from the ETT.

IX. **Hyperoxygenation may help to reduce the incidence of hypoxemia and ensuing bradycardia associated with suctioning.** FiO_2 is increased by 10–20% above baseline for approximately 2 minutes prior to suctioning and is continued until the infant returns to the presuctioning oxygen saturation level after suctioning is completed.

X. **Sustained inflation is thought to decrease the atelectasis associated with suctioning and restore functional residual capacity after suctioning.**

    A. Increasing tidal volumes by 1–1½ times above baseline is thought to be adequate.

    B. This may be difficult to measure.

    C. The practice of increasing the peak pressure by 10–20% above baseline should adequately raise tidal volume to accomplish inflation and restore collapsed alveoli.

XI. **Hyperventilation can be accomplished manually by using a resuscitation bag, or mechanically by using the ventilator.** Increasing respiratory rate by 5–10 breaths above baseline ventilator rate before and after endotracheal suctioning may help in preventing harmful side effects of suctioning especially when used in conjunction with hyperoxygenation and sustained inflation.

XII. **Associated procedures such as handling, repositioning, and feeding may exhaust the infant's oxygen reserve and lead to hypoxemia, cyanosis, apnea, and bradycardia.**

    A. A recuperation period of up to 30 minutes may be necessary to ensure adequate recovery from suctioning.

    B. A return to baseline heart rate, respiratory rate, and oxygen saturation are indicators that the infant has recovered adequately and the caregiver may resume activities.

XIII. **Suctioning is generally performed using sterile technique to avoid the introduction of microorganisms into the respiratory tract.**

    A. The two-person method of suctioning is preferred.

    B. In this method, one person remains sterile and performs the suctioning while the second person instills saline drops, if indicated, and ventilates the infant between passes with the suction catheter.

Suggested Reading

Evans JC: Incidence of hypoxemia associated with caregiving in premature infants. Neonat Network 1991; 10:17–24.

Feaster SC, West C, Ferketich S: Hyperinflation, hyperventilation, and hyper-oxygenation before tracheal suctioning in children requiring long-term respiratory care. Heart Lung 1985; 14:379–384.

Hodge D: Endotracheal suctioning and the infant: a nursing care protocol to decrease complications. Neonat Network 1991; 9:7–14.

Quinn W, Sandifer L, Goldsmith JP: Pulmonary care. In Goldsmith JP, Kartokin EH (Eds.): *Assisted Ventilation of the Neonate, 3rd Edition.* Philadelphia, W.B. Saunders Co., 1996, pp. 101–123.

Tolles CL, Stone KS: National survey of neonatal suctioning practices. Neonat Network 1990; 9:714.

SECTION XIV

Special Procedures

Chapter 64

Laryngoscopy and Endotracheal Intubation

Sam W.J. Richmond

I. **Endotracheal (ET) Tube Diameter**

   A. Size of tube (internal diameter), as per infant weight

≤1,000 g	2.5 mm
1,001–2,000 g	3.0 mm
2,001–3,000 g	3.5 mm
>3,000 g	4.0 mm

   B. Depth of insertion, at lip (orotracheal intubation)

≤1,000 g	7 cm
1,001–2,000 g	8 cm
2,001–3,000 g	9 cm
>3,000 g	10 cm

II. **Anesthesia or analgesia should be provided except in emergent situations.**

III. **Laryngoscopy and Oral Intubation**

   A. Position all the equipment you need close by and prepare a means of securing the ET tube once it is in place.

   B. Position the baby on a firm flat surface. Place a small roll or towel under the baby's shoulders so as to lift the shoulders approximately 1.5 inches (3 cm) off the surface. Extend the baby's neck **slightly** beyond the neutral position.

   C. Open the baby's mouth with the index finger of your right hand and push the tongue across to the left side of the baby's mouth.

   D. Holding the laryngoscope in your left hand, insert the blade carefully into the baby's mouth while looking along the blade.

   E. Position yourself so you can see comfortably along the laryngoscope blade. If the blade is pushed in too far, all you will see is the esophagus; you must then withdraw the blade slightly to allow the larynx to drop into view from above. Alternatively, if the blade is not in far enough you may see little except the tongue and the roof of the mouth. Advance the blade slightly until you can see the epiglottis.

F. Once you have found the epiglottis, place the tip of the blade at the base where it meets the tongue (into the vallecula). Lift the laryngoscope gently upward. This will open the mouth further and gently compress the tongue and will bring the larynx into view from behind the epiglottis. Slight external downward pressure on the cricoid should bring the larynx into the center of the field of view. Never lever the laryngoscope blade forward by pressing backward on the baby's upper jaw, as this may damage the alveolus and developing teeth.

G. Bring the ET tube in from the right-hand corner of the mouth and keep the curve of the tube horizontal so as not to obscure the view of the larynx. If necessary, wait for the cords to relax. Insert the tube 1–2 cm through the cords.

H. Tape or otherwise fix the ET tube in place immediately while it is still optimally positioned. Most tracheal tubes are marked in centimeters from the tip; make a note of the length at the upper lip.

I. If this is taking place at birth, then inflate the lung using a controlled inflation device. Watch the chest to check that it is moving appropriately and listen at the mouth to check that there is no significant leak around the ET tube.

IV. **Oral Intubation Without a Laryngoscope**
Oral intubation using a finger rather than a laryngoscope is possible. Skilled practitioners can place an ET tube in a baby with normal anatomy in 3–5 seconds.

A. Insert the index finger of the left hand into the baby's mouth, with the palmar surface sliding along the tongue. Use the little finger if the baby is small.

B. Slide the finger along the tongue until it meets the epiglottis. This feels like a small band running across the root of the tongue.

C. Slide the finger a little further until its tip lies behind and superior to the larynx and the nail touches the posterior pharyngeal wall.

D. Slide the ET tube into the mouth between your finger and the tongue until the tip lies in the midline at the root of the distal phalanx of your finger.

E. At this point place your left thumb on the baby's neck just below the cricoid cartilage in order to grasp the larynx between the thumb on the outside and the fingertip on the inside.

F. While the thumb and finger steady the larynx, the right hand advances the ET tube a short distance, approximately 1–2 cm.

G. A slight give can sometimes be felt as the tube passes into the larynx *but no force is needed for insertion.*

H. When the ET tube is in the trachea, the laryngeal cartilages can be felt to encircle it. If it has passed into the esophagus, it can be felt between the finger and the larynx.

V. **Nasal intubation is not normally used for emergency intubation but many neonatal intensive care units prefer to place ET tubes nasally for ventilation. Nasal intubation is therefore most commonly carried out as an elective procedure in an orally intubated baby.**

   A. Ensure that the baby is well oxygenated in preparation for the procedure.

   B. Give pain relief (e.g., morphine) and prepare a suitable paralyzing agent (e.g., atracurium).

   C. Position the baby supine with the shoulders supported on a small roll or towel (see above) with the neck **slightly** extended beyond the neutral position.

   D. Give the paralyzing agent (optional).

   E. Choose an appropriately sized tube, cut it to an appropriate length and attach the appropriate connector.

   F. Lubricate the end of the ET tube and insert it into the nostril and into the nasopharynx.

   G. Loosen the attachments of the oral ET tube and have an assistant prepared to remove it when requested.

   H. Visualize the larynx with the oral ET tube in place using a laryngoscope. Identify the nasal tube within the nasopharynx.

   I. Ask an assistant to remove the oral ET tube. Pick up the nasal ET tube with a small pair of Magill forceps or a similar instrument and position the end of the tube in the laryngeal opening.

   J. It may not be possible to advance the tip of the nasal ET tube directly into the larynx. Take hold of the tube connector at the nose and gently twist it clockwise about 120° while maintaining some forward pressure. The tube will usually slip gently through the cords.

   K. Fix the ET tube in place and continue ventilation.

VI. **Confirm ET Tube Position**

   A. Clinically

      1. Equality of breath sounds

      2. Good chest excursions, symmetrical

      3. Appropriate physiologic responses (heart rate, respiratory rate, arterial oxygen saturation)

   B. Radiologic

      1. Should always be obtained for initial intubation

      2. Obtain with head and neck in **neutral** position

      3. Optimal position is midway between glottis and carina.

   C. Capnography may also be helpful.

Suggested Reading

Donn SM, Faix RG: Special procedures used in resuscitation. In Donn SM (Ed.): *The Michigan Manual: A Guide to Neonatal Intensive Care, 2nd Edition.* Armonk, NY, Futura Publishing Co., 1997, pp. 10–11.

Donn SM, Kuhns LR: Mechanism of endotracheal tube movement with change of head position in the neonate. Pediatr Radiol 1980; 9:37–40.

Donn SM, Blane CE: Endotracheal tube movement in the preterm infant: oral versus nasal intubation. Ann Otol Rhinol Laryngol 1985; 94:18–20.

Woody NC, Woody HB: Direct digital intubation for neonatal resuscitation. J Pediatr 1968; 73:47–58.

Chapter 65

Replacing the Endotracheal Tube

Sunil K. Sinha, Jonathan P. Wyllie, Steven M. Donn

I. Despite meticulous postextubation care, use of methylxanthines, and a trial of continuous positive airway pressure (CPAP), approximately 20–25% of babies require reintubation. The immediate goal is to reintubate and provide assisted ventilation in order to stabilize their cardiopulmonary status.

II. The following factors, singularly or in combination should alert the caregiver that a trial of extubation is failing:

A. Clinical manifestation of respiratory muscle fatigue, such as progressive hypercapnia or apnea

B. Major cardiovascular collapse

C. Increasing base deficit and developing respiratory or metabolic acidosis

D. Increasing FiO_2 requirement (>0.6) to achieve PaO_2 or oxygen saturation in the normal range

III. Suggested Protocol for Reintubation

A. Stabilization with preoxygenation and bag and mask ventilation

B. Select optimal size (and length) of the endotracheal tube (ETT).

C. For technique, see Chapter 64.

D. Before fixation, determine for correct placement by assessing air entry, chest wall movement, and improvement in oxygenation saturation and heart rate. If in doubt, obtain a chest radiograph.

E. Use of premedication (see Chapter 54)

1. Sedation

2. Muscle relaxants should only be used with experienced neonatologists present. Do not paralyze the baby unless you are confident the airway can be maintained and manual ventilation provided.

3. When practical, premedication prior to intubation in the newborn offers the following potential advantages:

   a. Increased hemodynamic stability
   b. Faster intubation
   c. Less hypoxemia
   d. Less rise in intracranial pressure
F. Adjunctive or reversal agents
   1. Atropine – given prior to anesthesia to reduce secretions and prevent bradycardia and hypotension. Intravenous bolus will produce an effect in 30 seconds that will last for up to 12 hours.
   2. Neostigmine – reverses the effects of nondepolarizing muscle relaxants

IV. Changing an Indwelling Tube

A. Prepare new ETT and adjunctive equipment (e.g., tape, stylet, adhesives).
B. Remove tape and adhesive from existing ETT but stabilize tube position manually while doing so.
C. Visualize the glottis by direct laryngoscopy.
D. Hold new tube in the right hand.
E. Ask assistant to remove old ETT and quickly insert new ETT to desired depth.
F. Secure new ETT when successful placement is confirmed clinically.
G. A radiograph is necessary only if there is a question of suitable placement.

Chapter 66

Transillumination

Kim K. Tekkanat, Steven M. Donn

I. **Description**
Transillumination is the use of a high-intensity light to help define normal or abnormal structure or function. Using transillumination, the density and composition of tissue is assessed by its diffusion of light.

II. **Clinical Applications**
   A. Diagnosis of airleaks
   B. Distinguishing cystic from solid masses
   C. Finding veins and arteries for blood sampling or catheter insertion
   D. Initial diagnosis of central nervous system abnormalities which involve formation of fluid collections

III. **Technique**
   A. Prepare light source
      1. Check power supply
      2. Connect fiberoptic cable if necessary
      3. Practice good infection control by disinfecting light probe with antiseptic solution.
   B. Darken room as much as possible.
   C. Apply light probe to infant's skin surface in area to be examined; use contralateral side as control.
   D. Normally, extent of visible light corona around probe tip is 2–3 cm; presence of air (or fluid) in light path will substantially increase the degree of lucency. A significant collection of air will enable the entire hemithorax to "glow."
   E. Pneumomediastinum
      1. Suggested if cardiac pulsations are clearly evident in lucent area
      2. Best seen if light probe is placed next to costal margin
      3. High predictive value if >20 cc air (94%)

F. Pneumothorax
1. Generally expand uniformly in anterior direction
2. Best demonstrated if light probe is placed on anterior chest wall
3. Can be diagnosed with >95% accuracy under favorable conditions
G. Pneumopericardium
1. Place light probe in third or fourth intercostal space in left midclavicular line.
2. Angle light probe toward xiphoid process
3. When the probe is moved over thorax, corona will appear brightest over the pericardial sac, and silhouette of heartbeat may be seen.
H. All three collections may be aspirated under transillumination guidance.

IV. **Special Considerations**
A. The procedure is most effective in a darkened room with time allowed for visual adaption to darkness.
B. Care must be taken to avoid burning the patient with the high-intensity light. This is accomplished by using a red filter inserted in front of the light source and limiting contact of the light with skin.
C. Cross-contamination of patients is avoided by covering light with cellophane.

Suggested Reading

Cabatu EE, Brown EG: Thoracic transillumination: aid in the diagnosis and treatment of pneumopericardium. Pediatrics 1979; 64:958–960.

Donn SM, Kuhns LR: *Pediatric Transillumination.* Chicago, Year Book Medical Publishers, 1983.

Donn SM: Transillumination. In Donn SM (Ed.): *The Michigan Manual: A Guide to Neonatal Intensive Care, 2nd Edition.* Armonk, NY, Future Publishing Co., 1997, pp. 27–28.

Wyman ML, Kuhns LR: Accuracy of transillumination in the recognition of pneumothorax and pneumomediastinum in the neonate. Clin Pediatr 1977; 16:323–324.

Chapter 67

Evacuation of Airleaks

Kim K. Tekkanat, Steven M. Donn

I. **Pneumothorax**

   A. Nitrogen washout is a controversial, but sometimes effective way of eliminating a small pneumothorax.

   1. Technique

      a. Baby is placed in a 1.0 FiO_2 oxygen hood for 12–24 hours.

      b. Vital signs including oxygen saturation, heart rate, and blood pressure are continuously monitored.

   2. Precautions

      a. Should not be used in preterm infant

      b. Do not use if pneumothorax is under tension.

   B. Needle aspiration can be used to treat a symptomatic pneumothorax. It frequently is curative in infants who are not mechanically ventilated, and may be a temporizing treatment in infants who are mechanically ventilated.

   1. Technique

      a. Attach a 23-gauge butterfly needle to a 50-cc sterile syringe by way of a 3-way stopcock.

      b. Locate the second or third intercostal space in the midclavicular line on the affected side.

      c. Prepare the area with antiseptic solution.

      d. Under sterile conditions, if possible, locate the intercostal space *above* the rib (to avoid lacerating intercostal vessels located on the inferior surface of the rib). Insert the needle through the skin and into the pleural space, applying continuous suction with the syringe as the needle is inserted. A rush of air is usually experienced when the pleural space has been entered.

      e. Once the pleural space has been entered, stop advancing the needle to avoid the risk of puncturing lung.

      f. Apply slow, steady suction to the syringe until resistance is felt, indicating that no more air remains in the area surrounding the needle.

g. Air is evacuated from the syringe by turning the stopcock off to the baby and evacuating air from the sideport.

h. Once all possible air is evacuated, the needle is removed and the site is dressed, if necessary.

2. Complications

a. Infection

b. Laceration of intercostal vessels

c. Incomplete evacuation of airleak

d. Lung puncture

e. Damage to other intrathoracic structures (e.g., phrenic nerve, thoracic duct)

f. Recurrence of airleak

C. Chest tube (thoracostomy) drainage is usually needed for continuous drainage of pneumothoraces that develop in infants receiving positive pressure ventilation as the airleak may be persistent under these conditions.

1. Technique

a. Select a chest tube of appropriate size for infant. For very small infants, 10 French chest tubes are adequate while for larger infants, 12 French chest tubes function better. Be sure the trocar is freely mobile inside the chest tube.

b. Locate the fifth intercostal space in the anterior axillary line on the affected side.

c. Prepare the site with antibacterial solution.

d. Administer an analgesic to the patient.

e. Cover the site with sterile drapes.

f. Inject the area with a small amount of 1% lidocaine solution.

g. Make a small incision (approximately 1 cm) *directly over* the sixth rib. Avoid breast tissue and the nipple.

h. With a curved hemostat, dissect subcutaneous tissue above the rib. Make a subcutaneous track to the third or fourth interspace.

i. Applying continuous, firm pressure, enter the pleural space with the closed hemostat. Widen the opening by spreading the tips of the hemostat.

j. Carefully insert the chest tube. If a trocar is used, insert it to only 1.0–1.5 cm to avoid puncturing the lung. Advance chest tube a few centimeters to desired location while withdrawing trocar. The anterior pleural space is usually most effective for infants in a supine position. Be certain sideports of the chest tube are within the pleural space. Vapor is usually observed in the chest tube if it is in the pleural space.

k. Attach the chest tube to an underwater drainage system under low (-10 to -20 cm H_2O) continuous suction.

l. Suture the chest tube in place and close the skin incision using

3-0 or 4-0 silk. The chest tube is best held in place with a "purse string" stitch encircling it. Taping of the tube is also recommended

m. Cover the area with sterile petrolatum gauze and a sterile, clear plastic surgical dressing.

n. Confirm proper chest tube placement radiographically. If residual air remains, the chest tube may need to be readjusted, or a second tube placed until air is evacuated or no longer causing compromise.

2. Complications are the same as those seen in needle aspiration.

II. **Pneumomediastinum is often of little clinical importance and usually does not need to be drained.** Rarely, cardiovascular compromise occurs if the air accumulation is under tension and does not decompress. Treatments include:

A. Nitrogen washout, as described above

B. Needle aspiration (using technique described above for pneumothorax). Insert the needle in midline immediately subxiphoid and apply negative pressure as the needle is advanced in a cephalad direction.

C. A mediastinal tube is rarely needed, but if necessary, should be placed by a qualified surgeon.

III. **Pneumoperitoneum often will not adversely affect the patient's clinical status, but when respiratory compromise does occur treatment is warranted.** Upward pressure on the diaphragm may compromise ventilation because of decreased lung volumes and may reduce blood return to the heart by exerting pressure on the inferior vena cava.

A. Distinguishing the cause of a pneumoperitoneum is very important and will drastically change patient management. Pneumoperitoneum caused by a transthoracic airleak can be differentiated from pneumoperitoneum caused by bowel perforation by measuring the oxygen from a gas sample obtained from the peritoneum. Baseline gas concentration is measured and compared to gas concentration obtained from a peritoneal sample when ventilator FiO_2 is set at 1.0. If the PaO_2 from the latter sample is high, the source of the airleak is likely thoracic.

B. Needle aspiration can be used as a temporizing measure or, in some cases, is used to treat pneumoperitoneum. Following the general procedure for needle aspiration of pneumothorax, the needle is inserted in the midline approximately 1 cm below the umbilicus. Negative pressure is applied while the needle is advanced through peritoneum and air is evacuated.

C. Peritoneal drain placement may relieve a continuous peritoneal airleak.

IV. Pneumopericardium occurs when air from the pleural space or mediastinum enters the pericardial sac through a defect that is often located at the reflection near the ostia of the pulmonary veins. The majority of cases occur in infants ventilated with high peak inspiratory pressure (>32 cm H_2O), high mean airway pressure (>17 cm H_2O), and/or long inspiratory time (>0.7 sec). Cardiac tamponade is a life-threatening event that may result from airleak into the pericardial sac. A symptomatic pneumopericardium should be drained immediately.

   A. Needle aspiration via the subxiphoid route may be used as a temporizing measure or to treat symptomatic pneumopericardium.

   1. Prepare the subxiphoid area with an antiseptic solution.

   2. Attach a 20- or 22-gauge intravenous catheter to a short piece of IV tubing that is then attached via a stopcock to a syringe.

   3. Locate the subxiphoid space and insert the catheter with needle at a 30°–45° angle pointed toward the infant's left shoulder.

   4. Aspirate with the syringe as the catheter is advanced.

   5. Stop advancing the catheter once air is aspirated. Remove the needle, sliding the plastic catheter into the pericardial space. Reattach the syringe and remove the remaining air, then remove the catheter, or alternatively, place it to water seal if the leak is continuous.

   6. Complications of pericardiocentesis include hemopericardium and laceration of the right ventricle or left anterior descending coronary artery.

   7. The procedure can be facilitated by transillumination guidance.

   B. Pericardial tube placement and drainage may be necessary if the pericardial air reaccumulates. The pericardial tube can be managed like a chest tube except that less negative pressures are used for suction (−5 to −10 cm H_2O).

   C. Prevention of further pericardial airleak by appropriate ventilator management is very important.

Suggested Reading

Cabatu EE, Brown EG: Thoracic transillumination: aid in the diagnosis and treatment of pneumopericardium. Pediatrics 1979; 64:958–960.

Donn SM, Faix RG: Special procedures used in resuscitation. In Donn SM (Ed.): *The Michigan Manual: A Guide to Neonatal Intensive Care, 2nd Edition.* Armonk, NY, Futura Publishing Co., 1997, pp. 10–15.

Donn SM, Kuhns LR: *Pediatric Transillumination.* Chicago, Year Book Medical Publishers, 1983.

Donn SM, Faix RG: Delivery room resuscitation. In Spitzer AR (Ed.): *Intensive Care of the Fetus and Neonate.* St. Louis, Mosby Year Book, 1996, pp. 326–336.

Zak LK, Donn SM: Thoracic air leaks. In Donn SM, Faix RG (Eds.): *Neonatal Emergencies.* Mount Kisco, NY, Futura Publishing Co., 1991, pp. 311–325.

Chapter 68

Vascular Access

Steven M. Donn, Kim K. Tekkanat

I. **Umbilical Artery Catheterization (UAC)**

   A. Indications
      1. Monitoring arterial blood gases
         a. $FiO_2 \geq 0.4$
         b. Unreliable capillary samples
         c. Continuous monitoring
      2. Need for invasive blood pressure monitoring

   B. Procedure
      1. Elective procedure
      2. Use sterile technique
      3. Catheterize vessel after cutdown technique using 3.5 French (<1,500 g) or 5 French catheter
      4. Preferred position of tip
         a. High (T_7–T_{10})
         b. Low (L_3–L_4)
      5. Confirm position radiographically
      6. Secure with tape bridge and (optional) sutures

   C. Complications
      1. Blood loss
      2. Infection
      3. Thromboembolic events
         a. Digit necrosis
         b. Necrotizing enterocolitis
         c. Renal artery thrombosis
         d. Spinal cord injury (rare)
      4. Vasospasm
      5. Vessel perforation
      6. Air embolus

D. Removal
1. When FiO_2 <0.4 and decreasing
2. When noninvasive blood pressure monitoring is adequate
3. At first signs of complication

E. Comments
1. Confirm position. A malpositioned UAC can have life-threatening consequences.
2. Remember that samples obtained from the UAC are postductal.
3. Never infuse pressor agents through a UAC.
4. When removing, withdraw last 5 cm **very slowly**. Watch for pulsations to stop.
5. Controversy still exists regarding infusion of total parenteral nutrition and certain medications through a UAC.

II. **Umbilical Vein Catheterization**

A. Indications
1. Emergent need for vascular access (i.e., resuscitation)
2. Need for central venous line
    a. Pressure monitoring
    b. Total parenteral nutrition or hypertonic glucose administration
    c. Frequent blood sampling in unstable patient without other access
3. Exchange transfusion

B. Procedure
1. Sterile technique should be used
2. Direct cutdown approach
3. Use umbilical catheter (5.0 French; 8.0 French for exchange transfusion in term infant); do not use feeding tube except as last resort.
4. Preferred positions
    a. Low-insert 4–6 cm to achieve blood return if using for resuscitation or exchange transfusion
    b. High-tip should be above diaphragm and below right atrium in the vena cava for indwelling use
5. Confirm position radiographically.
6. Secure with tape and (optional) sutures.

C. Complications
1. Blood loss
2. Infection
3. Vessel perforation
4. Thromboembolic events
5. Air embolus
6. Liver necrosis (see below)

7. Necrotizing enterocolitis (may be more related to procedures such as exchange transfusion than to catheter itself)

D. Removal

1. When no longer needed or when other central venous access is achieved
2. At first signs of complications
3. When procedure is completed
4. May be pulled directly

E. Comments

1. Avoid infusion or injection of hypertonic solutions (e.g., sodium bicarbonate) unless catheter tip is above diaphragm. This may cause hepatic necrosis.
2. Central venous pressure monitoring may provide useful trend data regarding intravascular fluid status and hemodynamics.
3. Recent trend in increased longer-term use in extremely low birth-weight infants

III. **Peripheral Artery Catheterization**

A. Indications generally same as for UAC when umbilical access is un-available or cannot be achieved

B. Procedure

1. Preferred sites
   a. Radial artery
   b. Posterior tibial artery
2. Assess for adequate collateral circulation
3. Prepare site thoroughly using antiseptic solution.
4. Cannulate vessel percutaneously.
5. Secure catheter with tape.
6. Check for blood return, pulse waveform, and adequacy of distal circulation.

C. Complications

1. Infection
2. Blood loss
3. Thromboembolic events
4. Ischemic injury

D. Removal

1. At first sign of complications
2. When no longer indicated

E. Comments

1. Transillumination may be very helpful in locating vessel.
2. Keep patency by infusing continuously, but slowly. Use low tonicity

fluid (i.e., 0.45% sodium chloride). Many centers prefer use of low-dose heparin (0.5–1.0 units/mL) to decrease risk of clotting.

3. Brachial artery should not be cannulated (inadequate collateral circulation) and femoral artery should be used only as a last resort.

4. Cerebral infarction has been reported following superficial temporal artery cannulation, and thus this vessel is also not used.

IV. Peripheral Intravenous Catheters

A. Indications

1. To provide partial or total fluids and/or nutrition when gastrointestinal nutrition is not possible.

2. Used when central access is unnecessary or unattainable.

B. Procedure

1. Visualize, palpate, and/or use transillumination to select vessel for cannulation. Suggested order of preference for vessels to cannulate:

   a. Dorsal venous plexus of back of hand

   b. Median antebrachial, accessory, or cephalic veins of forearm

   c. Dorsal venous plexus of foot

   d. Basilic or cubital veins of antecubital fossa

   e. Small saphenous, or great saphenous veins of ankle

   f. Supratrochlear, superficial temporal or posterior auricular veins of scalp

2. Apply tourniquet if placing in extremity.

3. Clean area with antiseptic.

4. Attach syringe to cannula and test patency by passing small amount of saline through, then detach syringe.

5. Hold needle parallel to vessel, in direction of blood flow.

6. Introduce needle into skin a few millimeters distal to the point of entry into the vessel. Introduce needle into the vessel until blood flashback appears in the cannula.

7. Remove stylet and advance needle into vessel.

8. Remove tourniquet.

9. Infuse a small amount of saline to assure patency, then attach IV tubing.

C. Special considerations

1. Placement should not be near area of skin loss or infection, or across joints, if possible, because of problems with joint immobilization.

2. Care should be taken to assure that vessel is actually a vein and not an artery.

   a. Note color of blood obtained from vessel.

   b. Look for blanching of skin over vessel when fluid is infused suggesting arterial spasm.

    c. When attempting scalp vein cannulation, shave area of head where IV is to be placed. Avoid sites beyond hairline.

D. Complications

    1. Phlebitis

    2. Infection

    3. Hematoma

    4. Embolization of formed clot with vigorous flushing

    5. Air embolus

    6. Infiltration of subcutaneous tissue with IV fluid. Infiltration may cause

        a. Superficial blistering

        b. Sloughing of deep layers of skin that may require skin grafting

        c. Subcutaneous tissue calcification from infiltration of calcium containing IV solutions

Suggested Reading

Donn SM, Faix RG: Vascular catheters. In Donn SM (Ed.): *The Michigan Manual: A Guide to Neonatal Intensive Care, 2nd Edition*. Armonk, NY, Futura Publishing Co., 1997, pp. 20–23.

Feick HJ, Donn SM: Vascular access and blood sampling. In Donn SM, Faix RG (Eds.): *Neonatal Emergencies*. Mt. Kisco, NY, Futura Publishing Co., 1991, pp. 31–50.

Workman EL, Donn SM: Intravascular catheters. In Donn SM, Fisher CW (Eds.): *Risk Management Techniques in Perinatal and Neonatal Practice*. Armonk, NY, Futura Publishing Co., 1996, pp. 531–549.

Chapter 69

Bronchoscopy

Neil N. Finer

I. **Equipment**
  A. Rigid bronchoscope
  B. Flexible (2.2 mm) bronchoscope
    1. Will pass through 2.5-mm endotracheal tube (ETT)
    2. Optional equipment includes a video camera and recorder as well as a microphone (allows determination of phase of respiration).
    3. Does not have suction channel

II. **Patient Preparation**
  A. Suction airway thoroughly.
  B. Medications
    1. Atropine can be used to decrease secretions and block vagal-mediated bradycardia.
    2. Morphine (0.1 mg/kg) or meperidine (1.0–1.5 mg/kg) may be given for analgesia 10–15 minutes prior to procedure.
    3. For unintubated patients, apply topical Xylocaine to nares.
    4. For intubated infants, inject Xylocaine (4–7 mg/kg) at tip of ETT, using a feeding catheter, 3 minutes prior to procedure. Suction again just prior to procedure.
  C. Follow principles of conscious sedation; monitor continuously.
    1. Pulse oximetry
    2. Blood pressure
    3. Heart rate
    4. Respiratory rate

III. **Indications: Emergent (can be done in under 2 minutes by experienced operator)**
  A. Acute/subacute suspected airway obstruction
    1. Mucus
    2. Blood
    3. Dislodged ETT
  B. Evaluation of airway obstruction in recently extubated baby

C. To assist intubation in conditions with associated airway anomalies:
   1. Pierre-Robin
   2. Goldenhar's
   3. Treacher Collins
D. Procedure
   1. Premedicate
   2. Monitor
   3. Visualize larynx via nares
   4. Pass bronchoscope through vocal cords to carina

IV. Indications: Elective

A. Confirm ETT placement.
B. Stridor
C. Persistent or recurrent atelectasis or wheezing in an intubated patient
D. Evaluation of known or suspected tracheoesophageal fistula
E. Assist placement of Fogarty catheter for unilateral ventilation for pulmonary interstitial emphysema

V. Practical Clinical Hints

A. Prepare patient (and staff) adequately.
B. Always preoxygenate patient and provide continuous oxygen during procedure.
C. Video camera recording can decrease procedure time.
D. Consult with pediatric otolaryngologist.

Table 35
Common Neonatal Diagnoses Amenable to Bronchoscopy

Upper Airway Lesions	*Lower Airway Lesions*
Unilateral and bilateral choanal atresia	Tracheomalacia
Laryngomalacia	Bronchomalacia
Subglottic narrowing, secondary to edema, web, stenosis	Tracheal or bronchial granulations, Mucus plugs, blood clots
Vocal cord paralysis, unilateral or bilateral	(especially in ECMO patients) Obstructed or dislodged
Laryngeal hemangioma, cystic hygroma	endotracheal or tracheotomy tube
Laryngeal edema and/or inflammation	Tracheoesophageal fistula
Laryngotracheoesophageal cleft	Tracheal stenosis or web
	Abnormal tracheal anatomy, tracheal bronchus

ECMO = extracorporeal membrane oxygenation.

Suggested Reading

Berkowitz RG: Neonatal upper airway assessment by awake flexible laryngoscopy. Ann Otol Rhinol Larngol 1998; 107:75–80.

Bloch ED, Filston HC: A thin fiberoptic bronchoscope as an aid to occlusion of the fistula in infants with tracheoesophageal fistula. Anesth Analg 1988; 67:791–793.

Etches PC, Finer NN: Use of an ultrathin fiberoptic catheter for neonatal endotracheal tube problem diagnosis. Crit Care Med 1989; 17:202.

Finer NN, Etches PC: Fibreoptic bronchoscopy in the neonate. Pediatr Pulmonol 1989; 7:116–120.

Finer NN, Muzyka D: Flexible endoscopic intubation of the neonate. Pediatr Pulmonol 1992; 12:48–51.

Reeves ST, Burt N, Smith CD: Is it time to reevaluate the airway management of tracheoesophageal fistula? Anesth Analg 1995; 81:866–869.

Rotschild A, Chitayat D, Puterman ML, et al: Optimal positioning of endotracheal tubes for ventilation of preterm infants. Am J Dis Child 1991; 145:1007–1017.

Shinwell ES, Higgins RD, Auten RL, Shapiro DL: Fiberoptic bronchoscopy in the treatment of intubated neonates. Am J Dis Child 1989; 143:1064–1065.

Vauthy PA, Reddy R: Acute upper airway obstruction in infants and children: evaluation by the fiberoptic bronchoscope. Ann Otol Rhinol Laryngol 1980; 89:417–418.

Chapter 70

Tracheostomy

Steven M. Donn

I. **Description**
Creation of an artificial airway through the trachea for the purposes of establishing either airway patency below an obstruction or an airway for prolonged ventilatory support.

II. **Indications**
  A. Emergent
    1. Upper airway malformations
    2. Upper airway obstructions
  B. Elective
    1. Prolonged ventilatory support
      a. Chronic lung disease
      b. Neurologic or neuromuscular dysfunction
    2. Subglottic stenosis following endotracheal intubation

III. **Preparation**
  A. Rare need for emergent tracheostomy because of obstructive lesion which precludes endotracheal intubation first
  B. Baby should be intubated.
  C. Should generally be performed in operating room because of availability of:
    1. General anesthesia
    2. Optimal lighting
    3. Available suction
    4. Proper exposure
    5. All necessary equipment

IV. **Technique**
  A. Baby placed supine with head and neck maximally extended. Use towel roll or sandbag.
  B. Cricoid cartilage is identified by palpation of tracheal rings.

C. Short (1.0 cm) transverse skin incision made over second tracheal ring

D. Incision dilated with hemostat

E. Incision deepened by needle point cautery

F. Maintain meticulous hemostasis.

G. Strap muscles separated by fine hemostat

H. Trachea exposed by dividing isthmus of thyroid gland by cautery, if necessary

I. Longitudinal incision made in trachea (by cautery) through second and third tracheal rings. Do not excise tracheal cartilage, which would lead to loss of tracheal support and stricture formation.

J. Place silk ties on each side to facilitate placement of tracheostomy tube and postoperative replacement.

K. Withdraw endotracheal tube until it is visualized just proximal to incision.

L. Insert tracheostomy tube. Choose a size that requires minimal pressure to insert; avoid metal tubes. Remove endotracheal tube.

M. Assess proper fit by manual ventilation through tracheostomy tube. If leak is large, replace with bigger tube.

N. Secure tube with tapes around neck. These should be padded and can be tightened during neck flexion.

O. Trachea may be irrigated with 2.0 mL saline and suctioned.

P. Auscultate chest; obtain radiograph.

V. **Postoperative Care**

A. Minimize movement of head and neck for 3–5 days to establish stoma. Sedation and analgesia are strongly recommended.

B. Frequent suctioning and humidification required until stoma established

C. Caretakers must know how to replace tube if it becomes dislodged or occluded.

D. Removal should be accomplished in intensive care unit setting.

Suggested Reading

Coran AG, Behrendt DM, Weintraub WH, et al: *Surgery of the Neonate.* Boston, Little, Brown and Company, 1978, pp. 31–35.

Coran AG: Tracheostomy. In Donn SM, Faix RG (Eds.): *Neonatal Emergencies.* Mount Kisco, NY, Futura Publishing Co., 1991, pp. 247–251.

SECTION XV

Pharmacologic Agents Used in Respiratory Care

Chapter 71

Surfactants

Dharmapuri Vidyasagar

I. Background

A. VanNeergard described the presence of surface-active material in the lungs that retain air at the end of expiration (1939).

B. Pattle demonstrated low surface tension in lung extracts (1955).

C. Clements isolated the substance responsible for lowering the surface tension in the lung.

D. Avery and Mead were first to show surfactant deficiency in infants dying of respiratory distress syndrome (RDS).

E. Surfactant replacement in clinical condition was first tried by Robillard using dipalmitoylphosphatidylcholine (DPPC) by aerosol technique with no clinical improvement (1964).

F. Chu et al. showed transient improvement in compliance in infants treated with aerosolized DPPC, but no success in clinical outcome (1967), leading to a halt in clinical applications of surfactant therapy. Experimental and laboratory research continued.

G. The importance of surfactant proteins was described by King and Clements (1970).

H. Fujiwara reported the first successful clinical trial of tracheal applications of surfactant in infants with RDS (1980).

I. The trials of surfactant replacement therapy in the USA began (1983).

J. Commercial preparations of surfactant was approved by FDA in the USA (1989).

II. Pulmonary Surfactants

A. Surfactants are phospholipids synthesized in type II cells lining the alveoli.

B. They form the thin air/liquid interfaces of the alveoli.

C. Surfactants play an important role in maintaining the alveolar stability at the end of expiration.

D. The absence of surfactants, or diminished surfactant levels, leads to atelectasis of lung, leading to RDS.

Table 36
Surfactant

Biochemical Composition of Pulmonary Surfactant

Lipid	85%–90%
Phospholipids	75%–85%
PC	60%–70%
DSPC	40%–45%
PG PI PE	10%–15%
Lyso-PC SM	5%–10%
Neutral lipids	5%–10% (predominantly cholesterol)
Protein	5%–10%
Carbohydrate	5%

PC = phosphatidylcholine; DSPC = disaturated phosphatidylcholine; PG = phosphatidylglycerol; PI = phosphatidylinositol; PE = phosphatidylethanolamine; Lyso-PC = lysophosphatidylcholine; SM = sphingomyelin; DPPC = dipalmitoylphosphatidylcholine.

E. The composition of pulmonary surfactant is shown in Table 36. The DPPC constitutes the major portion of surfactant. It contributes to the important function of lowering surface tension of alveoli. Surfactant proteins found in natural surfactants play a very important role in maintaining surface-active properties. Synthetic surfactants do not have surfactant-associated proteins.

III. **Surfactant Source**

A. Surfactant is synthesized in type II cells lining the alveoli.
B. Surfactant is identifiable in fetal lung as early as 16 weeks.
C. Surfactant secretion begins after 24 weeks.
D. Surfactant is released into alveoli in large quantities soon after the lungs are distended with the first few breaths.
E. Surfactant synthesis and release is enhanced by antenatal maternal steroid therapy.

IV. **Surfactant Pool Size**

    A. In preterm infants, alveolar and tissue pools are low.

    B. Infants with RDS have 2–10 mg/kg of surfactant.

    C. Rate of accumulation is slow.

    D. Amniotic fluid (at term) has 100 mg/kg of surfactant.

    E. There is a slow catabolic rate.

    F. There is no feedback mechanism.

    G. Infants recovering from RDS show steady increase in phosphatidyl-choline, which reaches a normal level in 4–5 days.

    H. The slow secretion and alveolar accumulation is balanced by slow catabolism and clearance.

    I. The half-life of surfactant is 30 hours.

    J. Treatment with exogenous surfactant increases alveolar and tissue pools.

    K. The metabolism of surfactant proteins is less well known.

V. **Surfactant Preparations**

    A. Table 37 lists the commercially available surfactants. As of this writing, two surfactants, Exosurf Neonatal® (Glaxo Wellcome, Inc., Research Triangle Park, NC, USA) and Survanta® (Ross Products Division, Abbott Laboratories, Columbus, OH, USA) are approved by the Food and Drug Administration for clinical use in the USA. Other preparations are widely used outside the USA.

    B. The compositions of Survanta and Exosurf are also listed in Table 37. The important difference between these two surfactants is the lack of surfactant proteins in Exosurf.

VI. **Surfactant Proteins (Table 38)**

    A. SP-A

        1. Water soluble, molecular wt 36,000 kDa

        2. Gene located on chromosome 6

        3. Regulator of alveolar surfactant metabolism

        4. Host defense properties, activates macrophage function, facilitates phagocytosis of pathogens

    B. SP-B

        1. Hydrophilic, molecular wt 8,000 kDa

        2. Gene located on chromosome 2

       3. Critical to surface lowering property of surfactant

       4. Helps absorption of surfactant

       5. Genetic absence – manifests lethal RDS soon after birth

       6. Essential component of surfactant

Table 37
Commercially Available Surfactants

Surfactant			
Generic name	Trade name	Preparation	Manufacturer
Beractant	Survanta	Bovine lung mince extract with added DPPC, tripalmitin, and palmitic acid	Abbott Laboratories, Columbus, OH, USA
Colfosceril palmitate, hexadocanol, tyloxapol	Exosurf	DPPC with 9% hexadecanol and 6% tyloxapol	Glaxo Wellcome, Inc., Research Triangle Park, NC, USA
Calf lung surfactant extract (CLSE) SF-RI 1	Infasurf	Bovine lung wash; chloroform-methanol	Forest Laboratories, Inc., St. Louis, MO, USA
Peptide (KL$_4$)	Surfaxin	KL$_4$, peptide	Discovery Laboratories, Inc., Doylestown, PA, USA
Surfactant-TA	Surfacten	Bovine lung mince extract with added DPPC, tripalmitoglycerol, and palmitic acid	Tokyo Tanabe, Tokyo, Japan
Lipid-extracted bovine surfactant	Alveofact	Bovine lung wash; chloroform-methanol extract	Boehringer Ingelheim, Inc., Ingelheim, Germany
Porcine surfactant	Curosurf	Porcine lung mince; chloroform-methanol extract; liquid-gel chromatography	Chiesi Farmaceutici, Parma, Italy
Artificial lung expanding compound (ALEC)	Pneumactant	DPPC and phosphatidyl	Britannia Pharmaceuticals, Ltd., Surrey, UK

DPPC = dipalmitylphosphatidylcholine.

Table 38
Surfactant Proteins

Type	Monomer Size (kDa)	Predominant Oligomer
SP-A	28,000–36,000	Trimer
SP-B	8,000	Dimer
SP-C	3,800	Dimer
SP-D	43,000	Trimer

    C. SP-C
        1. Hydrophilic protein, molecular wt 3,800 kDa
        2. Gene located on chromosome 1
        3. Lines the developing airway in the developing lung
        4. Absence of SP-C leads to disrupted lung development
        5. Facilitates absorption of surfactant
        6. No SP-C specific deficiency disease has been identified
    D. SP-D
        1. Hydrophilic protein of molecular wt 43,000 kDa similar to SP-A
        2. Present in soluble form
        3. Localized in type II cells and clear cells
        4. Functions as host defense molecule by binding to pathogen

VIII. **Surfactant Deficiency**
    A. The appearance of surfactant in lung is gestational age-dependent
    B. Risk of RDS is also gestational age-dependent; lower gestational age has higher risk.
    C. Preterm infants are at risk of developing RDS.
    D. Leads to development of RDS
    E. Various factors influence surfactant production (Table 39)
        1. Only natural surfactants have SP proteins. Survanta has both SP-B and SP-C.
        2. Amniotic fluid-derived surfactant has SP-A.
        3. Synthetic Exosurf does not have any proteins.

VIII. **Surfactant Function**
    A. Surfactant molecules, once released, spread to line the alveolar surface.
    B. The molecules are pushed together during expiration and lower the surface tension.

Table 39
Clinical Factors that Influence Lung Maturation

Clinical Conditions

Accelerated maturation	Chronic maternal hypertension
	Maternal cardiovascular disease
	Placental infarction
	Intrauterine growth retardation
	Severe pregnancy-induced hypertension
	Prolonged rupture of membranes
	Incompetent cervix
	Hemoglobinopathies
Hormones and other factors	Corticosteroids
	Thyroid hormones
	Thyroid releasing hormone
	Methylxanthines
	β-agonists
	Prolactin
	Estrogens
	Epidermal growth factor
	Transforming growth factor
Delayed maturation	Diabetes mellitus
	Rh isoimmunization with hydrops fetalis
Hormones and other factors	Insulin
	Transforming growth factor-β
	Androgens
	Bombesin

C. Prevent alveolar collapse

D. Maintain residual lung volume

E. Allow the lungs to expand easily during next inspiration

F. Improve lung compliance

G. Allow better oxygenation and ventilation

H. Prevent leakage of fluid from alveolar capillary membranes

I. Lack or inadequate surfactant causes alveolar collapse with each expiration leading to difficulty in reexpansion with inspiration. In essence, each breath becomes a "first breath" requiring very high inspiratory pressure for each subsequent breath (Figure 73).

J. Surfactant deficiency leads to increased work or breathing.

K. Nonpulmonary functions include host defense mechanisms against infections.

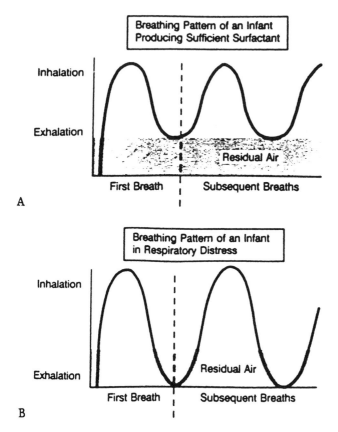

Figure 73. Role of surfactant in pulmonary mechanics. **A.** Breathing pattern of an infant producing sufficient surfactant. Shaded area represents residual air in lungs after expiration (functional residual capacity [FRC]). **B.** Breathing pattern of an infant in respiratory distress (surfactant-deficient). Lack of surfactant leads to alveolar collapse at end-expiration and severely decreased FRC. **C.** Pressure-volume curves for normal and surfactant-deficient (hyaline membrane disease) lungs. Note the severely decreased compliance in the latter.

IX. **Clinical Effects of Surfactant Deficiency**

   A. Lack of inadequate surfactant leads to generalized alveolar collapse and various degrees of atelectasis.

   B. Requires higher inspiratory pressure (increase in negative pleural pressure) leading to retractions of the chest wall

   C. Increased work of breathing

   D. Tachypnea

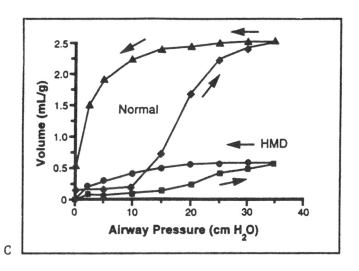

C

E. Radiographic findings
  1. Reticulogranular pattern in early and mild disease representing microatelectasis
  2. Air bronchograms (because of atelectasis of lung surrounding the airways in moderate to severe disease)
  3. Complete white-out of the chest with minimal distinction of cardiopulmonary shadows in severe RDS
F. Resultant hypoxia, hypercarbia, and acidosis

X. **Surfactant Deficiency and Pulmonary Function**
    Infants with RDS show the following changes in pulmonary function:

A. Tachypnea
B. Decreased tidal volume
C. Decreased functional residual capacity
D. Decreased residual volume
E. Decreased compliance
F. Airway resistance may be increased
G. $\dot{V}/\dot{Q}$ mismatch
H. Progressive deterioration if untreated

XI. **Short-Term and Long-Term Effects of Surfactant Deficiency**

A. Pulmonary interstitial emphysema
B. Pneumothorax

C. Lung collapse and lung edema

D. Development of bronchopulmonary dysplasia (BPD)

E. Progressive interstitial fibrosis – alveolar rupture and coalescence to cyst formation seen on radiography or at autopsy

F. Long-term oxygen and/or ventilatory dependence

G. Nonpulmonary complications, including patent ductus arteriosus (PDA)

H. Intraventricular hemorrhage/periventricular leukomalacia

I. Retinopathy of prematurity

J. Necrotizing enterocolitis

K. Infection

XII. **Treatment of Infants with Surfactant Deficiency**

A. General support

B. Oxygen therapy

C. Continuous positive airway pressure (CPAP)

D. Surfactant therapy: prophylaxis or treatment strategy

E. Ventilatory support

XIII. **Indications for Surfactant Administration**

A. The primary indication is surfactant deficiency to either prevent (prophylaxis) or treat (rescue) RDS.

B. Contraindications: there are no major contraindications except that infants with pneumothorax may lose surfactant into chest drainage.

XIV. **Techniques of Administration**

A. The two available surfactants (USA) are given in somewhat different ways. Both require the following:

1. Endotracheal intubation

2. Localization of endotracheal tube (ETT) in proper position above the carina

3. Clearance (suction) of trachea prior to administration of surfactant

4. Liquid form of surfactant

5. Stabilization of infant's status if in shock, acute episode of pneumothorax, or severely acidotic requiring life-saving cardiopulmonary resuscitation.

B. Survanta (beractant)

1. Administered only intratracheally

2. Use a 5 French catheter with end hole.

3. Draw into syringe at appropriate dose (4 mL/kg).

4. Attach catheter (step 2) and fill catheter to the tip.
5. Insert catheter directly into tracheal tube or via a sideport of previously attached adapter.
6. The length of catheter should be shorter than the tip of the ETT.
7. Direct instillation will require brief detachment of infant from respirator. Sideport will allow continuation of mechanical ventilation while administering surfactant.
8. To ensure homogenous distribution, the manufacturer recommends change of infant's position as follows:
   a. Head and body reclined to 5–10°; head turned to right first and then to left
   b. Head and body inclined to 5–10°; head turned to right first and then to left
9. The procedure requires two people.

C. Exosurf
1. The company supplies different sized ETT adapters with a sideport for catheter insertion.
2. The adapter should be used as described by the manufacturer.
3. Prepare the solution as follows:
   It is provided in a powder form; each vial contains powder for DPPC. It should be reconstituted **only with the liquid supplied by the manufacturer** along with the powder. **Do not use any other solution.**
4. Draw 8 mL of solution provided with Exosurf vial into a syringe.
5. Inject one-third solution into the vial containing the Exosurf powder.
   a. Draw the solution back into the syringe and release the plunger.
   b. Repeat 2–3 times to mix the powder.
   c. The reconstituted solution should be particle free.
   d. Shake gently – **do not form bubbles or flakes.**
6. Once the solution is prepared and the right amount drawn into the syringe, attach the proper catheter and fill it to the tip. The dose is 4 mL/kg.
7. Insert the catheter via the sideport of the adapter.
8. The following steps are used for installation:
   a. Keep infant supine with head in neutral position.
   b. Inject ½ dose slowly over 1–2 minutes while on mechanical ventilation in small bursts to coincide with inspiration.
   c. After the instillation, turn infant's head/body 45° to the right and for 30 seconds while ventilation continues.
   d. Return head/body to midline.
   e. Inject the second half of the dose.

    f. Turn infant's head/body to the left 45° and continue ventilation for 30 seconds.

    g. Return head/body to midline.

    h. Withdraw the catheter and close the port; continue ventilation.

  9. Studies have shown that slow continuous administration of surfactant solutions leads to poor, nonuniform distribution (mostly to dependent areas of lung) and is not recommended.

D. Monitoring of vital signs

  1. Although a steady improvement in SaO_2 and/or $TcPO_2$ is usually observed during administration or immediately thereafter, the following adverse reactions may be encountered:

    a. Reflux of solution

    b. Decrease in $TcPO_2$

    c. Increase in $TcPCO_2$

    d. Bradycardia and/or hypotension

    e. Increase in mucus or secretions

    f. Gagging

  2. Each event is usually transient. However, cessation of treatment and ventilation with 10–15% increase in FiO_2 is recommended to overcome >20% decrease in oxygen saturation, apnea, or bradycardia. Once stabilized, readminister the remaining solution – similarly make changes in ventilatory parameters.

E. Postadministration monitoring

  1. Stay with the infant for at least 30 minutes to closely observe the changes in vital signs.

  2. Watch for proper chest expansion.

  3. Watch for trends in SaO_2, $TcPO_2$, and $TcPCO_2$ if used, or obtain arterial blood gases.

  4. Titrate ventilatory settings and FiO_2 according to response, to avoid pneumothorax. Pulmonary mechanics monitoring is also very helpful.

  5. Obtain a chest radiograph.

XV. **Response to Treatment**

A. There is a uniform improvement in oxygenation in 80% of infants.

B. In some, the response may be poor because of existing acidosis, severe hypoxia, or myocardial failure.

C. In another small percentage, a poor response may result from the presence of PDA.

D. Infant with cyanotic congenital heart disease will also show no response.

E. Initial good response followed by reversal may result from inappropriate ventilatory management following surfactant therapy (e.g., not changing peak pressure with subsequent development of pneumothorax).

XVI. Single Versus Multiple Doses

A. Prophylactic studies

1. Surfactant prophylaxis studies with single dose given soon after birth of infants 750–1,250 g showed:

   a. Decreased incidence of RDS

   b. Decreased need for oxygen

   c. Decreased death from RDS

   d. Decreased complications from RDS (pneumothorax and pulmonary interstitial emphysema [PIE])

2. Multiple dose studies also showed similar results

B. Rescue studies

1. Most studies gave surfactant treatment within 4-8 hours of birth.

2. These studies also showed overall:

   a. Decrease in deaths from RDS

   b. Improved PaO_2

   c. Decrease in mean airway pressure (Pāw)

   d. Decreased need for ventilation

   e. Decreased incidence of PIE and pneumothorax

3. Multiple doses are indicated if the response is inadequate as noted by:

   a. No improvement in PaO_2, the arterial/alveolar (a/A) ratio, or mean Paw from the baseline in 4–6 hours

   b. Drop in PaO_2 or increased need for oxygen or mean Paw

   c. Further worsening changes on chest radiography

4. Inactivation of surfactant during alveolar protein leak or development of PDA are major causes of poor response to multiple doses. In large infants with RDS not responding to multiple doses of surfactant, genetic defect of SP-B protein synthesis must be considered.

5. In general, there may be no advantage to giving more than two doses of treatment.

6. The need for additional doses is determined by the clinical course. Clinical studies using a three-dose schedule have shown significant improvement in outcome and a decrease in complications.

   a. Indications include continued requirement of intubation and ventilation, FiO_2 >0.3 to maintain PaO_2 >80 torr (10.7 kPa). Dose need not be repeated sooner than every 6 hours.

   b. Response to surfactant is improved if infant is exposed to antenatal steroid treatment.

C. Dosage

1. Survanta is available in liquid form dispersed in 0.9 NaCl solution. Each milliliter of Survanta contains 25 mg of phospholipid. The recommended dose is 4 mL/kg (100 mg/kg) per single dose.

2. Exosurf is available in lyophilized form. When reconstituted with 8 mL of sterile water, each milliliter will contain 13.5 mg/mL of DPPC. The dose is 5 mL (67.5 mg)/kg per single dose.

D. Timing of administration

1. Extensive studies have been conducted to assess the benefits of "prophylactic" treatment within minutes in the delivery room or "rescue" treatment within 6–8 hours of birth.

2. It is generally accepted that surfactant administered within 1–2 hours of birth and diagnosis of RDS is appropriate.

3. Routine prophylactic administration to all high-risk infants (<28 weeks gestation) may result in unnecessary treatment of many infants who would not in fact develop RDS.

4. It is also suggested that infants not be intubated only for administration of surfactant if other clinical or radiographic criteria are lacking.

XVII. **Other Uses of Surfactants**

A. Surfactants have been anecdotally used successfully to treat:

1. Meconium aspiration syndrome

2. Full-term infants with respiratory distress

3. Pulmonary hemorrhage

4. Congenital diaphragmatic hernia

5. Severe pneumonia

6. Because of the important role of SP-A in host defense mechanism, surfactant may be very important in pulmonary infections.

B. In conditions where there is loss of surfactant and lung volume

XVIII. **Overall Effects of Surfactant Therapy**

A. Increased survival from RDS

B. Decreased pneumothorax

C. Increased need for oxygen and ventilatory support

D. Decreased incidence/severity of BPD

XIX. **Follow-Up Data**

A. Long-term studies for detection of antibodies to surfactant protein (when natural surfactants were used), and development of allergic and atopic reactions, showed no persistence of antibodies or any increase in atopic allergies.

B. Neurodevelopmental assessment did not show a greater incidence of deficiencies in infants treated with surfactant compared with infants who did not receive surfactant.

XX. **Cost Analysis**

    A. Surfactant use has resulted in:

        1. Decreased length of stay (LOS) in hospital for survivors, especially in infants >1,250 g

        2. In infants <1,250 g, LOS has increased with increased survival.

        3. Overall, there is a decrease in utilization of ancillary services, and thus an increase in cost savings.

        4. The increase in the cost of care for infants <1,250 g is minimal when prorated over 70 years of life expectancy.

    B. The current cost of any commercial surfactant, however, is prohibitive for routine "free" use in developing countries. In many countries, cost of one dose of surfactant for each affected infant may equal or exceed its gross national product.

    C. Each country must make its own policy for the use of surfactant.

Suggested Reading

Corbet A: Clinical trials of synthetic surfactant in respiratory distress syndrome. Clin Perinatol 1993; 20:737–760.

Jobe AH, Ikegami M: Surfactant metabolism. Clin Perinatol 1993; 20:683–696.

Kattwinkel J: Surfactant: evolving issues. Clin Perinatol 1998; 25:17–32.

Mercier CE, Soll RF: Clinical trials of natural surfactant extract in respiratory distress syndrome. Clin Perinatol 1993; 20:711–736.

Merritt TA, Hallman M, Vaucher Y, et al: Impact of surfactant treatment on cost of neonatal intensive care: a cost-benefit analyis. J Perinatol 1990; 10:416–419.

Morley CJ: Surfactant treatment for premature babies: a review of clinical trials. Arch Dis Child 1991; 66:445–450.

Chapter 72

Adjunctive Pharmacologic Agents

Sam W. J. Richmond

I. **Analgesics**

A. Fentanyl

1. A short-acting opioid analgesic used for perioperative pain relief. The short action is more a function of rapid redistribution into fat and muscle depots because the elimination half-life is actually quite long – 4 hours in the adult and probably twice as long in the newborn. Morphine may be a better alternative for sustained pain relief.

2. Anesthetic doses, 5–10 micrograms/kg IV, will provide good pain relief for about 1 hour in the newborn. Respiratory drive will usually be abolished and artificial ventilation will be needed. Respiratory depression may also occur unexpectedly presumably following redistribution from fat or muscle depots. Continuous infusions of 3 micrograms/kg per hour are effective for a period but tolerance develops rapidly and, if the infusion is continued for more than 4–5 days, serious withdrawal symptoms may follow discontinuation.

B. Morphine

1. This is the most well-studied opiate analgesic for use in the newborn period. Respiratory depression, urinary retention, and constipation can occur with normal doses, and hypotension, bradycardia, and seizures with overdose.

2. For relief of severe pain, such as in necrotizing enterocolitis or following surgery, a loading dose of 240 micrograms/kg followed by an infusion of 20 micrograms/kg per hour is probably required. This dose will cause respiratory depression and artificial ventilation will be needed. For sedation of a ventilated baby, a loading dose of 120 micrograms/kg and an infusion of 10 micrograms/kg per hour will usually be sufficient. For less severe pain in the nonventilated baby, a dose of 100 micrograms/kg once every 12 hours may be sufficient. For the treatment of opiate withdrawal, oral doses of 40 micrograms/kg initially every 4 hours are advised, with increases in dosage interval resulting in withdrawal over 6–10 days.

   3. For elective intubation, give a dose of 120–200 micrograms/kg at least 2 minutes (preferably 5 minutes) before intubation, optionally followed by a suitable muscle relaxant. This dose may produce apnea.
  C. Acetaminophen (paracetamol)
   1. Analgesic and antipyretic with no anti-inflammatory properties. Well absorbed by mouth and, less predictably, rectally. Conjugated in the liver and excreted in urine. Half-life is about 4 hours.
   2. 24 mg/kg as an oral loading dose followed by a maintenance dose of 12 mg/kg orally every 4 hours. Consider measuring plasma levels if regular dosage is continued at this level for more than 24 hours. Rectal administration is less predictable, but a dose not exceeding 30 mg/kg every 6 hours is likely to be sufficient.

II. **Bronchodilators and Respiratory Stimulants**
  A. Aminophylline/theophylline
   1. An effective remedy for apnea of prematurity. Toxic effects include tachycardia, hyperactivity, and seizures. Therapeutic ranges for treatment of apnea of prematurity are 7–12 micrograms/mL, and for treatment of bronchospasm in older infants are 10–20 micrograms/mL.
   2. A loading dose of 6 mg/kg followed by 2.5–3.5 mg/kg IV every 12 hours will generally abolish apnea of prematurity in most babies. Treatment can be continued with oral theophylline. A loading dose of 9 mg/kg is followed by 4 mg/kg every 12 hours.
  B. Caffeine
   1. For many clinicians, caffeine is the drug of choice for the treatment of apnea of prematurity. Its safe therapeutic range is wider than theophylline, is well absorbed by mouth, and only needs to be given once daily. It is most commonly given as caffeine *citrate,* 1 mg of which is equivalent to 0.5 mg of caffeine *base.* Doses are usually quoted as doses of the citrate.
   2. Give a loading dose of 20 mg/kg of caffeine citrate orally or IV, followed by a once daily dose of 5 mg/kg. Both the loading dose and the maintenance dose can be safely doubled if necessary.
  C. Albuterol (USA)/salbutamol (UK)
   1. Selective β_2-adrenergic agonist, bronchodilator. Adult half-life is 6 hours. Can cause tachycardia, tremor, irritability. Well absorbed orally.
   2. 100–500 micrograms/kg nebulized 4–8 times daily. 100–300 micrograms/kg orally 3–4 times daily.
  D. Ipratropium – an anticholinergic bronchodilator synergistic with β-agonists. A synthetic derivative of atropine, given as 125 micrograms nebulized, q6–8h.
  E. Epinephrine (for stridor)
   1. Direct acting sympathomimetic agent with a more marked effect on β-adrenoreceptors than on α-adrenoreceptors.

2. Can be used (nebulized) to treat stridor.

3. Dose is 50-100 micrograms/kg prn.

III. **Diuretics**

A. Acetazolamide

1. A sulfonamide derivative which can cause agranulocytosis, aplastic anemia, skin toxicity, and crystalluria in addition to the more common problems of hypokalemic acidosis and gastrointestinal disturbances. Of questionable value in slowing the progress of posthemorrhagic hydrocephalus in patients unsuitable for immediate surgery.

2. 8 mg/kg orally every 8 hours increasing to a maximum of 32 mg/kg every 8 hours. Consider giving 4 mmol/kg of sodium bicarbonate orally prophylactically once daily to avoid metabolic acidosis.

B. Bumetanide (UK)

1. Loop diuretic more potent than furosemide and with similar mechanism of action

2. Causes very significant urinary salt loss as well as calcium and bicarbonate

3. Half-life in newborns: 2–6 hours

4. Dose: 5–50 micrograms/kg q6h IV, IM, or PO

C. Chlorothiazide (do not confuse with hydrochlorothiazide)

1. Benzothiazide diuretic usefully combined with spironolactone for additional effect. This is probably the safest diuretic combination for long-term control of fluid retention in congestive cardiac failure and chronic lung disease in the newborn, though it can result in considerable urinary calcium losses.

2. 10 mg/kg (usually combined with 1 mg/kg of spironolactone) orally twice daily. This dose can be safely doubled. Potassium supplements may not be needed if both drugs are given together.

D. Furosemide

1. A loop diuretic that inhibits active chloride reabsorption in the loop of Henle and the distal tubule, resulting in reduced passive sodium reabsorption and diuresis. There is some evidence for a direct effect on the lung improving lung function in bronchopulmonary dysplasia (BPD). Causes significant urinary losses of sodium, chloride, potassium, bicarbonate, and calcium. Stimulates renal synthesis of prostaglandin E_2 and may increase the incidence of patent ductus arteriosus. It is ototoxic and enhances the ototoxic effect of aminoglycosides. Chronic use may cause nephrolithiasis or nephrocalcinosis.

2. 1 mg/kg IV or 2 mg/kg orally given once or twice daily. Patients on long-term treatment should receive potassium chloride to pre-

vent hypokalemia. In renal failure, a single 5 mg/kg dose may help to reduce ischemic tubular damage. In BPD, 1 mg/kg of the IV preparation diluted in 2 mL of 0.9% saline and given by nebulizer once every 6 hours may improve pulmonary compliance without affecting renal function.

E. Spironolactone

1. Competitive inhibitor of aldosterone resulting in potassium-sparing diuresis. Usually used in combination with a thiazide diuretic such as chlorothiazide.

2. 1 mg/kg orally twice daily (combined with chlorothiazide, 10 mg/kg twice daily). Double this dose (of both drugs) may be safely used if necessary.

IV. **Inotropes**

A. Dobutamine

1. A synthetic inotropic catecholamine with primarily β_1-adrenergic activity, but in high doses it exhibits both α and β_2 effects. It stimulates myocardial contractility and increases cardiac output. Because it has less effect than dopamine on systemic vascular resistance, it has less effect in raising blood pressure (however, effectively increasing tissue perfusion is likely to be a more important goal than reaching a specific blood pressure target). Tachycardia may occur at high dosage and tissue ischemia may occur if the infusion infiltrates.

2. Start with a dose of 5 micrograms/kg/min by continuous IV infusion, increasing to 10–20 if needed. Do not give bicarbonate or other alkaline solutions through the same line, as this will inactivate dobutamine. Never give this through an arterial catheter.

B. Dopamine

1. A naturally occurring catecholamine precursor of noradrenaline

2. Generally speaking, at low doses (2–5 micrograms/kg/min), dopamine causes coronary, mesenteric, and renal vasodilatation, while at high doses (6–15 micrograms/kg/min) it causes vasoconstriction. It is best given via a central vein and it is inactivated by bicarbonate or other alkaline solutions. Never give this through an arterial catheter.

C. Noradrenaline (norepinephrine)

1. Sympathomimetic vasoconstrictor. Mainly causes increased cardiac contractility, increased heart rate, and increased myocardial oxygen consumption (β_1 stimulation). High-dose infusion can also increase peripheral vasoconstriction (α_1 stimulation), resulting in significantly increased cardiac afterload and a decrease in cardiac output.

2. Dosage calls for careful judgment. Give 0.1 micrograms/kg/min of noradrenaline base via a central vein. This may be increased to a maximum of 1.5 micrograms/kg/min as long as limb perfusion

and urine output are carefully monitored. Never give this through an arterial catheter.

V. Skeletal Muscle Relaxants

A. Atracurium

1. Atracurium besylate is a nondepolarizing competitive antagonist of acetylcholine at the motor end plate of voluntary muscle. Its effect can be reversed by anticholinesterases such as neostigmine. Its main advantage in the newborn period is that it does not depend on either renal or hepatic function for degradation. In the newborn, the effect lasts about 20–30 minutes.

2. 500 micrograms/kg IV will cause complete paralysis lasting about 20 minutes. For sustained paralysis, give an infusion of 400 micrograms/kg/h. Babies older than 1 month of age may require 500 micrograms/kg/h.

B. Pancuronium

1. Pancuronium is a nondepolarizing competitive antagonist of acetylcholine similar to atracurium. This effect extends to autonomic cholinergic receptors as well as those in skeletal muscle. It is partially metabolized in the liver and excreted by the kidneys and has a variable duration of action in the newborn of approximately 2–4 hours. Its effects can be reversed with atropine and neostigmine.

2. Give 100 micrograms/kg to produce complete paralysis within a couple of minutes and adjust repeat doses (50–150 micrograms/kg) based on the duration of the observed effect.

C. Suxamethonium (succinylcholine)

1. Suxamethonium acts as a depolarizing competitive agonist of acetylcholine. Brief muscle contraction is seen before paralysis occurs. These contractions are reported as painful by adults.

2. 2 mg/kg will provide paralysis for 5–10 minutes. 15 micrograms/kg of atropine is often given before any dose of suxamethonium and should certainly be given before a second dose.

D. Vecuronium

1. A nondepolarizing competitive antagonist of acetylcholine similar to pancuronium. Metabolized by the liver and excreted in urine.

2. 30–150 microgram/kg bolus will cause complete paralysis lasting 1–2 hours.

VI. Steroids

A. Betamethasone

1. Potent glucocorticoid used to enhance lung development in fetuses of mothers at risk for preterm birth

2. Give the mother 12 mg IM, repeated once after 24 hours.

B. Dexamethasone

    1. Potent glucocorticoid similar to betamethasone, and also used to encourage fetal lung development. Though it appears to be beneficial in treating severe BPD, the ideal treatment regimen has not yet been established. Treatment of babies with dexamethasone causes increased protein catabolism, which affects growth. Hypercalcuria, hypertension, hyperglycemia, gastrointestinal hemorrhage, left ventricular outflow tract obstruction, hypokalemia, and increased risk of infection are other well-recognized adverse effects.

    2. Standard regimen: 500 micrograms/kg base orally or IV once daily for 7 days followed, if necessary, by a 9-day course of tapering dosage.

    3. Pulse regimen: 250 micrograms/kg orally or IV twice daily for 3 days, repeated at 10-day intervals if necessary.

    4. Postintubation airway edema: 200 micrograms/kg orally or IV at 8-hour intervals starting 4 hours before extubation. Three doses are recommended.

C. Hydrocortisone

    1. Glucocorticoid with minimal mineralocorticoid effect. Primarily used for physiologic replacement, but can also be useful in the treatment of acute hypotension.

    2. Standard replacement treatment requires a dose of 6–9 mg/m^2/day. Three times this dose may be needed during acute illness. Start with 1–2 mg orally every 8 hours.

    3. Doses of 2.5 mg/kg IV every 4 hours have been shown to be as effective as dopamine in some cases of acute hypotension.

VII. Sedatives

A. Chloral hydrate

    1. Sedative, well-absorbed orally, metabolized in the liver and excreted in urine. Acts within 30 minutes, half-life of active metabolite is 36 hours.

    2. 45 mg/kg as a single dose. Higher doses (75 mg/kg) have been used for sedation for imaging, but can produce hypoxemia.

    3. 30 mg/kg orally every 6 hours can be helpful in babies with cerebral irritability. Usage for more than 2 days risks drug accumulation.

B. Midazolam

    1. Benzodiazepine anxiolytic and sedative. Metabolized in the liver and excreted in urine. Drug accumulation may occur with repeated doses. IV infusion or rapid bolus dosage has been reported to produce seizures in some babies.

    2. 150 micrograms/kg IV, IM, or intranasally produces rapid sedation and can be used for induction of anesthesia. (Midazolam does not relieve pain.)

3. 10–60 micrograms/kg/h IV infusion can be used for sedation of ventilated babies for 3–4 days. This dose should be halved after the first day for babies <33 weeks gestational age to prevent accumulation.

VIII. Pulmonary Vasodilators

A. Nitric oxide

1. Given as a gas by inhalation. Acts on receptors within the muscle of blood vessel walls to produce vasodilation. Rapidly inactivated by hemoglobin producing methemoglobin. Half-life <5 seconds. Vasodilator effect is therefore limited to the pulmonary circulation. Methemoglobin levels need to be monitored and kept below 2.5%.

2. In term babies and those >34 weeks gestation, start at 20 parts per million (ppm). If this produces a rise in postductal PaO_2 of at least 20 torr (3 kPa) with no alteration in ventilator settings, reduce the concentration to the lowest level possible. Once started on nitric oxide, babies are extremely sensitive to any interruption in supply.

B. Tolazoline

1. Vasodilator affecting both pulmonary and systemic vessels with an adrenergic blocking effect. Seems to work best when severe acidosis has been corrected. Cardiotoxic in high dosage and accumulates in renal failure.

2. 1–2 mg/kg given as a rapid bolus ideally into a **peripheral or central vein that drains into the superior vena cava.** If a positive response is seen, an infusion of 200 micrograms/kg/h may be helpful.

3. 200 micrograms/kg given as an intratracheal bolus instillation has been reported anecdotally to be effective.

Suggested Reading

Northern Neonatal Network: *Neonatal Formulary.* London, BMJ Books, 1998.

Young TE, Mangum OB (Eds.): *A Manual of Drugs Used in Neonatal Care, 11th Edition.* Raleigh, NC, Acorn Publishing, Inc., 1998.

SECTION XVI

Transport of Ventilated Babies

Chapter 73

Transport Equipment

Steven M. Donn, Molly R. Gates

I. **Goals of Neonatal Transport**
   A. Optimally, all infants requiring neonatal intensive care should be delivered at a facility capable of providing such services. Unfortunately, numerous circumstances arise which prevent this, including geographical and economic constraints, and unexpected complications of labor, delivery, or the neonatal period.
   B. The next best option is maternal transport when time and circumstances permit the transfer of a mother with an identified high-risk pregnancy to a facility able to care for the infant.
   C. When neither of these options is possible, transport of a critically ill newborn must be accomplished in a manner that maximizes safety and minimizes complications to the infant. Neonatal transport must be considered an extension of the neonatal intensive care unit (NICU), and the same philosophy of care as implemented in the NICU should be practiced in the transport vehicle.

II. **Transport Vehicles**
   A. Ground ambulance
      1. The most frequently used vehicle
      2. Provides the most access to the patient during transport
      3. Enables the largest number of transport team members
      4. Easy to stop vehicle in the event of patient deterioration and need for medical intervention
      5. Subject to traffic delays, road conditions, and weather (though to a lesser extent than airborne vehicles)
      6. Should be adaptable to special needs of neonatal transport
   B. Helicopter
      1. Provides a rapid means of transport
      2. Not subject to traffic or road conditions, but weather conditions may preclude use
      3. Size of vehicle may limit number of team members
      4. Landing pad may not be adjacent to hospital, requiring extra time and possible ambulance use

5. Virtually no access to patient en route
6. Must land in event of patient deterioration
7. Requires special training of crew
8. Expensive

C. Fixed-wing aircraft
1. Enables long distance transport
2. Subject to weather conditions
3. Size of vehicle may limit number of team members
4. Rapid, although travel time to and from airport and hospitals must be considered
5. Intermediate access to patient en route; deterioration may be problematic
6. Special problems at higher altitudes (see Chapter 75)
7. Expensive

D. Combination
At times it may be advantageous to combine modes of transport, such as the "fly-drive" method. Transport team and only essential emergency equipment is flown to referring hospital, helicopter returns to tertiary facility immediately, while ambulance is dispatched with the remainder of transport equipment. This eliminates helicopter "down time" while infant is stabilized and allows for use of a more stable environment for transport of infant.

III. Transport Incubator and Related Equipment

A. Several commercial types are available.
1. Self-contained types include virtually all necessary components as "built-ins" which may result in a reduced cost, although repairs may be costlier and may require that the device be out of service for a longer period of time.
2. More basic models are available, to which specific components can be added according to the specific needs of an institution.

B. Basic necessities
1. The incubator must be able to maintain the infant in a thermoneutral environment, and for small infants, infant servo-controlled heaters are recommended. This is especially important for winter climates that have a significantly low ambient temperature. Additional heat-conserving or heat-generating devices are necessary in colder climates.
   a. Heat shield or thermal blanket
   b. Exothermic chemical mattress
2. An electronic cardiorespiratory monitor, which should work well despite vehicle vibration or electrical interference
3. A pulse oximeter is strongly recommended.

4. A means of recording the temperature of the incubator and the baby
5. A source of air and oxygen, including a blender and an analyzer, and the means to deliver increased FiO_2 to the infant
6. A self-contained power source (battery) and the ability to be run by an external power source (e.g., wall electricity, vehicle generator)
7. Easy accessibility to the infant (e.g., portholes, front and side doors)
8. A means of securely anchoring the incubator within the transport vehicle
9. All necessary resuscitative equipment, including
   a. Bag and masks (assorted sizes)
   b. Laryngoscope and endotracheal tubes (assorted sizes)
   c. Vascular access devices
   d. Emergency medications and the means to deliver them

Table 40
Typical Transport Equipment

Adapters	Microbore tubing
Adhesive tape: ½" and 1"	Needles: 18 g, 21 g, 25 g
Alcohol wipes	Nasogastric tubes: 5 and 8 French
Antiseptic ointment	Occlusive dressing
Antiseptic swabs	Paperwork (extra)
Blood culture bottle	Platelet infusion set
Blood supplies	Pneumothorax aspiration set
Blood pressure transducer	Replogle tubes: 6 and 8 French
Bulb syringe	Saline squirts
Butterflies: 23 g, 25 g	Scalpel
Camera with film	Scissors, sterile
Catheters: 22 g, 24 g	Stopcocks
Chest tubes #10	Stopcock plugs
Connectors	Suction catheters: 6 and 8 French
Cotton balls	Suture: 4-0 silk
DeLee suction tube	Syringes: tuberculin, 3 cc, 5 cc, 10 cc,
Dextrose 10% in water: 250 mL bag	20 cc, 30 cc, 60 cc
Dressings: 4 × 4 and 2 × 2	T-connectors
Forceps, sterile	Tape, plastic: ½" and 1"
Gauze squares: see dressings	Tape measure, sterile
Gloves, sterile	Thermometer
Glucose screening strips	Toumey syringe: 60 cc
Heimlich valves	Umbilical artery catheters
Hemostats, sterile	UAC double lumen
Labels	UAC tray
Lancets	Umbilical tape
Large bore tubing	Waterproof adhesive tape
Lubricating gel	

C. Recommended options
1. Transport ventilator, especially if transporting critically ill infants or transporting long distance
2. Communications device
   a. Vehicle radio system
   b. Cellular telephone
3. Vascular infusion pump(s)
4. Blood pressure monitoring device, either invasive or noninvasive
5. Transcutaneous $TcPO_2/PCO_2$ device or portable blood gas analyzer for long distance transport of critically ill infant

IV. **Transport Equipment (Tables 40 and 41)**
Equipment should be readily available to treat any emergency that might occur either at the referring hospital or en route.

Table 41
Respiratory Care Transport Equipment

Hood and aerosol tubing (include extra tubing)	Endotracheal tube stylets (2)
Venturi mask	Pulse oximeter
Stethoscope	Pulse oximetry probes with elasticized wrap (2)
Infant restraints	Laryngoscope handle with spare batteries and bulb
Chemical exothermic mattress	
Resuscitation bag	Laryngoscope blades: Miller #0 and Miller #1
Flashlight	
Cargo netting	Magill forceps
Wrench for medical gas "E" tanks	Hemostats and scissors
Surfactant administration devices	Adhesive tape
Electronic cardiorespiratory monitor	Adhesive solution
	Cotton swabs
ECG electrode patches and leads	Adhesive remover
Blood pressure cable	Nasal CPAP prongs, assorted sizes
Neonatal mask	Sterile water soluble lubricant
Infant mask	Oxygen tubing (2)
Manometer	Oxygen tubing connectors (2)
PEEP valve	Flowmeter nipples (2)
22 mm connectors (2)	Suction catheters, 6 French (2)
15 mm connectors (2)	Air and oxygen connectors
Rubber connector	Nasal cannula, newborn
Endotracheal tubes: 2.5 mm (2); 3.0 mm (2); 3.5 mm (2); 4.0 mm (2)	Nasal cannula, premature
	Aluminum oxygen tank
Endotracheal tube adapters	Aluminum air tank

Table 42
Typical Transport Medications

Adenosine 3 mg/mL	Isoproterenol 1 mg/5 mL
Albumin 5%	Lidocaine 1%
Ampicillin 250 mg	Lidocaine 2%
Aquamephyton 10 mg/mL	Lorazepam 2 mg/mL
Atropine 0.1 mg/mL	Midazolam 1 mg/mL
Calcium Gluconate 10%	Morphine 0.5 mg/0.5 mL
Dexamethasone 4 mg/mL	Narcan 0.4 mg/mL
Dextrose 25%	Pancuronium 1 mg/mL
Diazepam 5 mg/mL	Phenobarbital 30 mg
Digoxin 25 mcg/mL	Phenobarbital 60 mg
Dobutamine	Potassium chloride
Dopamine 40 mg/mL	Prostaglandin E
Epinephrine 1:10,000	Sodium bicarbonate, 42% (0.5 mEq/mL)
Furosemide 10 mg/mL	Sodium chloride
Gentamicin 10 mg/mL	Sterile water
Glucagon and diluent	Survanta
Heparin	Tris-hydroxyaminomethane (THAM)

V. **Transport Medications (Table 42)**
Medications should also be readily available, as well as the means for administration (e.g., syringes, diluents, catheter connectors). Medications must be secured and checked regularly for condition and expiration date.

VI. **Miscellaneous Issues**

A. An instant camera is useful, both to give the parents a picture of the infant and to document any unusual physical findings.

B. All necessary documents for the medical record, as well as printed information given to the parents, should be prepared in advance. A clipboard is useful to keep the documents together.

C. Team members must protect themselves at all times.

1. Dress appropriately for the weather.

2. Use flame-retardant clothing for air transport.

3. Use approved helmets for air transport.

4. Have provisions (i.e., snacks) for long distance transports, especially if there is a likelihood of missing meals.

5. Always use seat belts.

6. Maintain current knowledge of transport supplies and procedures.

D. Packs or containers for miscellaneous transport gear should be lightweight, sturdy, well labeled, and secure. It is useful to store all supplies needed for a given procedure in one compartment.

Chapter 74

Stabilization of the Transported Newborn

Steven M. Donn, Molly R. Gates

I. **Basic Stabilization Upon Arrival**

  A. Respiratory

    1. Assess the adequacy of gas exchange

      a. Clinical assessment

        (1) Breath sounds

        (2) Chest excursions

        (3) Skin color

        (4) Presence of distress

      b. Laboratory assessment

        (1) Blood gas analysis

        (2) Chest radiograph

    2. Airway management

      a. Patency (suction if necessary)

      b. If already intubated and the tube position is satisfactory, secure tube adequately.

      c. If not intubated, consider elective intubation if there is any chance that this might become necessary en route. It is safer (and easier) to do this under controlled conditions at the referring hospital than in the back of an ambulance or while in flight.

    3. Insert an orogastric tube (especially important for air transport).

  B. Cardiac

    1. Assess tissue perfusion, and treat if inadequate.

      a. Blood pressure

      b. Capillary refill time

      c. Urine output

    2. Auscultation

      a. Murmur

      b. Abnormal heart sounds

      c. Abnormal rhythm

3. Chest radiograph

4. If cyanotic congenital heart disease is suspected, consider starting infusion of prostaglandin E (consult with neonatologist or cardiologist before doing so).

C. Hematologic

1. Check for sites of active bleeding.

2. Assure all vascular connections are secure.

3. Check hematocrit if not already done. Consider transfusion if low and infant is critical, and transport is anticipated to be long.

D. Metabolic

1. Perform glucose screen. If low, check serum glucose and treat.

2. Assure adequate glucose load during transport. Stress may increase consumption.

3. Check baby's temperature and maintain thermoneutrality. Prewarm transport incubator before transferring baby to it.

E. Vascular access

1. It is generally best to achieve vascular access prior to departing the referring hospital in the event that an emergency arises en route.

2. A well-placed peripheral venous line is usually sufficient.

3. If there is difficulty in securing peripheral venous access, consider placing an umbilical venous catheter. Confirm position radiographically before infusing medications through it (see Chapter 68).

4. An umbilical artery catheter (see Chapter 68) is generally not needed for transport unless no other vascular access can be achieved. It is an elective procedure that can be time-consuming and can significantly delay the departure and prolong the transport. Many community hospitals are ill-equipped to handle a complication. As a rule, this procedure is best left until the infant is admitted to the neonatal intensive care unit (NICU).

F. Miscellaneous issues

1. Make sure the infant is secured within the transport incubator. Retaining straps should be used but must not be too tight to impair thoracic excursions.

2. Tighten all connections (e.g., endotracheal tube adapter, ventilator circuit, vascular catheter connections, power lines) before departing. Label all lines.

3. Consider the use of infant "ear muffs" to decrease noise exposure for air transports.

4. Always have spare batteries for equipment that requires them.

5. Give the parents an opportunity to see and touch the infant before departing the referring hospital.

6. Be sure baby is properly identified.

7. Collect records from referring hospital to accompany infant.

II. Stabilization During Transport

A. If the infant was well stabilized in the referring hospital, there should be little else necessary once under way.

B. Check to be sure all of the vehicle equipment is functioning at the time the move from incubator to vehicle is made.

1. Power (generator or inverter)
2. Gas (air and oxygen) sources
3. Suction source

C. Be sure the transport incubator is securely anchored and that there is no loose equipment or tanks which could cause a hazard en route.

D. Monitoring of the infant during the transport should be no different than that which is done in the NICU.

E. Should the infant unexpectedly deteriorate en route, it is generally best to stop the vehicle (this may mean landing if in a helicopter) while attending to the infant. It is extremely difficult to perform resuscitative procedures and draw up and administer medications in a moving vehicle; attempting to do this places both the patient and the transport team members at risk for injury.

III. After the Transport

A. A thorough transport note should be written in the medical record to document the events of the transport, as well as any treatments rendered, and how the baby tolerated the procedure.

B. All supplies should be promptly replenished.

C. Any mechanical problems (vehicle, equipment, or other) should be reported and corrected immediately.

D. Give feedback to the referring physician and notify the parents that the baby arrived safely.

Chapter 75

Special Considerations

Steven M. Donn, Molly R. Gates

I. Intensive Care

   A. Although transport vehicles are an attempt at extending intensive care services to referring hospitals, they are not intensive care units. One of the most difficult decisions during neonatal transport is deciding whether a specific procedure should be performed in the referring hospital/transport vehicle or deferred until admission to the neonatal intensive care unit (NICU). Some aspects to consider include:

   1. Urgency of the procedure in light of the patient's condition (i.e., elective, semi-elective, or emergent)
   2. Availability of experienced personnel to assist
   3. Suitability of available equipment
   4. Ability to handle a major complication if it occurs
   5. Adequacy of monitoring the patient during the procedure

   B. Some procedures that are of an elective nature should be considered in view of the difficulty with which they are performed in a transport vehicle.

   1. Endotracheal intubation. Control of the airway in a baby with respiratory distress is crucial. Do not wait until the baby is in marked distress to intubate.
   2. Vascular access. Placement of a peripheral intravenous line *prior to departure* from the referring hospital is strongly advised. This is an extremely difficult procedure in a dimly lit and moving vehicle, especially if the baby is hypotensive. It also enables prompt treatment of problems such as hypoglycemia.

II. Effects of Altitude

   A. Impact on respiratory status

   1. The partial pressure of oxygen decreases as altitude increases; thus, the availability of oxygen to the baby decreases and alveolar hypoxia increases. The baby must work harder to achieve satisfactory gas exchange.

2. The cabins of fixed-wing aircraft are either pressurized or nonpressurized. If nonpressurized, this effect of altitude will occur early. Pressurized cabins generally have a pressure equivalent to that at 8,000 feet rather than atmospheric pressure at sea level.

3. These effects must be considered in the management of respiratory insufficiency. They underscore the need for close monitoring (i.e., pulse oximetry) as well as anticipating the need for increasing support as altitude is increased.

B. Impact on contained gases

1. As altitude increases, and thus barometric pressure decreases, the volume of contained gases also increases.

2. This effect must also be taken into consideration in the management of the infant.

a. Gas in the stomach and bowel will expand, potentially aggravating respiratory distress by impinging on the diaphragm. Ensure that an orogastric or nasogastric tube is in place to vent the stomach.

b. Abnormal accumulations of gas in the chest (e.g., pulmonary interstitial emphysema, pneumomediastinum) can also expand, leading to pneumothorax. Observe closely and be ready to intervene.

3. The effects of altitude must be considered in treatment as well.

a. Medications and fluids are packaged at sea level, and thus are at higher pressure at altitude. Take caution when drawing up medications from vials.

b. As the aircraft descends, carefully observe gravity drip infusions; external pressure may create a gradient which causes reversal of flow from the baby with subsequent blood loss.

III. **Miscellaneous Effects on the Infant**

A. Noise and vibration. While not totally avoidable, some measures can be taken to minimize their effects.

1. Muffle noise by using "ear muffs" or cotton inserts.

2. Make sure vehicle suspension is in good order.

3. Avoid excessive speed or poorly maintained roads, if possible

B. Cold stress (see Chapters 73 and 74)

C. Position infant optimally for clinical support and to maximize caregivers' ongoing assessment.

IV. **Miscellaneous Effects on the Transport Team**

A. Motion sickness, aversion to exhaust fumes

B. Stress

C. Safety issues

V. Effects on the Family

    A. Separation from the infant (especially for the mother)

    B. Economic hardship

    C. Psychosocial stress

VI. Systems Issues

    A. Organized procedures must be in place and communicated to all potential participants for requesting, accepting, dispatching, and conducting neonatal transports.

    B. Periodic review of transports enables identification and correction of system problems.

    C. Contingency planning and prior consideration of unusual circumstances improves response and lessens stress.

Suggested Reading (Chapters 73–75)

Donn SM, Faix RG, Gates MR: Emergency transport of the critically ill newborn. In Donn SM, Faix RG (Eds.): *Neonatal Emergencies.* Mt. Kisco, NY, Futura Publishing Co., 1991, pp. 75–86.

Donn SM, Faix RG, Gates MR: Neonatal transport. Curr Prob Pediatr 1985; 15:1–63.

Gates MR, Geller S, Donn SM: Neonatal transport. In Donn SM, Fisher CW (Eds.): *Risk Management Techniques in Perinatal and Neonatal Practice.* Armonk, NY, Futura Publishing Co., 1996, pp. 563–580.

SECTION XVII

Alternative Therapies for Intractable Respiratory Failure

Chapter 76

Extracorporeal Membrane Oxygenation

Robert E. Schumacher

I. **Description**

    A. Extracorporeal membrane oxygenation (ECMO) is a means for an infant (usually term) with reversible lung failure to have a period of "lung rest" by use of an artificial lung. This "rest" period may allow for lung recovery and ultimately survival of the infant.

    B. Oxygen delivery is determined by ECMO pump flow ("cardiac output").

    C. Ventilation is determined by gas flow though the artificial lung.

II. **ECMO Circuit**

    A. For venoarterial bypass, venous blood is passively drained via the right atrium and passed via a roller pump to a venous capacitance reservoir (bladder box), a membrane lung, a heat exchanger, and an arterial perfusion cannula. The right internal jugular vein and common carotid artery are used as access points and are often ligated as part of the bypass procedure.

    B. For venovenous bypass, a double lumen cannula is used. In this, isovolemic procedure blood is removed from and returned to the right atrium, the remainder of the circuit being the same as in venoarterial ECMO.

    C. To prevent thrombotic complications while on ECMO, the patient is treated with systemic heparinization.

III. **Patient Selection**

    A. For standard neonatal ECMO the patient should:

        1. Be ≥35 weeks gestation (intracranial hemorrhage remains a significant concern for premature infants)

        2. Have a cranial sonogram with no intraventricular hemorrhage > grade I

3. Have no major bleeding problem
4. Not have an irreversible condition, uniformly associated with poor outcome such that attempts to prolong life are futile or not in the best interests of the infant (e.g., pulmonary hypoplasia, trisomy 18)
5. Be <1 week old (relative contraindication, used as a marker for infants with a significant component of irreversible respiratory failure)
6. Be failing conventional medical management

B. Failure of conventional medical management is a definition that should be individualized for each ECMO center.

1. Guidelines (based on experience with populations) are used, but the ultimate decision is up to those caring for the individual infant. Cutpoint values (i.e., ECMO/no ECMO) should be chosen taking into account not only mortality statistics but also long-term morbidity.

2. Oxygenation index (OI) criteria:

   a. $$OI: \frac{\text{mean airway pressure} \times FiO_2}{P_aO_2 \text{ (postductal)}} \times 100$$

   b. **After** stabilization, if the patient has OI values $\geq$40 on 3 of 5 occasions (each value separated by >30 and <60 minutes), ECMO criteria have been met (University of Michigan criteria).

   c. Venovenous ECMO may not provide the same cardiac support that venoarterial ECMO does.

      (1) Infants with severe cardiac compromise may not tolerate venovenous ECMO. Identification of these patients is difficult.

      (2) Because the risk of carotid artery ligation is not present, consideration for venovenous ECMO is made at lower OI values (25–40).

3. Other criteria include alveolar-arterial oxygen tension gradient (A-aDO$_2$), acute deterioration, intractable airleaks, and "unresponsive to medical management."

IV. Management

A. Initial bypass problems

1. Hypotension

   a. Hypovolemia. ECMO circuit has high blood capacitance; treat this with blood volume expanders. The technician should have packed red blood cells (PRBCs) or colloid available from circuit priming procedure.

   b. Sudden dilution of vasopressors, especially with venovenous ECMO: treat by having separate pressor infusion pumps to infuse into circuit.

   c. Hypocalcemia from stored blood: circuit can be primed with calcium to prevent this.

2. Bradycardia – from vagal stimulation by catheter(s)
3. Consequences of catheter misplacement. Correct catheter placement should be documented radiographically.

B. Initial management

1. Venoarterial bypass. Wean ventilator rapidly (10–15 min) to "rest" settings (FiO_2, 0.3; pressure, 25/4 cm H_2O; rate, 20 bpm; inspiratory time, 0.5–1.0 sec). Use SvO_2 as guide. Continuous positive airway pressure/high positive end-expiratory pressure (CPAP/high PEEP) (10–12 cm H_2O) may shorten bypass time. Inotropes can usually be quickly discontinued.

2. Venovenous bypass. Wean with caution; infant is still dependent on innate myocardial function for O_2 delivery. SvO_2 useful only for trends at same pump flow rate. Innate lung still provides gas exchange. High CPAP with venovenous ECMO may impede cardiac output; if desired, use end-tidal carbon dioxide ($ETCO_2$) to optimize PEEP. Inotropes must be weaned with caution.

3. Infants have self-decannulated; restraints are mandatory.

4. Head position is critical; head turned too far left will functionally occlude the left jugular vein (right is already ligated). Such a scenario may lead to central nervous system (CNS) venous hypertension.

5. Analgesia and sedation are usually required. Narcotic used for analgesia; if patient needs additional sedation, benzodiazepines or phenobarbital are reasonable choices.

6. Heparin management
   a. Prior to cannulation, the loading dose is 100 U/kg.
   b. Drip concentration is 60 U/mL (6 mL heparin [1,000 U/mL] in 94 mL dextrose 5% in water).
   c. Usual consumption is 20–40 U/kg/h. Affected by blood-surface interactions in circuit, infant's own clotting status, and heparin elimination (renal excretion).
   d. Titrate heparin to keep activated clotting time (ACT) in desired range (usually 180–200 sec).

C. Daily management, patient protocols, problems

1. Chest radiograph – daily

2. Cranial sonogram – obtain the first day after cannulation, after every change in neurologic status, and minimally every third day.
   a. Brain hemorrhage. Includes both typical and atypical (including posterior fossa) hemorrhages. If present, and patient is able to come off ECMO, do so. If patient is likely to die if removed from bypass, has stable hemorrhage, or is neurologically stable, consider keeping patient on bypass with strict attention to lower ACT values (e.g., 160–180 sec), and keeping platelet counts higher (e.g., 125,000–200,000/mm^3).
   b. Cranial sonography is not as effective as computed tomography (CT) for demonstrating peripheral/posterior fossa lesions.

3. Fluids – follow input/output, weights; the membrane lung provides an additional area for evaporative losses.
   a. Total body water (TBW) is high: a common problem, etiology is probably multifactorial. A problem arises when TBW is high but intravascular volume is low (capillary leak); vigorous attempts at diuresis in this instance will not help and can be harmful. Aggressive diuresis may allow for more caloric intake. Some argue that vigorous attempts at diuresis can hasten lung recovery; others state that diuresis is a marker for improvement and attempts to hasten it are of no avail. If diuresis is deemed advisable, use diuretics first, hemofilter last. (Furosemide in combination with theophylline may be helpful.) Expect decreased urine output when hemofilter is used.
   b. K^+: serum values often low and require replacement, check for alkalosis.
   c. Pump is primed with banked blood; ionized Ca^{2+} can be low, priming the circuit prevents this.
4. Hemostasis/hemolysis
   a. Obtain fibrinogen, fibrin split products, serum hemoglobin, and platelet counts daily.
   b. Clots are common especially in venous capacitance reservoir (bladder). Prelung clots are usually left alone. Those postlung are handled by the ECMO technician. When clots appear, review platelet/heparin consumption, fibrin split products, etc.
   c. Bleeding
      (1) From neck wound: treat with cannula manipulation (by surgeon), light pressure, or fibrin glue
      (2) Hemothorax/pericardium will present with decreased pulse pressure and decreased pump filling. Treat with drainage first.
      (3) A more common problem if previous surgery has been done (e.g., congenital diaphragmatic hernia, thoracostomy tube)
      (4) Treat with blood replacement, keep platelet counts high ($>150,000/mm^3$), lower acceptable ACT values.
5. Total parenteral nutrition (TPN): a *major* benefit of ECMO can be immediate provision of TPN and adequate caloric/low volume intake (use high dextrose concentrations).
6. Blood products
   a. Minimize donor exposures, give only when indicated.
   b. Excessive PRBCs administration without increasing pump flow leads to lower aortic PO_2 but has little impact on oxygen delivery.
7. Hypertension is a known complication. The final mechanism by which it is achieved is usually high total body water. It is almost

always transient and resolves near the end of a run. A working definition is mean arterial pressure >75 mm Hg. Initial treatment is with diuretics.

8. White blood cells (WBCs) often low, probably from peripheral migration.

9. Infections are not a common problem. Suspect infection if unanticipated increased ECMO support is required. Fungal infection is a concern.

10. Bilirubin can be elevated especially with sepsis or long ECMO runs. A cholestatic picture is typical; plastic tubing may be hepatotoxic. Hepatosplenomegaly is common.

11. Cardiac stun. Once on ECMO, a dramatic decrease in cardiac performance is seen in up to 5% of patients. May be ECMO induced from increased afterload. The stun phenomenon usually resolves, but these patients do have higher overall mortality rates. Treatment is supportive.

D. Selected, more common, circuit problems

1. Air in circuit – treatment depends upon location; can often be aspirated

2. Pump cutouts – kinked tube, malposition, low volume, low filling pressure (pneumothorax, hemopericardium), agitated infant

3. Pump
   a. Electric failure – can be cranked by hand
   b. Occlusion set too loose – false high flow readings; too tight – hemolysis

4. Lung pathophysiology – the membrane lung can get "sick," and have pulmonary embolus, edema, etc. Treatment depends upon specific problem.

E. Weaning

1. Follow S_vO_2; wean by preset parameters

2. Chest radiograph is very helpful.
   a. Usually shows initial complete opacification
   b. Starts to clear prior to "reventilating" the lungs and serves as a marker for lung recovery

3. Pulmonary mechanics tests – compliance becomes poor hours after beginning bypass and improvement is an early marker of lung recovery.

4. ETCO$_2$ – increasing expired CO_2 is indicative of return of lung function.

F. Trial off bypass

1. Lung conditioning – lungs are periodically (hourly) inflated using a long (≥ 5 sec) sustained inflation.

2. Turning up the ventilator FiO$_2$ and following SvO$_2$ will give a feel for whether or not there is any effective pulmonary gas exchange.

3. Increased ventilator settings to achieve adequate tidal volumes 30–60 minutes before trial off appears to allow for recruitment of lung units.

4. Venoarterial: obtain blood gas q10 min. Wean FiO_2 aggressively per pulse oximetry.

5. Venovenous: halt gas flow to membrane lung; keep pump flowing. Since infant is still on bypass but with no effective gas exchange through membrane, use venous line SvO_2 to wean FiO_2 as it is now a true venous saturation.

6. A successful trial off depends upon the individual patient. Patient should be stable on FiO_2 ≤ 0.4, settings as per trial off.

G. Decannulation

1. Notify surgeon as soon as possible.

2. Infant will be paralyzed to prevent air embolism.

3. Need for repair of carotid artery or jugular vein controversial

V. **Post-ECMO Follow-Up**

A. Neck sutures removed in 7 days

B. Platelets will continue to fall post-ECMO. Serial counts are necessary until stable (24–48 hr).

C. CNS

1. Electroencephalogram (EEG) – if normal on ECMO (if obtained), no need to repeat

2. EEG is a sensitive (too sensitive?) screening test for CNS problems. Focal abnormality correlates with structural findings and computed tomagraphy/magnetic resonance imaging (CT/MRI) is needed.

3. CT/MRI – obtained because of relative insensitivity of sonography for posterior fossa and "lateral" parenchymal lesions

4. Brainstem audiometric evoked responses (BAER) – because of the high incidence of sensorineural hearing loss with persistent pulmonary hypertension of the newborn, hearing screening is recommended. Delayed onset loss has been described and repeated screening is advised.

D. Airway
Vocal cord paresis seen in approximately 5% of infants post-ECMO; acute respiratory deterioration has occurred. If persistent stridor is noted, flexible bronchoscopy is recommended. Hoarseness has always resolved clinically within a period of days to months.

E. Long-term follow-up

1. Neurodevelopmental: 10–20% of patients show major problems post-ECMO.

2. Medical problems include lower respiratory tract infections in many of these patients.

Suggested Reading

Bartlett RH: Extracorporeal life support for cardiopulmonary failure. Curr Probl Surg 1990; 27:621–705.

Bartlett RH, Zwischenberger JB (Eds.): *ECMO: Extracorporeal Cardiopulmonary Support in Critical Care.* Ann Arbor, MI, Extracorporeal Life Support Organization, 1995.

Glass P, Wagner AE, Papero PH, et al: Neurodevelopmental status at age five years of neonates treated with extracorporeal membrane oxygenation. J Pediatr 1995; 127:447–557.

UK Collaborative ECMO Trial Group: UK collaborative randomised trial of neonatal extracorporeal membrane oxygenation. Lancet 1996; 348:75–82.

Chapter 77

Inhaled Nitric Oxide Therapy

Martha Nelson

I. **Background**

A. Historic importance

1. Originally thought of as merely an atmospheric pollutant

2. 1980: a tangible endothelial-derived relaxing factor (EDRF) is first described.

3. 1987: EDRF is discovered to be nitric oxide (NO).

4. 1992: the initial reports of clinical efficacy of inhaled nitric oxide (iNO) therapy for treatment of persistent pulmonary hypertension of the newborn (PPHN) are published.

5. 1992: NO is named Science Magazine's "Molecule of the Year."

6. 1997: The Inhaled Nitric Oxide Study Group reports the results of its large, randomized, multicenter, controlled trial of NO.

B. Generalized physiologic functions attributed to endogenous NO

1. Synthesis of NO by vascular endothelium is thought to be responsible for maintaining the vascular tone essential for regulating blood pressure.

2. In the central nervous system, NO acts as a neurotransmitter.

3. A variety of peripheral nerves operate through an NO-dependent mechanism to mediate some forms of neurogenic vasodilation (gastrointestinal, respiratory, and genitourinary tract functions).

4. NO contributes to control of platelet aggregation and inhibits platelet (and leukocyte) adhesion to vessel walls (and increases bleeding time in animals and adults).

5. NO contributes to the regulation of cardiac contractility.

6. NO is produced in large quantities during host defense, and is thought to have a nonspecific role in immunity.

7. NO is a bronchodilator.

II. **Mechanisms for Activity and Metabolism**

A. Vascular relaxation mediated by nitric oxide

1. Shear stress on vessel endothelium (e.g., increased blood flow) or endothelial receptor activation by bradykinin or acetylcholine leads to a cellular influx of calcium.

2. Increased intracellular calcium stimulates activity of *nitric oxide synthase* (NOS) enzyme systems.
3. NOS induces the conversion of intracellular L-arginine to L-citrulline; this reaction generates free NO.
4. Free NO diffuses into nearby smooth muscle cells where it stimulates soluble guanylate cyclase (sGC).
5. This enzyme system (sGC) stimulates conversion of guanosine triphosphate (GTP) to cyclic guanosine monophosphate (cGMP).
6. cGMP initiates a cascade of intracellular events (e.g., efflux of cellular potassium through calcium-dependent channels) leading to smooth muscle relaxation.
7. cGMP is then rapidly hydrolyzed and inactivated in the smooth muscle cell by phosphodiesterase enzyme systems; continuous tonic release of NO with ongoing production of cGMP is necessary to maintain basal tone in several vascular beds.

B. Pathologic release of NO
1. A calcium-independent isoform of NOS can be induced in the vasculature by certain cytokines and endotoxin lipopolysaccharides (at the vascular endothelium and smooth muscle).
2. This induces vascular relaxation resistant to vasoconstrictors.
3. This phenomenon can be prevented with glucocorticoids and inhibitors of NOS.
4. It is well established that NO released by this inducible enzyme system accounts for the persistent vasodilation and resistance to vasoconstrictors seen in septic shock.

C. Metabolism and potential toxicity of NO
1. Endogenous metabolism of NO in mammals produces plasma and urinary nitrite and nitrate, but the precise mechanism for the breakdown into these forms is unknown.
   a. NO will dissolve in water in the absence of oxygen; the molecule is very stable under these conditions.
   b. In water, ultrafiltrate, and plasma, NO is oxidized to nitrite, and is very stable in this form for several hours.
   c. In whole blood, nitrite is rapidly converted to nitrate (basal nitrite concentration in blood is very low, but nitrate levels in blood are 100 times higher).
   d. NO has a very high affinity for hemoglobin (roughly 3,000 times greater than that of oxygen); nitrosylhemoglobin is rapidly oxidized to **methemoglobin,** which is in turn reduced by the NADH-dependent *methemoglobin reductase* enzyme system to the benign nitrate form. (Methemoglobinemia is not recognized as a significant complication for term infants at iNO doses of ≤20 ppm.)
2. Exposure of appreciable amounts of NO to air can lead to formation of more toxic metabolites.

    a. In air, NO reacts quickly to form nitrogen dioxide (NO_2), which is a toxic, brown gas capable of causing significant tissue damage.

    b. At very low concentrations, NO will be somewhat more stable, even in the presence of oxygen.

    c. NO is also very rapidly oxidized to higher oxides of nitrogen (e.g., peroxynitrites), which rapidly decompose to form hydroxyl radicals and other cytotoxic compounds with the ability to damage cells and denature surface proteins. Laboratory data show low-dose iNO does not cause such tissue injury to lung parenchyma.

  3. NO is a carcinogen in very high doses.

III. Fetal and Neonatal Vascular Tone

  A. Fetal circulation

    1. Characterized by high pulmonary vascular resistance

    2. Pulmonary blood flow accounts for <10% of combined ventricular output in the fetus because blood is shunted away from the lungs ($R \rightarrow L$ shunt).

    3. Precise mechanisms for maintaining high pulmonary vascular resistance during fetal life, and those causing sustained vascular dilation after birth, are unknown.

  B. Some mediators of vascular tone

    1. Endogenous vasoconstrictors

      a. Hypoxia

      b. Acidosis

      c. Endothelin-1 (vasoactive peptide produced by vascular endothelium)

      d. Leukotrienes

      e. Thromboxanes

      f. Platelet-activating factor

      g. $PGF_{2\alpha}$

    2. Mechanical factors inducing pulmonary vasoconstriction

      a. Over- or underinflation of the lung

      b. Excessive arterial muscularization and vascular remodeling

      c. Altered mechanical properties of smooth muscle

      d. Pulmonary hypoplasia

      e. Ventricular dysfunction

      f. α-adrenergic stimulation

    3. Endogenous vasodilators

      a. Oxygen

      b. NO

      c. PGI_2, PGE_2, PGD_2

      d. Adenosine, adenosine triphosphate, magnesium

   e. Bradykinin

   f. Atrial natriuretic factor

   g. Histamine

   h. Acetylcholine

  4. Mechanical factors mediating vasodilation

   a. β-adrenergic stimulation

   b. Vagal nerve stimulation

   c. Lung inflation

   d. Vascular cell structural changes

   e. Interstitial fluid and pressure changes

   f. Shear stress

 C. PPHN (see Chapter 43)

  1. Syndrome characterized by marked pulmonary hypertension and altered vasoreactivity, which leads to R $\rightarrow$ L shunting of blood across the patent ductus arteriosus and foramen ovale

  2. Often associated with an underlying process that has caused poor ventilation, hypoxia, and/or acidosis at or near term (e.g., meconium aspiration syndrome, respiratory distress syndrome, congenital diaphragmatic hernia, sepsis, pneumonia)

  3. "Idiopathic" PPHN occurs when no other definitive, underlying cause of lung disease is identified.

  4. Exact pathophysiology remains unclear; infants dying from PPHN show marked distal extension of vascular smooth muscle, thickening of the arterial media and adventitia, and excessive accumulation of matrix protein in pulmonary blood vessel walls.

 D. NO as treatment for PPHN

  1. Given by inhalation, it *selectively* dilates the pulmonary vasculature (the excess is quickly bound to hemoglobin and inactivated).

  2. The exact mechanism by which iNO works is unknown; it is presumed to diffuse through the pulmonary interstitium and the vascular adventitia to activate the smooth muscle guanase cyclase system.

  3. The exact site of pulmonary vasculature actually affected by NO remains unknown (there are some data indicating pulmonary veins are more sensitive to NO than are pulmonary arteries).

IV. Clinical Applications

 A. Term infants

  1. PPHN

   a. Echocardiographic evidence of pulmonary hypertension including R $\rightarrow$ L (or bidirectional) shunting across the patent ductus arteriosus and/or foramen ovale, tricuspid regurgitation, and increased right ventricular pressures

   b. Pre- and postductal PaO_2 gradient of ≥ 20 torr (2.7 kPa) by arterial blood gas measurement or transcutaneous oxygen monitoring

    c. Pre- and postductal SaO_2 measurement gradient of $\geq 10\%$

    d. Significant clinical lability with profound hypoxemia (e.g., PaO_2 <70 torr [9.3 kPa], or SaO_2 $\leq 80\%$ in an infant receiving FiO_2 of 1.0)

  2. Increased pulmonary vascular resistance with congenital heart disease

  3. iNO therapy for infants with congenital diaphragmatic hernia remains an unproven treatment (results of clinical trials are mixed).

B. Preterm infants

  1. No randomized controlled trials of iNO therapy in preterm infants have been reported to date.

  2. Preliminary data suggest iNO improves oxygenation in preterm infants and support a potential role for low-dose iNO therapy; the clinical outcomes for safety (intraventricular hemorrhage) and efficacy are not yet fully elucidated.

C. Dosage

  1. Current data support the use of iNO doses beginning at 20 ppm in term infants with PPHN. The University of Michigan initiates treatment at a dose of 80 ppm and quickly (within an hour) weans this to 40 ppm. Doses are further weaned to 20 ppm as tolerated. Once at 20 ppm, the dose is weaned in 5–10 ppm decrements as tolerated. (Administration of FiO_2 of 1.0 is not possible with concurrent administration of NO because of the dilutional effect of NO in the inspiratory circuit.)

  2. The lowest effective starting dose for iNO in term newborns with PPHN has not been determined.

  3. Long-term, low-dose iNO appears to be safe for infants; inability to tolerate weaning from iNO has been postulated to result from exogenous NO down-regulation of endogenous NO production.

  4. Once clinically stable, attempts to wean the infant from NO therapy should be attempted daily. A compensatory increase in supplemental FiO_2 may be required when first discontinuing iNO therapy.

D. Other management strategies

  1. Support systemic blood pressure with volume expansion and inotropic therapy.

  2. Attempt alkalosis with systemic buffer, and/or hyperventilation strategies.

  3. Fully sedate the infants to minimize oxygen expenditure; consider elective paralysis.

  4. Use optimal ventilatory strategies with real-time pulmonary graphics to assure provision of appropriate lung expansion; consider use of high-frequency oscillatory ventilation (HFOV) as needed to achieve satisfactory lung expansion; iNO administered through the

INOvent® Delivery System (Ohmeda, Inc., Madison, WI, USA) enables gas delivery with conventional, high-frequency oscillatory, or manual ventilation.

5. Close, continuous monitoring of vital signs, ventilatory status (frequent blood gas measurements), and changes on physical examination are necessary. Infants who do not respond to iNO therapy may require extracorporeal membrane oxygenation (ECMO).

E. Adjunctive therapies under investigation

   1. HFOV: as above, current data suggest HFOV may be more effective in delivering iNO in certain clinical settings (e.g., severe lung disease with low lung volumes).

   2. Pharmacologic augmentation of iNO therapy with phosphodiesterase inhibitors (dipyridamole) has been studied, and preliminary results are variable.

   3. Exogenous surfactant has been studied, and some early data are consistent with favorable results, linking surfactant use and iNO with sustained clinical improvement and decreased need for ECMO in term infants with pneumonia and PPHN.

F. Clinical evaluation during use

   1. The INOvent Delivery System offers continuous on-line monitoring of NO, NO_2, and O_2 levels; other systems are also available.

   2. Methemoglobin levels are measured on initiation of therapy (baseline); levels are followed every 12 hours until the iNO dose ≤ 20 ppm, then measured daily; at a level of $>5\%$ consider treatment with methylene blue (1–2 mg/kg/dose IV infused over 5 minutes), and attempts to wean NO further.

   3. The infant should be carefully monitored for signs of left ventricular dysfunction and pulmonary edema (iNO is not recommended for use in infants with signs of pulmonary *venous* hypertension that is associated with mitral insufficiency and increased left atrial pressure).

Suggested Reading

Davidson D, Barefield E, Kattwinkel J, et al: Inhaled nitric oxide for the early treatment of persistent pulmonary hypertension of the term newborn: a randomized, double-masked, placebo-controlled, dose-response, multicenter study. Pediatrics 1998; 101:326–334.

Finer NN, Barrington KJ: Nitric oxide in respiratory failure in the newborn infant. Sem Perinatol 1997; 21:426–440.

Kinsella JP, Abman SH: Controversies in the use of nitric oxide therapy in the newborn. Clin Perinatol 1998; 25:203–217.

Shaul PW: Ontogeny of nitric oxide in the pulmonary vasculature. Sem Perinatol 1997; 21:381–392.

The Inhaled Nitric Oxide Study Group: Inhaled nitric oxide in full-term and nearly full-term infants with hypoxic respiratory failure. N Engl J Med 1997; 336:597–604.

Chapter 78

Liquid Ventilation for Neonatal Respiratory Failure

David S. Foley, Ronald B. Hirschl

I. **Description.** Liquid ventilation refers to the process of enhancing pulmonary function through the instillation of perfluorocarbon liquid into the lungs.

   A. Total liquid ventilation (TLV) – the achievement of gas exchange through the delivery of tidal volumes of perfluorocarbon liquid to the lungs using a specialized mechanical liquid ventilator

   B. Partial liquid ventilation (PLV) – the achievement of gas exchange through the delivery of gas tidal volumes to lungs which have been filled with perfluorocarbon liquid

II. **Physiology of Perfluorocarbon Ventilation**

   A. Perfluorocarbons (PFCs) – inert liquids that are produced by the fluorination of common organic hydrocarbons. These liquids have high solubilities for the respiratory gases and low surface tensions.

   B. Physical properties of perfluorocarbons

   1. Density – much more dense than hydrocarbon counterparts with levels approaching twice that of water (1.75–1.95 g/mL @ 25°C)

   2. Surface tension – have weak intermolecular forces and remarkably low surface tensions (15–20 dynes/cm @ 25°C)

   3. Respiratory gas solubility – solubilities of the respiratory gases in perfluorocarbons are significantly greater than their corresponding solubilities in water or nonpolar solvents.

   a. O_2 solubility @ 37°C = 44–55 mL gas/100 mL liquid

   b. CO_2 solubility @ 37°C = 140–210 mL gas/100 mL liquid

   4. Some perfluorocarbons, such as perflubron (C8F17Br) (Liquivent®, Alliance Pharmaceutical Corp., San Diego, CA, USA), are radiopaque.

   C. Basis for the use of liquid ventilation in neonatal ventilator-dependent respiratory failure

   1. Gas exchange

a. Dependent portion of the lungs tends to be collapsed or filled with inflammatory exudate during severe pulmonary inflammation leading to $\dot{V}/\dot{Q}$ mismatching and hypoxemia.

b. Densities of the perfluorocarbon liquids facilitate their distribution to the dependent portions of the lungs where atelectatic lung appears to be recruited.

c. Perfluorocarbons have also been shown to redistribute pulmonary blood flow to the better-inflated nondependent segments.

d. These effects, combined with the high respiratory gas solubilities of perfluorocarbons, lead to improvements in $\dot{V}/\dot{Q}$ matching and arterial oxygenation.

2. Pulmonary compliance

a. Perfluorocarbons lead to an increase in pulmonary compliance secondary to their density-related recruitment effect on collapsed, inflamed alveoli.

b. They act as an artificial surfactant and increase the stability of small airways.

c. The regions of the lung that are filled with perfluorocarbon liquid (all regions for TLV, the dependent regions for PLV) exhibit a reduction of the gas-liquid interface in the distal airway which also reduces surface active forces favoring alveolar collapse.

d. The result of these effects is enhanced alveolar recruitment at lower inflation pressures.

3. Reduction of lung injury

a. Effects may relate to improved alveolar inflation and better displacement and lavage of inflammatory mediators and debris from the affected portions of the lungs, or to a limitation of excessive ventilator pressures from improvements in compliance.

b. Perfluorocarbons have recently been shown to have *in vitro* anti-inflammatory activities, such as reductions in neutrophil chemotaxis and nitric oxide production, as well as decreased lipopolysaccharide-stimulated macrophage production of cytokines. Neutrophil infiltration also appears to be reduced following lung injury in liquid ventilated animals.

D. Uptake, distribution, elimination, and toxicology

1. Uptake – PFCs are absorbed in small quantities from the lungs during liquid ventilation, reaching a steady state at 15–30 minutes of liquid breathing.

2. Distribution – PFCs have preferential distribution to tissues with high lipid content. These compounds are cleared most quickly from vascular, lipid-poor tissues such as muscle.

3. Elimination – PFCs do not undergo significant biotransformation or excretion. PFCs are primarily eliminated by evaporation from the

lungs and are scavenged by macrophages in both the lungs and other tissues.

4. Toxicology – pulmonary, metabolic, hematologic, and clinical effects of liquid ventilation have been studied extensively in laboratory animals with no significant pulmonary or systemic toxicity noted. Clinical studies have identified the development of pneumothorax and transient hypoxemia during PFC dosing as potential short-term complications of liquid ventilation in humans.

III. Total Liquid Ventilation

A. The delivery of tidal volumes of perfluorocarbon liquid to the lungs for the purpose of gas exchange

1. Because the lungs are completely filled with PFC during TLV, the process is completely dependent upon the PFCs for gas exchange and centers around the tidal regeneration of warmed PFC with a high O_2 and low CO_2 content.

2. Because of densities of the PFC liquids, spontaneous breathing during TLV is impaired by increased resistance and rapidly leads to hypercarbia and respiratory acidosis.

3. Secondary to the above, achievement of unchanged models for the study of TLV has been dependent on the development of specialized mechanical liquid ventilators for fluid regeneration and assistance with tidal flow.

4. Because of the flow and diffusional limitations of PFCs, TLV is usually performed at low respiratory rates (3–9 breaths/min) and with relatively high tidal volumes (14–25 mL/kg).

B. Liquid ventilators

1. Gravitational assistance (original method employed by Greenspan)

    a. PFC reservoir elevated above patient to deliver liquid to the lungs during inspiration and lowered below the patient during expirations to drain fluid by gravity.

    b. Perfluorocarbon was oxygenated and warmed by a bubble oxygenator and heater.

    c. Limited beyond short-term usage by inefficiency with respect to both fluid regeneration and tidal volume assistance

2. Demand-regulated liquid ventilator (a mechanical assist device)

    a. Demand-regulated system. Pressure changes created by the subject's spontaneous respiratory efforts are sensed at the trachea and used to electrically trigger the movement of rubber diaphragms to assist with both inspiratory and expiratory fluid movement.

    b. A double-limb system with inspiratory and expiratory lines, so a "fresh" tidal volume of PFC is warmed and oxygenated in a bubble oxygenator while a separate tidal volume is distributed to the lungs

    c. The mechanical assistance and improved efficiency of fluid regeneration allowed less subject effort and improved CO_2 clearance.

3. Modified extracorporeal membrane oxygenation circuit ventilator-simplified design

    a. Closed circuit inspiratory and expiratory lines with tidal movement accomplished by a roller pump and fluid regeneration achieved with a membrane oxygenator

    b. The original ventilator had check valves that directed flow in an inspiratory or expiratory direction. The system was later simplified by stopping the roller pump during expiration and achieving gravitational drainage to a siphon reservoir.

    c. Has been used successfully in neonatal animal models and is more compact. Expiratory flow is assisted only by gravity, which does not provide optimal control over this phase of ventilation.

4. Piston-driven ventilator based on the improved efficiency of expiratory flow during piston driven vs. roller pump-driven ventilation

    a. A double-piston pump system with piston movement controlled by computer software

    b. During inspiration, warmed, oxygenated fluid moves from the inspiratory piston to the subject, while expired fluid from the previous breath moves from the expiratory piston to a bubble oxygenator. During expiration, fluid is withdrawn from the subject to the expiratory piston and withdrawn from the oxygenator to the inspiratory piston for the next cycle.

    c. Better control of ventilator parameters such as rate, tidal volume, and flow is obtained through the use of computer software to direct piston movement.

C. Clinical studies of TLV. Limited at this point by the technical complexity of the ventilators needed to employ TLV beyond brief periods.

IV. Partial Liquid Ventilation (PLV)

A. A hybrid method of gas exchange, achieved through the delivery of conventional gas tidal volumes to perfluorocarbon-filled lungs

1. Methods

    a. Lungs are filled to an estimated fraction of functional residual capacity (approximately 5–20 mL/kg, depending on disease process, age, and weight) with perfluorocarbon liquid, and conventional ventilation superimposed to achieve gas exchange.

    b. Adequate filling of the lungs is judged by the presence of a fluid meniscus in the endotracheal tube at zero positive end-expiratory pressure, by the opacification of the dependent portions of the lungs on lateral chest radiography, and by the adequacy of gas tidal volumes. Fluid may be added or withdrawn.

2. Theoretical basis for use of PLV in respiratory distress syndrome (RDS)

   a. PLV has relative simplicity as the need for a complex mechanical liquid ventilator is eliminated.

   b. The presence of dense perfluorocarbon fluid in the dependent regions of the lungs allows the recruitment of severely inflamed airways for the purpose of gas exchange. Oxygenation during PLV can occur either by the gas ventilation of these airways directly, or by the oxygenation of the liquid as it equilibrates with the inspired gas.

   c. Ventilation may be increased because of PFC-induced alveolar recruitment.

   d. Compliance is enhanced secondary to alveolar recruitment and the surfactant-like activity of the PFCs. Because the gas-liquid interface is not completely eliminated during PLV, compliance improvement is not as dramatic as is seen during TLV and can actually deteriorate if the lungs are overfilled with perfluorocarbon liquid.

B. Clinical studies of PLV in neonatal ventilator-dependent respiratory failure

   1. Hirschl et al. used PLV as an adjunctive therapy to extracorporeal life support (ECLS) in 1995. Five neonatal patients with severe ventilator-dependent respiratory failure (four with congenital diaphragmatic hernia, one with pulmonary hypertension) were included in the trial. As a whole, the group demonstrated significant decreases in alveolar-arterial oxygen gradients and increases in pulmonary compliance after institution of PLV.

   2. Leach et al. reported significantly improved gas exchange and pulmonary compliance during PLV in 13 premature infants (24–34 weeks gestation at birth) with refractory RDS, as part of a multicenter noncontrolled trial. Significant complications that occurred during the trial were limited to the development of grade IV intraventricular hemorrhage in one patient. Of the 10 patients completing at least 24 hours of PLV, survival to a corrected gestational age of 36 weeks was 60%.

   3. Leach et al. compared the use of PLV to exogenous surfactant administration in premature infants with RDS, demonstrating improved gas exchange and pulmonary compliance in the PLV group.

   4. Pranikoff et al. evaluated the use of PLV in four newborn patients maintained with ECLS for respiratory failure secondary to congenital diaphragmatic hernia. During 5–6 days of PLV therapy, patients exhibited significant increases in arterial oxygen tension and static pulmonary compliance compared with pretreatment values. The therapy was well tolerated and significant complications were limited to the development of pulmonary hemorrhage in one patient 4 days after the final dose of PFC.

Suggested Reading

Furhman BP, Paczan PR, DeFancisis M: Perfluorocarbon-assisted gas exchange. Crit Care Med 1991; 19:712–722.

Greenspan JS, Wolfson MR, Rubenstein SD, et al: Liquid ventilation of human preterm neonates. J Pediatr 1990; 117:106–111.

Hirschl RB, Pranikoff T, Gauger P, et al: Liquid ventilation in adults, children and neonates. Lancet 1995; 346:1201–1202.

Leach CL, Greenspan JS, Rubenstein SD, et al: Partial liquid ventilation with perflubron in infants with severe respiratory distress syndrome. N Engl J Med 1996; 335:761–767.

Pranikoff T, Gauger P, Hirschl RB: Partial liquid ventilation in newborn patients with congenital diaphragmatic hernia. J Pediatr Surg 1996; 31: 613–618.

Shaffer TH, Douglas PR, Lowe CA, et al: The effects of liquid ventilation on cardiopulmonary function in preterm lambs. Pediatr Res 1983; 17:303–306.

Shaffer TH, Moskowitz GD: Demand-controlled liquid ventilation of the lungs. Appl Physiol 1974; 36:208–213.

Shaffer TH, Wolfson MR, Clark C: Liquid ventilation: state of the art review. Pediatr Pulmonol 1992; 14:102–109.

Wolfson MR, Shaffer TH: Liquid ventilation during early development: theory, physiologic processes and application. J Appl Physiol 1990; 13:1–12.

Wolfson MR, Tran N, Bhutani VK, et al: A new experimental approach for the study of cardiopulmonary physiology during early development. J Appl Physiol 198; 65:1436–1443.

SECTION XVIII

Outcome of Neonatal Intensive Care

Chapter 79

Discharge Planning of the NICU Graduate

Win Tin, Unni Wariyar

I. **Introduction**
Hospitalization of an ill newborn is not only one of the most costly of all hospital admissions, but also a very stressful event for a family. Discharging the neonatal intensive care unit (NICU) graduate early has several advantages, including enhancement of family/infant bonding, provision of a better environment for infant development, and a decrease in cost. Too early discharge, however, can impose some risk of deterioration of an infant, and can create hospital readmissions and further strain on the family. Effective discharge planning is an important factor to make the discharge of NICU graduates as positive and stress-free as possible.

II. **Essential Features of Effective Discharge Planning**
   A. Educates parents from the early stages and forms a team between the parents and NICU service providers
   B. Customized to meet the needs of an individual infant and family
   C. Involves multidisciplinary agencies as appropriate
   D. Avoids duplication of services and minimizes disruption to the family
   E. Provides for good communication between the NICU and community-based primary care providers
   F. Simplifies the care of an infant prior to discharge; **does not** effect major changes in infant's management immediately before discharge
   G. Identifies unresolved medical issues and specifies arrangements for appropriate follow-up

III. **Assessment of Readiness for Discharge**
   A. Assessment of infant
      1. Healthy infants can be considered ready for discharge if they:
         a. Maintain normal temperature in an open bed or crib
         b. Feed well by mouth and maintain appropriate weight gain

      c. Do not need any cardiac or respiratory monitoring

  2. Infants with specific ongoing problems need individualized discharge plans; they should be considered ready for discharge only when the specific needs can be provided at home by the parents, with the support of care providers in the community.

  3. Common problems among NICU graduates include bronchopulmonary dysplasia, need for home oxygen therapy, and long-term feeding problems requiring nasogastric tube feeding. Community nurse specialists or nurse practitioners play a vital role in these circumstances.

B. Family assessment should start from the time of the admission of an infant to the NICU or may be even earlier. Family factors that will influence readiness for discharge include:

  1. Parenting skills and the willingness to take responsibility

  2. Parents' experience and understanding of routine infant care and their ability to cope with specific problems

  3. Family structure

  4. Parents' medical and psychological history

  5. Home environment

  6. Financial concerns

  7. Cultural differences and language difficulties

IV. Predischarge Evaluation and Examination

A. Specific evaluation and screening of NICU graduates

  1. Ophthalmologic examination

    a. Routine retinopathy of prematurity (ROP) screening for all infants with risk factors, according to the agreed upon guidelines (see Chapter 52).

    b. Specific eye examination should be arranged for infants with congenital infections, congenital eye abnormalities, chromosomal abnormalities, and those with absent red reflex on routine newborn examination.

  2. Hearing screening. There are no agreed upon guidelines for hearing screening in the NICU, but it is generally accepted that hearing assessment is necessary in infants with a family history of sensorineural hearing loss, neonatal meningitis or encephalitis, severe hyperbilirubinemia, congenital infection, congenital malformation of the ear, and hypoxic-ischemic injury. Prematurity *per se* is also considered a high-risk factor, and some centers also use this as a criterion.

  3. Cranial ultrasound screening for hemorrhagic and/or ischemic brain injuries in high-risk infants – according to individual NICU guidelines. However, a structurally normal cranial sonogram does not entirely rule out long-term neurodevelopmental problems and

---

Discharge Checklist

| Name |
| Address |
| Date of Birth |

Check box
when completed

1. Discharge examination ☐

2. Parents' child health record ☐

3. Discharge summary ☐

4. Follow-up appointment ☐

5. Retinopathy of prematurity screening and follow-up ☐
   ($<$32 weeks and/or $<$1,500 g)

6. Hearing screening and follow-up (as per NICU criteria) ☐

7. Referral to other teams of specialists (e.g., orthopedics, ☐
   surgical, etc.)

8. Liaison with community nurse (e.g., home tube feeding, ☐
   home oxygen, etc.)

9. Oral vitamin K course and instructions ☐

10. Check metabolic screening and TSH (date sent and ☐
    result obtained)

11. Parent education ☐

12. Discharge medications and instructions to parents ☐

13. Discharge date and time entered into admission book ☐

Figure 74. Example of a discharge checklist.

parents need to be aware that follow-up of these NICU graduates
(see Chapter 80) remains the most important part of the ongoing
assessment.

4. Immunization should be administered based on chronological age
   (i.e., no need to correct for prematurity) with the same dosage as
   their full-term counterparts.

B. Predischarge examination remains a routine practice in many NICUs,
   and mainly serves to ensure that good general health and growth have
   been maintained in a healthy infant who is ready for discharge. It also

serves as a problem-finding approach in some infants who need further evaluation (e.g., heart murmur, unstable hip). However, a normal predischarge examination does not give complete reassurance and the parents need to be aware of this.

V. Discharge Information/Letter and Checklist

A. Written information should be made available to the primary care providers and, ideally, also to the parents. All the medical terminology contained in the letter should be explained to the parents by NICU staff. The information should include:

1. Infant's name, address, date of birth
2. Date of admission and discharge
3. List of important medical problems
4. Brief clinical summary
5. Outstanding problem(s) at the time of discharge
6. Specific medications and instructions
7. Immunization instructions
8. Plans for follow-up and further assessment

B. A checklist to ensure that all the appropriate arrangements have been made for the infant can be very useful for all NICU discharges, and should be designed to suit the needs of individual NICUs (Figure 74).

Suggested Reading

Damato EG: Discharge planning from the neonatal intensive care unit. Perinatal Neonatal Nurs 1991; 5:43.

Edwards M: Discharge planning. In Avery G, Fletcher M, MacDonald M (Eds.): *Neonatology: Pathophysiology and Management of the Newborn.* Philadelphia, J.B. Lippincott, 1994, pp. 1349–1354.

Fielder AR, Levene MI: Screening for retinopathy of prematurity. Arch Dis Child 1992; 67:860–866.

Lefebvre F, Bard H: Early discharge of preterm newborn infants. In Davis JA, Richards MPM, Roberton NRC (Eds.): *Parent-Baby Attachment in Premature Infants.* London, Croom Helm, 1983, pp. 281–287.

Chapter 80

Follow-Up of the NICU Graduate

Unni Wariyar, Win Tin

With a better understanding of neonatal pathophysiology and recent advances in medical technology, there has been an increase in long-term survival for very ill neonatal intensive care unit (NICU) graduates over the past two decades. As this group of babies has a high risk of adverse neurodevelopmental outcome, it is of importance that carefully planned follow-up for these NICU graduates becomes an essential part of NICU service provision.

I. **Importance/Objectives of Follow-Up**
   A. For the child
      1. To identify early on major problems of perinatal origin (e.g., cerebral palsy, developmental delay, major hearing or visual impairment). This will facilitate further diagnostic testing, assessment, and involvement of other appropriate professionals and agencies.
      2. To screen for other medical problems, e.g., squint, speech delay, and growth failure, so that early remedial measures can be implemented
      3. To maintain optimum health in order to achieve the utmost potential for growth and development
   B. For the parents/caregivers
      1. To provide support to the families/caregivers of babies with special needs. It is important that one "lead" clinician coordinate the infant's care with the help and support of other professional agencies and services, to avoid or minimize confusion and to provide consistency of care and advice.
      2. To counsel caregivers regarding the baby's condition, its relationship to perinatal events, and the probable prognosis, and to discuss appropriate diagnostic testing and the results of various assessment
      3. To provide instructions regarding immunization, medications, diet, and the need for involvement of other specialists/therapists
      4. To reassure caregivers and address concerns regarding the baby's condition and progress
   C. For other involved professionals/institutions – follow-up studies/ programs (hospital-based or population-based) are very useful as an audit process:

1. To evaluate and improve the standards of neonatal intensive care
2. To monitor changing patterns of prognosis (mortality and morbidity) over time
3. To evaluate newer modalities of management methods and interventions where long-term neurodevelopment is used as the primary outcome measure
4. Audit information is extremely important for an evidence-based approach to parental counseling. Population-based follow-up studies provide more reliable information than hospital-based studies, hence the importance of cooperation and standardization between NICUs. It is also important to achieve a high return for follow-up among survivors (ideally 100%) in order to get a reliable information on morbidity.

II. Selection of Appropriate Candidates for Follow-Up

A. This depends to a great extent on the resources available. We suggest the following criteria as indicative of appropriate candidates for follow-up:

1. Very preterm and very low birthweight infants (<32 weeks gestation and/or <1,500 g at birth). Accurately assessed gestation is a better predictor for long-term morbidity than birthweight.
2. All NICU graduates who required ventilatory support
3. Very small size for gestational age (<3rd percentile), which has been associated with an increased incidence of minimal cerebral dysfunction
4. Perinatal neurological problems, i.e., hypoxic-ischemic encephalopathy, known ischemic and/or hemorrhagic brain injury, or ventriculomegaly, and those with abnormal neurological behavior (neonatal convulsion, hypotonia, etc.)
5. Hydropic infants, from any cause
6. Intrauterine or severe perinatal infections
7. Metabolic derangements, i.e., persistent hypoglycemia, hyperbilirubinemia requiring exchange transfusion, etc.
8. Congenital abnormalities
9. Prior exposure to toxic agents, i.e., drugs *in utero*

III. Providers of Follow-Up to NICU Graduates

A. Who provides follow-up will vary from one unit to another depending on the structure and resources, but the follow-up team should ideally consist of:

1. The "lead" clinician (usually a developmental pediatrician) whose role is to coordinate communication between the families and other appropriate professionals/agencies

2. Community liaison nurse or specialist nurse practitioner
3. Pediatric physiotherapist
4. Pediatric nutritionist

B. The NICU follow-up team may often need support and consultation from other specialists, i.e., ophthalmologists, pediatricians, orthopedic surgeons, neurosurgeons, neurologists, geneticists, audiologists, speech and language therapists, psychologists, and play therapists. As described earlier, however, it is important that the family can communicate with a liaison whose role is to coordinate and communicate with other service providers involved in the care of the child.

C. Some NICU graduates may need regular follow-up at specialized clinics that provide multidisciplinary assessment of children, i.e., for:
1. Complex or multiple needs
2. Bronchopulmonary dysplasia (respiratory, cardiac, dietary, and developmental assessment)

IV. Components of Follow-Up Assessment

A. Listening to the parents/caregivers and addressing their concerns is probably the most important part of follow-up.

B. Anthropometric assessment: weight, length and head circumference should be regularly monitored. If updated consistently, the parents' child health records provide very good information on serial growth measurements.

C. System review: particularly any health problems, feeding, and bowel habits

D. Vision and hearing assessment: further referral for detailed assessment may be needed for some infants. Vision and hearing screening prior to discharge for the high-risk NICU graduate is discussed in Chapter 79.

E. Neurological/neurodevelopmental assessment:
1. Posture, tone, reflexes and presence of primitive reflexes after certain age. Multidisciplinary assessment by a physiotherapist and pediatrician may prove very useful.
2. Gait and detailed neurological examination in older children
3. Achievement of developmental milestones. It is appropriate to adjust for prematurity for children who are chronologically <24 months of age, especially if they were born extremely preterm.

F. Other systemic examination

G. Review of medications (including oxygen therapy): some medications may need to be discontinued whereas others may need adjustment of dosage

H. Check whether all immunizations have been administered (as appropriate), and whether all necessary screening tests have been completed as indicated on the discharge plan (see Chapter 79)

V. Frequency and Duration of Follow-Up

A. This determination depends on the needs of the child and family and also on the available resources. Minor cognitive and learning problems, clumsiness, and poor attention span are more common in NICU graduates than in their full-term "normal" counterparts; ideally, NICU graduates should be followed until they are in elementary school or even, it can be argued, until adulthood.

B. Most NICU graduates, however, do not need regular follow-up once their growth and development are determined to be progressing satisfactorily.

C. Communication between the follow-up team, the community pediatrician, and the school system is important if the child needs longer term follow-up, particularly because of potential learning difficulties.

VI. In summary, follow-up of NICU graduates is an essential part of perinatal services, to facilitate better care for the child and family, enhancement of perinatal services, and to ensure the provision of appropriate support services for these children.

Suggested Reading

Allen MC: The high risk infant. Pediatr Clin North Am 1993; 40:479–490.

Davies PA: Follow-up of low birthweight children. Arch Dis Child 1984; 39:794–797.

McCormick MC, Stuart MC, Cohen R, et al: Follow-up of NICU graduates: why, what and by whom? J Intens Care Med 1995; 10:213–225.

Tin W, Fritz S, Wariyar U, Hey E: Outcome of very preterm birth: children reviewed with ease at 2 years differ from those followed-up with difficulty. Arch Dis Child 1998; 79:F83–F87.

Tin W, Wariyar U, Hey E: Changing prognosis for babies of less than 28 weeks' gestation in the north of England between 1983 and 1994. BMJ 1997; 314:107–111.

SECTION XIX

Ethical Considerations

Chapter 81

Initiation of Life Support at the Border of Viability

Daniel G. Batton, M. Jeffrey Maisels

I. **Introduction**

For many years, parents and caregivers have had to make a decision about whether or not to resuscitate an infant at the border of viability. This dilemma is not new, and there are no infallible answers to these difficult questions.

II. **Definitions**

   A. Pre-viable infants – those born at a gestational age for which survival is currently very unlikely (<10%)

   B. Viable infants – those born at a gestational age for which survival is currently likely (>50%)

   C. Border of viability – gestational age at which survival is currently >10% but <50%

III. **Historical Morbidity and Mortality Trends of Premature Newborns**

   A. The gestational age at the border of viability has declined steadily over the last 30 years as survival for all premature babies has improved.

   B. The gestational age difference between pre-viable (survival <10%) and viable (survival >50%) infants has continued to decrease with improved survival. At many centers this difference is now as short as 1 week of gestation.

   C. Surviving infants born very prematurely have significantly more long-term medical and neurodevelopmental problems than do normal term infants. However, the majority of surviving infants, even those born at the earliest gestations, are free of significant neurosensory impairment.

   D. Recent institutional-specific statistics are needed before decisions about resuscitation can be made.

IV. **Ethical Guidelines for Making Decisions about the Resuscitation of Borderline Viable Infants**

   A. The decision should represent the best interests of the patient, not the parents or caregivers.

B. Whenever possible, the decision-making process should be deliberate. There should be sufficient time devoted to the process and parents should not feel pressured.

C. The decision should be made jointly by parents and caregivers and should not be unilateral. If desired, the parents should be encouraged to consult others.

D. The decision must be fully informed and all relevant data must be considered. This may require altering the process to allow time to collect more information.

E. The process should not be arbitrary. Using an absolute gestational age or birthweight limit can be hazardous as these limits have changed and continue to change over time.

F. It is important to avoid the problem of a self-fulfilling prophecy. If newborns at a given gestational age are not supported, they will all do poorly and the results can then be used to justify nonsupport. Comparison of the institution's outcome data with national data can help to avoid this situation.

G. Poor anticipated quality of life or impending (inevitable) death are acceptable reasons for not initiating resuscitation. However, it must be recognized that:

  1. These predictions have significant error rates.

  2. The perception of what is or is not an acceptable quality of life varies widely among individuals.

H. If there is **any** uncertainty, resuscitation should be initiated, and decisions regarding subsequent care reevaluated frequently (see Chapter 82). Initiating resuscitation in the delivery room does not preclude subsequent withdrawal of care and this should be emphasized in discussions with the parents.

V. Problems Involved in Decision Making

A. It is very difficult to make a prenatal decision not to resuscitate because the condition of the baby (by physical examination) and the birthweight are unknown, and this information is critical in determining the prognosis. Unless a poor outcome is certain, a prenatal decision not to resuscitate could be viewed as uninformed, because not all of the relevant facts are known.

B. Decisions in the delivery room are, of necessity, more or less instantaneous. This means that many decisions cannot be made in a deliberate manner and that all relevant data are not available.

C. There are no agreed upon guidelines for how poor the prognosis must be in order to justify withholding resuscitation. The most common developmental problems of extremely premature infants who survive are learning disabilities and behavior problems. However, these are not usually sufficiently severe to justify a nonaggressive approach.

VI. Conclusion

The approach to borderline viable newborns should be similar to that used for older children and adults who have a comparable prognosis.

Suggested Reading

American Academy of Pediatrics, Committee on Fetus and Newborn, American College of Obstetricians and Gynecologists, Committee on Obstetric Practice: Perinatal care at the threshold of viability. Pediatrics 1995; 96: 974–976.

American Academy of Pediatrics: Guidelines on forgoing life-sustaining medical treatment. Pediatrics 1994; 93:532–536.

American College of Obstetricians and Gynecologists: Perinatal care at the threshold of viability. ACOG Technical Bulletin 136. Washington, DC; ACOG, 1995; 163:1–4.

Batton DG, DeWitte DB, Espinosa R, Swails T: The impact of fetal compromise on outcome at the border of viability. Am J Obstet Gynecol 1998; 178:909–915.

Byrne PJ, Tyebkhan JM, Laing LM: Ethical decision-making and neonatal resuscitation. Semin Perinatol 1994; 18:36–41.

Hack M, Friedman H, Fanaroff AA: Outcomes of extremely low birth weight infants. Pediatrics 1996; 98:931–937.

Lantos JD, Tyson JE, Alexander A, et al: Withholding and withdrawing life sustaining treatment in neonatal intensive care: issues for the 1990s. Arch Dis Child 1994; 75:F218–F223.

Meadow W, Reimshisel T, Lantos J: Birth weight-specific mortality for extremely low birth weight infants vanishes by four days of life: epidemiology and ethics in the neonatal intensive care unit. Pediatrics 1996; 97:636–643.

O'Shea TM, Preisser JP, Klinepeter KL, Dillard RG: Trends in mortality and cerebral palsy in a geographically based cohort of very low birthweight neonates born between 1982 to 1984. Pediatrics 1998; 101:642–647.

Stevenson DK, Wright LL, Lemons JA, et al: Very low birth weight outcomes of the National Institute of Child Health and Human Development Neonatal Research Network, January 1993 through December 1994. Am J Obstet Gynecol 1998; 179:1632–1639.

Tin W, Wariyar U, Hey E: Changing prognosis for babies of less than 28 weeks' gestation in the north of England between 1983 and 1984. BMJ 1997; 314:107–111.

Whitfield MF, Eckstein Grunau RV, Holsti L: Extremely premature (≤800 g) school children: multiple areas of hidden disability. Arch Dis Child 1997; 77:F85–F90.

Chapter 82

Withdrawal of Ventilatory Support

Malcolm L. Chiswick

I. **Introduction**

    A. Assisted ventilation, from an ethical perspective, should be viewed not as a treatment but as a temporary support measure for infants with *potentially reversible* respiratory failure. In effect, this is a *trial of life,* and the desired outcome is survival with a reasonable chance of an independent existence in later childhood.

    B. Physicians who start assisted ventilation have *a duty* to consider with the parents withdrawal of ventilatory support if it seems that the desired outcome will not be achieved.

    C. The idea that life-support must be continued as long as an infant is alive, and that no one has the right to terminate assisted ventilation is an extremist view that few would defend.

II. **Withdrawing Ventilatory Support**

    A. A robust and coherent code of practice is needed to define the circumstances that permit the withdrawal of assisted ventilation. Otherwise, *ad hoc* ethical standards will be applied to each case and a decision will be justified only *after* it has been made.

    B. The code of practice should be derived from logical and moral concepts, based on a respect for human life that can be applied consistently across a broad range of individual circumstances. It should not be necessary to change the rules for each infant.

    C. In practice, there are two main circumstances where withdrawal of ventilatory support is a consideration:

        1. When it is considered that the infant has already entered the process of dying

        2. Where the continuation of assisted ventilation might well allow the infant to survive, but with a risk of severe neurodevelopmental disability.

III. **The Dying Infant**

    A. Physicians are not obliged to continue with treatments that serve no purpose, especially when the treatment is associated with discomfort.

B. The problem for the physician is to decide when assisted ventilation has ceased to become a trial of life and is simply prolonging the process of dying.

C. The infant's state is generally one of multiorgan system failure that may include hypotension and circulatory failure, renal failure, metabolic and electrolyte dysregulation, disseminated intravascular coagulopathy, and cardiac dysfunction, against a background of poor or no respiratory drive and often an impaired level of consciousness. Specific or supportive treatments directed at these complications will normally have been offered, but without success. In effect, the decision to withdraw ventilatory support is based on *medical indications* that further treatment is deemed pointless.

D. Withdrawal of ventilatory support in this situation gives some control over the timing and circumstances of the death. Instead of the parents and staff helplessly presiding over an infant who is surrounded by the technological trappings of failed intensive care, and who will die from cardiac standstill at an unpredictable time, a more acceptable alternative can be offered.

IV. **The "Quality of Life" Decision**

A. Here the judgment is that an infant might well survive as a result of continuing ventilatory support, but the potential quality of life is seriously called into question.

B. There are circumstances, albeit rarely, when it is ethically acceptable to withdraw assisted ventilation from such an infant. This may apply in the case of an infant whose life might be saved only by further prolonged discomfiture of neonatal intensive care, and in whom it is probable that substantial neurodevelopmental or physical handicap will radically limit the child's ability to participate in human experience and will render him or her forever dependent on a caregiver for everyday living.

C. The arguments surrounding quality of life decisions have been well rehearsed. Reservations include the following ideas:

1. "Quality of life" is a subjective notion.
2. We can rarely be certain about the extent of any predicted handicap.
3. The infant cannot take part in the decision making.
4. No one has the right to "act like God" and to judge whether death or survival with severe handicap is the better of the two.

D. On the other hand, faced with an intolerable existence, responsible adults may exert their right to end their own lives, and someone has to advocate on behalf of the infant.

E. The most common scenario for withdrawing ventilatory assistance on the basis of a quality of life decision is when an infant has bilateral gross white matter damage on a brain scan and persisting abnormal neurological signs including impaired level of arousal, seizures, and abnormal muscle tone. The approach to decision making will be guided by local practice. In the author's experience a trusting relationship between the parents and a designated physician under whose care the infant was admitted, together with a consensus view among senior and experienced staff, obviates the need for involvement of an ethics committee.

F. It is rare for parents to request thoughtfully and consistently that assisted ventilation be withdrawn against medical advice. On those occasions the physician must act in the best interests of the infant as professionally perceived.

G. It is more common for parents to request that ventilation be *continued* against medical advice. Here, the physician's duty to the infant is to ensure that the parents understand the facts so they are capable of acting on behalf of the infant. The author's stance is to continue to counsel the parents but certainly not to coerce them.

V. **Engaging Parents in Decision Making**

A. Parents of seriously ill infants need time to make their views known. When it is clear that their infant is seriously ill, parents should be led into the discussion early rather than later.

B. Do not place the burden of decision making on the parents. (*"These are the facts. What do you want us to do?"*)

C. Instead, *communicate your view clearly* and indicate that you are seeking the parents' support.

D. Most decisions involve infants in whom the continuation of ventilatory assistance is merely prolonging the process of dying, and it is unfair in those cases to burden parents with the complex issues surrounding quality of life decisions.

VI. **Deceptive Signals**

A. We need to guard against "giving up" on sick infants prematurely. There are deceptive signals that might erroneously persuade attendants that continuing ventilatory support is not justified:

1. Despair
2. Adverse appearance of infant
   a. Severe malnourishment
   b. Cholestatic jaundice
   c. Multiple skin trauma from infusion sites ("war wounds")
3. Biased impression of prognosis based on superficial comparisons with other infants
4. Nonvisiting parents

469

VII. Engaging Staff in Decision Making

A. Problems arise on neonatal units where there is no proper leadership, where staff does not work together as a team, and where there is no proper forum for discussing ethical issues. Staff may feel unable to discuss the possibility of withdrawing assisted ventilation from an infant and instead unspoken signals occur.

1. *Standing off on clinical rounds:* disgruntled staff turns away and shows a lack of interest in discussing the infant and contributing to further management.

2. *Exaggeration of clinical signs:* an infant with pallor might be described as appearing "white as a sheet"; skin peeling might be referred to as "peeling off in layers."

3. *Therapeutic nihilism:* all suggested treatments are rejected on the basis of their side effects.

4. *Incongruous search for the expert:* paradoxically, staff may suggest calling in an "expert" such as a nephrologist or cardiologist to advise on organ system failure.

5. *Group formation among staff:* small groups form among the staff and discuss among themselves the apparent futility of continuing ventilatory support.

6. *"The parents don't realize how sick the infant is":* in spite of the physician's discussions of the infant's progress with the parents at frequent intervals, the staff insist that the parents do not understand how ill the infant is.

B. These unspoken signals reflect desperation and despair among staff who cannot communicate their feelings to the senior physician. They are cries for help. It is essential that this situation is recognized and steps taken to improve the organization and communication on the neonatal unit. Unless this happens decisions about withdrawing assisted ventilation will generate a crisis each time and provoke additional suffering for parents and, indeed, for infants.

VIII. Care Following Withdrawal of Assisted Ventilation

A. The concept of withdrawing assisted ventilation should not be communicated to parents simply as a matter of "turning off the switch."

B. Parents should be prepared for events and offered a choice of how they would like their infant to be cared for during and after withdrawal.

C. A minority of parents want simply to bid farewell to their infant, depart from the neonatal unit, and leave the details to the staff. Their wishes should be respected.

D. At the other extreme, some parents wish to remove the endotracheal tube and intravascular lines themselves.

E. Facilities should be made available to allow parents to remain with their infant in a secluded room immediately after withdrawal. Some will wish to bathe and dress their infant even if death has already occurred.

F. There are some uncomfortable facts that we must be prepared to face together with the parents.

1. After withdrawal of assisted ventilation parents often want to know how long it will be before their baby dies. If the indication was that the baby had "already entered the process of dying" then one can anticipate that death will occur very soon after withdrawal. This is not always the case and parents should be made aware beforehand of the inherent uncertainty.

2. In the author's practice it is not necessary to reverse the effect of muscle relaxants or sedatives before assisted ventilation is withdrawn. However, it is treading on a legal tightrope to introduce these drugs prior to withdrawal in order to facilitate death once ventilation has been withdrawn. Moreover, the use of sedatives *after* withdrawal in order to facilitate death probably amounts to "falling off" that legal tightrope. If an infant breathes vigorously and with obvious distress for a prolonged period after withdrawal of ventilatory support, then the notion that he or she had "already entered the process of dying" was probably erroneous. Retrieving this situation is challenging and illustrates how important it is to assess infants accurately and thoughtfully before making decisions, rather than being misled by deceptive signals.

3. Even more challenging is the after-care of infants in whom ventilation has been withdrawn because of quality of life considerations. Often by the time agreement has been reached that ventilation should be withdrawn, the infant is no longer dependent on the ventilator and may well survive without it. In effect, the time taken for a quality of life decision may exceed the narrow window of opportunity to effect withdrawal of ventilation, and parents should be made aware of this in a sensitive way.

4. Withholding fluids, nutrition, and warmth during after-care is not a reasonable option for these infants. The logic behind this statement is that all infants are *expected* to breathe spontaneously and the use of assisted ventilation is an *extraordinary measure* of medical care. In contrast, all babies are *normally dependent* on a caregiver for the provision of fluid, nutrition, and warmth and so it is reasonable to continue to provide them.

Suggested Reading

Campbell AGM: Quality of life as a decision making criterion I. In Goldworth A, Silverman W, Stevenson DK, Young EWD (Eds.): *Ethics and Perinatology.* Oxford, Oxford University Press, 1995, pp. 82–98.

Chiswick ML: Withdrawal of life support in babies: deceptive signals. Arch Dis Child 1990; 65:1096–1097.

Delaney-Black V: Delivering bad news. In Donn SM, Fisher CW (Eds.): *Risk Management Techniques in Perinatal and Neonatal Practice.* Armonk, NY, Futura Publishing Co., 1996, pp. 635–649.

Kraybill EN: Ethical issues in the care of extremely low birth weight infants. Semin Perinatol 1998; 22:207–215.

Kuhse H: Quality of life as a decision making criterion II. In Goldworth A, Silverman W, Stevenson DK, Young EWD (Eds.): *Ethics and Perinatology.* Oxford, Oxford University Press, 1995, pp. 104–120.

Pierce SF: Neonatal intensive care decision making in the face of prognostic uncertainty. Nurs Clin North Am 1998; 33:287–297.

Roloff DW: Decisions in the care of newborn infants. In Donn SM, Faix RG (Eds.): *Neonatal Emergencies.* Mt. Kisco, NY, Futura Publishing Co., 1991, pp. 635–643.

Weil WB Jr, Benjamin M (Eds.): *Ethical Issues at the Outset of Life: Contemporary Issues in Fetal and Neonatal Medicine.* Boston, MA, Blackwell Scientific Publications, 1987.

SECTION XX

Ventilatory Case Studies

Chapter 83

Ventilatory Case Studies

Marie C. McGettigan, Jay P. Goldsmith

I. **CASE 1: Respiratory Distress Syndrome (RDS)**

   A. Prenatal information
Mother: 21-year-old, G1 P0 → 1

   B. Patient information

      1. 1,400 gm male born by spontaneous vaginal delivery

      2. Apgar scores of 3 (one minute) and 6 (five minutes)

   C. Findings

      1. Tachypnea

      2. Retractions

      3. Grunting

      4. Flaring

      5. Cyanosis

   D. Physical examination

      1. Decreased breath sounds bilaterally

      2. Rales heard in all lung fields

   E. Interventions

      1. Intubated with a 3.0-mm endotracheal tube (ETT) and hand ventilated during transport to the neonatal intensive care unit (NICU) where the infant was placed on pressure-limited, time-cycled conventional mechanical ventilator (CMV) with a peak inspiratory pressure (PIP) of 20, positive end-expiratory pressure (PEEP) of 5, rate of 40, FiO_2 0.5, inspiratory time (T_I) of 0.4 seconds, and flow of 8 LPM.

      2. Umbilical arterial catheter placed. Arterial blood gas initially acceptable

   F. Chest radiograph (Figure 75)

      1. Decreased lung volume

      2. Fluid in right horizontal fissure

      3. Air bronchograms

      4. Reticulogranular alveolar pattern

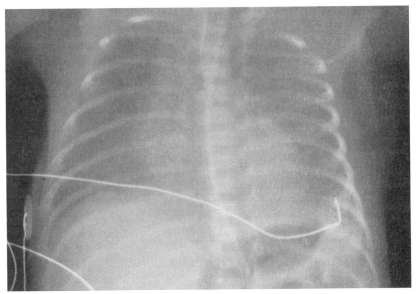

Figure 75. Typical chest radiograph of respiratory distress syndrome. Note decreased lung volume, fluid in the right horizontal fissure, air bronchograms, and the overall reticulogranular alveolar pattern.

G. Arterial blood gases at 12 hours of age: pH 7.18, $PaCO_2$ 58 torr (7.7 kPa), PaO_2 35 torr (4.7 kPa), base deficit -8, and bicarbonate 19

H. Differential diagnoses
1. Sepsis
2. Intraventricular hemorrhage
3. Patent ductus arteriosus (PDA)
4. Pulmonary airleak
5. Hypoventilation
6. RDS (progressive atelectasis)

I. Diagnosis – RDS, worsening with increasing atelectasis and inadequate ventilatory support

J. Therapies
1. Increase mean airway pressure (increase PIP)
2. Increase FiO_2
3. Give surfactant if a/A <0.22, or if FiO_2 >0.3 and PaO_2 <80 torr (10.7 kPa)

K. Denouement
1. Infant evaluated for repeat doses of surfactant
2. Infant stabilized after surfactant and weaned from maximal settings of PIP of 25, PEEP of 5, rate of 50, and FiO_2 1.0.

II. **CASE 2: Patent Ductus Arteriosus (PDA)**

   A. Prenatal information
   Mother: 21-year-old, Gl P0 → 1 with artificial rupture of membranes just prior to delivery

   B. Patient information
   1. Spontaneous vaginal delivery under epidural anesthesia
   2. Birthweight: 1,332 gm
   3. 30 weeks gestational age
   4. 10% placental abruption
   5. Apgar scores of 6 (one minute) and 8 (five minutes)
   6. Placed in oxyhood with increasing respiratory distress
   7. Transported to a level III unit where baby was intubated and given surfactant for RDS
   8. IV fluids
       a. First 24 hours: 80 mL/kg/day
       b. Second 24 hours: 100 mL/kg/day
       c. Third 24 hours: 140 mL/kg/day

   C. Signs (on 3rd day of life)
   1. Loud systolic murmur heard
   2. Increasing ventilatory support
   3. Bounding pulses
   4. Decrease in diastolic blood pressure

   D. Chest radiographs
   1. First 24 hours: air bronchograms, reticulogranular pattern. (Similar to that seen in Figure 75.)
   2. Second 24 hours: clearing (Figure 76A)
   3. Third 24 hours: white-out lung fields, increased heart size (Figure 76B)

   E. Ventilator settings on the 3rd day of life: on pressure-limited, time-cycled CMV, PIP 28, PEEP 5, rate 60, FiO_2 1.0, T_I 0.4 sec, and flow 10 L/min. Arterial blood gases: pH 7.35, $PaCO_2$ 55 torr (7.3 kPa), bicarbonate 24, base deficit −2, PaO_2 60 torr (8 kPa)

   F. Differential diagnosis
   1. Pneumonia
   2. Sepsis
   3. PDA
   4. Congenital heart disease with left-to-right shunt

   G. Diagnosis: PDA
   1. Echocardiographic signs
       a. Left atrial size/aortic root size >1.3
       b. Increased left atrial, left ventricular dimensions
       c. PDA seen on echocardiogram with Doppler flow study

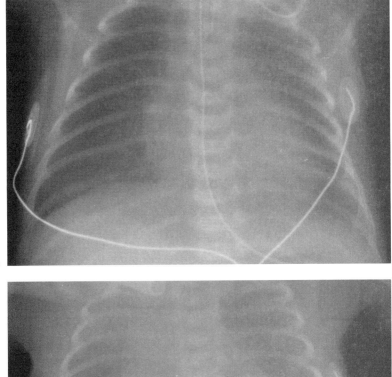

Figure 76. A. Clearing of chest radiograph following surfactant administration. **B.** White-out of lungs from pulmonary edema secondary to left-to-right shunting through a patent ductus arteriosus. The heart size can also increase.

H. Therapies
1. Restrict fluids to ≤130 mL/kg/day
2. Indomethacin for prostaglandin inhibition if platelets >50,000/mm³ (causes decreased platelet aggregation) and creatinine <1.8 mg/dL. (Dose: 0.1–0.3 mg/kg q8h × 3 IV.)
   a. With indomethacin, there is decreased urinary flow, glomerular filtration rate, and free water excretion; electrolytes must be monitored.
   b. Ensure adequate renal function (urine output >0.5–1.0 mL/kg/h)
   c. Do not use if bleeding diathesis
   d. Do not use with severe hyperbilirubinemia since indomethacin binds to albumin
3. Surgical ligation if patient is not a candidate for indomethacin or if pharmacologic closure fails
I. Preventative strategy – restrict fluids to 130 mL/kg/day

III. CASE 3: Persistent Pulmonary Hypertension of the Newborn (PPHN)
A. Prenatal information
1. Mother: 23-year-old, G2 P1 → 2, with spontaneous rupture of membranes 10 hours prior to delivery (meconium-stained fluid)
2. Pitocin-augmented labor
3. Variable heart rate decelerations seen on electronic fetal heart rate tracing
B. Patient information
1. Born by spontaneous vaginal delivery at 40 weeks with birthweight of 3,420 gm
2. Meconium-stained fluid suctioned from stomach but not from below vocal cords
3. Apgar scores of 5 (one minute) and 7 (five minutes)
C. Interventions
1. Placed in oxyhood at 0.5 FiO_2
2. Transported to tertiary center
3. Intubated with 3.5-mm ETT. Placed on pressure-limited, time-cycled CMV with settings of PIP 26, PEEP 5, FiO_2 0.5, rate 40, T_I 0.35 sec, and flow 8 L/min
4. Umbilical arterial and venous catheters placed
5. Blood culture drawn and antibiotics started
6. Preductal and postductal oximeters placed
D. Chest radiograph (Figure 77): lung fields clear with decreased pulmonary vascularity; "black" lungs
E. Arterial blood gases: pH 7.42, PCO_2 30 torr (4 kPa), PaO_2 32 torr (4.3 kPa), base excess 0, bicarbonate 21, and SaO_2 70%

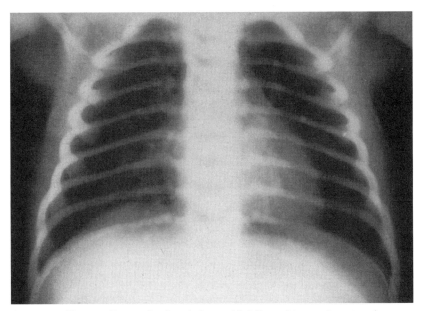

Figure 77. Chest radiograph of an infant with idiopathic persistent pulmonary hypertension of the newborn with decreased pulmonary vascularity ("black lung").

F. Differential diagnoses
   1. Congenital heart disease
   2. Sepsis
   3. PPHN
G. Diagnosis
   1. Perform hyperoxia test
   2. In 1.0 FiO_2, arterial blood gas results were pH 7.42, PCO_2 30 torr (4 kPa), PaO_2 32 torr (4.3 kPa), base excess 0, and HCO_3 21
   3. Echocardiography demonstrated normal cardiac function and structure, normal connections, flattening of interventricular septum, and tricuspid regurgitation jet (estimate of right heart pressures)
   4. Results: PPHN
H. Pathophysiology
   Muscular pulmonary arterioles are constricted *in utero* as 90% of cardiac output bypasses the lungs through shunts at the foramen ovale and PDA. If the pulmonary vessels are abnormally muscularized, fail to dilate at birth, or have prolonged constriction from intrapartum or postpartum event, persistent pulmonary hypertension ensues with elevation of right ventricular and atrial pressures.

479

I. Treatments
   1. Sedation with morphine sulfate and/or fentanyl infusion
   2. Minimal stimulation
   3. Supportive measures to maintain systemic blood pressure above the estimated right ventricular pressure, maintaining good cardiac output, and avoiding hypoxia and acidosis. (Some clinicians use alkalinization with sodium bicarbonate infusions to obtain a pH >7.50.)
   4. Different ventilator strategies (e.g., moderate hyperventilation, high frequency ventilation, selective pulmonary vasodilation with inhaled nitric oxide)
   5. Paralysis with neuromuscular blocking agents (e.g., pancuronium)
   6. Extracorporeal membrane oxygenation (ECMO) if oxygenation index (OI) ≥ 40 (× 3)

$$OI = \frac{FiO_2 \times Paw}{PaO_2 \ (torr)} \times 100$$

IV. **CASE 4: Meconium Aspiration Syndrome (MAS)**
   A. Prenatal information
      1. Mother: 33-year-old G2 P1 → 2 at 41 4/7 weeks, in labor
      2. Spontaneous rupture of membranes occurs with thick "pea soup" meconium-stained amniotic fluid.
   B. Patient information
      1. Variable decelerations of heart rate seen on the electronic fetal heart rate tracing
      2. Infant born vaginally, 6 hours after rupture of membranes, with forceps assistance, birthweight of 4,010 gm
      3. Apgar scores of 2 (one minute) and 5 (five minutes)
   C. Findings
      1. Macrosomia, green-stained nails and umbilical cord
      2. Cyanotic with no respiratory effort at birth
   D. Interventions
      1. Intubated with a 4.0-mm ETT and suctioned below the vocal cords with return of copious amounts of meconium-stained secretions
      2. Received bag ventilation, saline lavage, and gentle chest physiotherapy
      3. Brought to the NICU and placed on pressure-limited, time-cycled CMV with PIP 36, PEEP 5, rate 60, FiO₂ 1.0, T$_I$ 0.5 sec, and flow 10 LPM
      4. Umbilical arterial and venous catheters placed
      5. Blood culture drawn
      6. Antibiotics started

E. Arterial blood gases
   1. Infant sedated. T_I shortened to 0.4 seconds
   2. Results: pH 7.15, $PaCO_2$ 68 torr (9.1 kPa), bicarbonate 15, base deficit -8, PaO_2 47 torr (6.3 kPa). PIP increased to 39.
F. Chest radiograph (Figure 78): fluffy infiltrates in both lung fields, areas of atelectasis, as well as clearer areas of lung
G. Differential diagnoses
   1. Pneumonia
   2. Sepsis
   3. MAS
H. Diagnosis: MAS
   1. Meconium suctioned from trachea
   2. Classic radiographic appearance
I. Pathophysiology
   1. Meconium: viscous green liquid consisting of GI secretions, bile, mucus, pancreatic products, cellular debris, amniotic fluid, vernix caseosa, lanugo, and blood
   2. When meconium is aspirated, the respiratory distress that develops is directly correlated with the degree of viscosity.

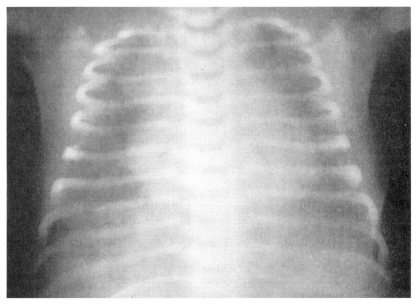

Figure 78. Typical chest radiograph of meconium aspiration syndrome showing fluffy infiltrates in both lung fields, areas of atelectasis/infiltrate, and clearer areas in the lungs.

3. Meconium can completely obstruct the airways, leading to atelectasis and $\dot{V}/\dot{Q}$ mismatch.

4. Partial obstruction can result in ball valve effect in which gas flows into the airway on inspiration but, because of smaller airway on exhalation, gas is trapped. This can lead to pneumothorax.

5. After several hours, since meconium is irritating and a good bacteriologic medium, inflammation and infection can result.

J. Treatment

1. Mechanical ventilation, short inspiratory times to minimize air trapping

2. Sedation

3. Pulmonary toilet with suctioning and gentle chest physiotherapy as needed

4. Intravenous antibiotics

5. Monitor for pulmonary hypertension and pneumothorax

V. **CASE 5: Bronchopulmonary Dysplasia (BPD)**

A. Prenatal information

1. Mother: 29-year-old, G4 P3 → 4

2. Premature, prolonged rupture of membranes prior to delivery

B. Patient information

1. 1,200 gm male infant at 28 weeks gestation

2. Spontaneous vertex vaginal delivery

3. Apgar scores of 3 (one minute) and 6 (five minutes)

4. Patient required increased oxygen and intubation for acute respiratory failure

5. Born in rural hospital. Received bag and mask ventilation with pressures of 44/5 and high rate. Transported to NICU for ventilation and surfactant.

C. Chest radiograph

1. Reticulogranular alveolar pattern with air bronchograms and pulmonary interstitial emphysema (PIE) (Figure 79A)

2. Initially placed on pressure-limited, time-cycled CMV at referral hospital

3. Oxygen requirements remained high despite surfactant therapy (two doses)

4. Maximum settings on CMV were PIP 36, PEEP 5, rate 60, FiO_2 1.0, T_I 0.5 sec, and flow 10 LPM

5. Switched to high-frequency oscillatory ventilation with mean airway pressure 16, delta P 36, FiO_2 1.0, rate 14 Hz. Remained in 0.8–0.9 FiO_2 for 2 weeks utilizing a low lung volume strategy for resolution of PIE

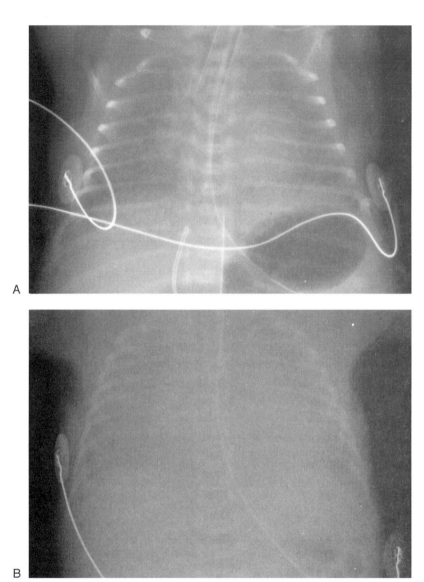

Figure 79. A. Chest radiograph demonstrating pulmonary interstitial emphysema (air leak through the terminal bronchioles) and respiratory distress syndrome, with small air cysts superimposed on a reticulogranular alveolar pattern with air bronchograms. **B.** Stage II (Northway) bronchopulmonary dysplasia showing a hazy appearance of both lung fields approaching a white-out. (*continued*)

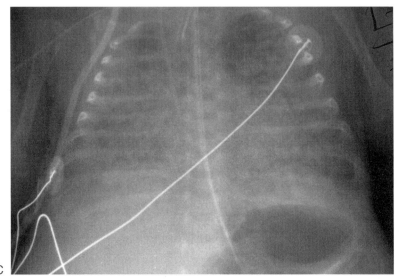

C

Figure 79. *(continued)* **C.** Stage III (Northway) bronchopulmonary dysplasia showing hyperinflated lung fields and developing cysts.

     6. At the end of 2 weeks on the oscillator, PIE had resolved – replaced by a hazy appearance of both lung fields approaching white-out (Figure 79B).

D. Diagnosis: BPD

E. Further treatment

     1. Despite methylxanthines, albuterol aerosols, and diuretic therapies, the infant remained in 0.8–0.9 FiO_2. Echocardiogram ruled out a silent PDA.

     2. Enteral feedings at 130 mL/kg/day, then increased to 150 mL/kg/day

     3. Started on corticosteroid protocol and gradually weaned oxygen and ventilator settings. Extubated to nasal continuous positive airway pressure (CPAP) by 30 days of age at 1,400 gm in 0.35 FiO_2

     4. Chest radiograph at 30 days of life: consistent with moderately severe BPD, hyperinflated lung fields, and small cysts (Figure 79C)

F. Pathophysiology

BPD is a multifactorial disease. Factors that contribute are baro/volutrauma to the lungs from mechanical ventilation and high oxygen use, fluid overload, PDA, pulmonary airleaks, poor nutritional status, infection and leukocyte invasion with resulting released toxic factors.

G. Trends in management

     1. To reduce pulmonary edema and improve compliance, methylxanthines, diuretics, beta-agonist aerosols, and steroids have been used.

2. Early use of high-frequency ventilation may reduce incidence of BPD in very low birthweight infants.
3. Steroids given to mother may decrease BPD incidence.

H. Denouement

1. Venous cortisol level was checked 1–2 weeks after "Avery protocol" was completed. Result: <5 mg/dL (indicating adrenal suppression)
2. Methylprednisone started at 8 mg/m² each morning
3. Prednisone discontinued at 38 weeks with demonstration of morning cortisol level >5 mg/dL.
4. The patient was gradually weaned from oxygen at a postconceptional age of 42 weeks.
5. At risk for pulmonary infection (especially respiratory syncytial virus) in first year of life and reactive airway disease
6. For 1 year – consider stress steroids for significant fever, if vomiting accompanies fever, or for surgical procedures

Appendix

Conversion Table A
torr → kPa

torr	kPa
20	2.7
25	3.3
20	4.0
35	4.7
40	5.3
45	6.0
50	6.7
55	7.3
60	8.0
65	8.7
70	9.3
75	10.0
80	10.7
85	11.3
90	12.0
95	12.7
100	13.3
105	14.0
110	14.7
115	15.3
120	16.0
125	16.7
130	17.3
135	18.0

Conversion Table B
kPa → torr

kPa	torr
2.5	19
3.0	22.5
3.5	26
4.0	30
4.5	34
5.0	37.5
5.5	41
6.0	45
6.5	49
7.0	52.5
7.5	56
8.0	60
8.5	64
9.0	67.5
9.5	71
10.0	75
10.5	79
11.0	82.5
12.0	90
12.5	94
13.0	97.5
13.5	101
14.0	105

Index

493